Immunopharmacology and the Regulation of Leukocyte Function

IMMUNOLOGY SERIES

Edited by NOEL ROSE
Professor and Chairman
Department of Immunology and Microbiology
Wayne State University
Detroit, Michigan

1. Mechanisms in Allergy: Reagin-Mediated Hypersensitivity
   Edited by Lawrence Goodfriend, Alec Sehon, and Robert P. Orange

2. Immunopathology: Methods and Techniques
   Edited by Theodore P. Zacharia and Sidney S. Breese, Jr.

3. Immunity and Cancer in Man: An Introduction
   Edited by Arnold E. Reif

4. *Bordetella pertussis:* Immunological and Other Biological Activities
   J. J. Munoz and R. K. Bergman

5. The Lymphocyte: Structure and Function (in two parts)
   Edited by John J. Marchalonis

6. Immunology of Receptors
   Edited by B. Cinader

7. Immediate Hypersensitivity: Modern Concepts and Development
   Edited by Michael K. Bach

8. Theoretical Immunology
   Edited by George I. Bell, Alan S. Perelson. and George H. Pimbley, Jr.

9. Immunodiagnosis of Cancer (in two parts)
   Edited by Ronald B. Herberman and K. Robert McIntire

10. Immunologically Mediated Renal Diseases:
    Criteria for Diagnosis and Treatment
    Edited by Robert T. McCluskey and Giuseppe A. Andres

11. Clinical Immunotherapy
    Edited by Albert F. LoBuglio

12. Mechanisms of Immunity to Virus-Induced Tumors
    Edited by John W. Blasecki

13. Manual of Macrophage Methodology: Collection, Characterization,
    and Function
    *Edited by Herbert B. Herscowitz, Howard T. Holden, Joseph A.
    Bellanti, and Abdul Ghaffar*

Other Volumes in Preparation

Immunopharmacology and the Regulation of Leukocyte Function

edited by DAVID R. WEBB

Roche Institute of Molecular Biology
Nutley, New Jersey

MARCEL DEKKER, INC.   New York and Basel

Library of Congress Cataloging in Publication Data
Main entry under title:

Immunopharmacology and the regulation of leukocyte function.

(Immunology series ; v. 19)
Includes indexes.
1. Leukocytes. 2. Immune response--Regulation.
3. Pharmacology. I. Webb, David R., [date].
II. Series. [DNLM: 1. Immunochemistry. 2. Immunity,
Cellular--Drug effects. 3. Immunocompetence--Drug
effects. W1 IM53K v.19 / QW 504.5 1335]
QR185.8.L48I47 1982   616.07'9   82-18224
ISBN 0-8247-1707-4

MARCEL DEKKER, INC.
270 Madison Avenue, New York, New York 10016

Current printing (last digit):
10   9   8   7   6   5   4   3   2   1

PRINTED IN THE UNITED STATES OF AMERICA

Foreword

During the past 3 years immunopharmacology has entered the immuno-logical thesaurus. One international congress has already been held and a second is just around the corner. Three new journals devoted to immunopharmacology appeared within a single year and are already filled with articles of both basic and clinical significance.

The term "immunopharmacology" denotes different things to different people. To some it means the application of drugs to modify the immunological response, to others it connotes the identification of immunologically generated factors that produce pharmacological actions. To the basic biologist, immunopharmacology implies the use of drugs to dissect the steps involved in the developing immunological reaction. To the clinician the term suggests the treatment of patients with immunological diseases. The editor and his contributors have taken the most generous view that immunopharmacology includes everything from studies of immunological modifiers to the characterization of colony-stimulating factors. The book emphasizes the almost limitless horizons of immunopharmacology.

As one contemplates the sudden emergence of pharmacology as a distinct subdiscipline, one gets the impression it sprang, fully armed, like Minerva from the head of Jove. Did it not have a gestation period? As one looks back over the history of immunology, the embryonic and fetal development of immunopharmacology becomes evident. It has long been with us, although not clearly delineated. What was the moment of its conception? Probably it should be dated just over a century ago from the studies of a young medical student, Paul Erhlich, on the effects of aniline dyes on cells. The story is told by his secretary, Martha Marquardt, that when Robert Koch was first introduced to the young student, he was told that "this 'little Erhlich' is very good at staining, but he will *never* pass his examinations." Like Ehrlich, immunopharmacology has now come of age and it has *passed* its examinations.

Noel R. Rose, M.D., Ph.D.
Professor and Chairman
Department of Immunology and Microbiology
Wayne State University Medical Center
Detroit, Michigan

Preface

Historically, the subject matter of research in immunology has moved
from the serological and biochemical analysis of immunoglobulins to a
consideration of the cellular components of the immune system. In the
last 15 years our understanding of the nature of the cells involved
in immunity and the complex cell interactions which occur has grown
enormously. Concomitantly, this has led to the opportunity for molecular geneticists, cell biologists, and pharmacologists to exploit the
immune system for their own interests. The molecular geneticists
have been particularly successful in unraveling the unique mechanisms used by immunoglobulin genes to generate diverse sequences. As
immunologists begin to dissect cell behavior and study the regulation
and physiology of immunocompetent cells, they are relying to an increasing degree on drugs and natural products to help dissect the
mechanisms which control immune responses. The usefulness of immune modulating agents in deciphering the cellular immune system has
led to an awareness of the power of a pharmacological approach to
research problems. Many immunologists now consider such an approach to be worthy of a specific subdisciplinary designation, hence
the name immunopharmacology. Insofar as this writer is concerned,
the name implies the use of drugs or natural products to modify the
function of immunocompetent cells in order to learn how such cells
function and what sort of regulatory mechanisms are operative in the
immune system. In the present volume I have asked a number of investigators whom I consider experts in the use of this approach to
present a review of their respective research areas. Few, if any,
would probably call themselves immunopharmacologists, yet I have
become increasingly persuaded that the term accurately reflects what
many of us practice.

The contributors to this volume cover several of the areas of interest in cellular immunology which have benefited from what is in
essence an immunopharmacological approach. Drs. Schreier and
Cammisuli and Watson et al. present their studies on the regulation
of T and B cell function using in vitro models. Cohen and Crnic give
a broad overview of the role glucocorticoids play as physiological
regulators of the immune system. There follow several chapters which
reflect my own biases and research interests, namely the regulation

of leukocyte function by products of arachidonic acid metabolism. These ubiquitous substances, the prostaglandins, the hydroxy-fatty acids, etc., seem to play a role in fine tuning an extraordinarily diverse range of cell and tissue activities. Macrophages and lymphocytes may be studied not only by using drugs but also through the use of a fascinating group of plant substances, the lectins. The results of studies using lectins are presented in the chapters by Edelson and Olfant and by myself and my associates. In addition to plant lectins, the bacterial lipopolysaccharides have provided an interesting group of substances with selective effects on the immune system. Dr. Rietschel and his associates provide a detailed account of the chemistry and biology of these substances, and this is complemented by the studies reported by Dr. Jacobs which focus more on the effects of lipopolysaccharides on lymphocyte function. Lastly, Dr. Reynard reviews the complex area of the complement system and the kinds of substances which can modulate the activity of the various complement components.

This volume is by no means complete in its coverage of topics which may be rightfully considered as immunopharmacology. Rather it is offered as a sampler of the kinds of approaches which can be taken which result in meaningful revelations concerning the functioning of the immune system.

David R. Webb, Ph.D.
Roche Institute of Molecular Biology
Nutley, New Jersey

Contributors

Marc Alfant, D.D.S., M.M.Sc.* Research Fellow, Department of
Periodontology, Harvard School of Dental Medicine, Boston,
Massachusetts

Salvatore Cammisuli, Ph.D.† Basel Institute for Immunology, Basel,
Switzerland

Louis Chedid, M.D. Professeur à l'Institut Pasteur, Service d'Immunothérapie Expérimentale, Institut Pasteur, Paris, France

J. John Cohen, Ph.D., M.D., C.M. Associate Professor, Department of Microbiology and Immunology, University of Colorado School
of Medicine, Denver, Colorado

Linda S. Crnic, Ph.D. Assistant Professor, Departments of Pediatrics and Psychiatry, University of Colorado School of Medicine,
Denver, Colorado

Paul J. Edelson, M.D.‡ Assistant Professor of Pediatrics, Harvard
Medical School, Boston, Massachusetts

Mark Barton Frank, Ph.D. Postdoctoral Scholar, Department of
Microbiology, University of California, Irvine, Irvine, California

Chris Galanos, Ph.D. Research Associate, Max-Planck-Institut für
Immunbiologie, Freiburg, Federal Republic of Germany

Steven Gillis, Ph.D. Assistant Member, Basic Immunology Program,
Fred Hutchinson Cancer Research Center, Seattle, Washington

Present affiliations:
*Assistant Professor, Department of Periodontics, University of
Florida College of Dentistry, Gainesville, Florida

† Pharmaceutical Division, Preclinical Research, Sandoz Ltd., Basel,
Switzerland

‡ Division of Infectious Diseases and Immunology, Department of
Pediatrics, Cornell Medical College, Ithaca, New York

Diane M. Jacobs, Ph.D.   Professor, Department of Microbiology, Schools of Medicine and Dentistry, State University of New York at Buffalo, Buffalo, New York

Otto Lüderitz, Ph.D.   Director, Max-Planck-Institut für Immunbiologie, Freiburg, Federal Republic of Germany

Diane Mochizuki, Ph.D.*   Department of Microbiology, University of California, Irvine, Irvine, California

Malcolm A. S. Moore, D.Phil.   Member and Laboratory Head, Developmental Hematopoiesis, Sloan-Kettering Institute for Cancer Research, New York, New York

Irene Nowowiejski, B.A.   Department of Cell Biology, Roche Institute of Molecular Biology, Nutley, New Jersey

Monique Parant, D.Sc. Maître de Recherche at the Centre National de la Recherche Scientifique, Service d'Immunothérapie Expérimentale, Institut Pasteur, Paris, France

Louis M. Pelus, Ph.D.   Research Associate, Developmental Hematopoiesis, Sloan-Kettering Institute for Cancer Research, New York, New York

Alan M. Reynard, Ph.D.   Professor, Department of Pharmacology and Therapeutics, State University of New York School of Medicine, Buffalo, New York

Ernst Th. Rietschel, Prof. Dr. rer. nat.†   Max-Planck-Institut für Immunbiologie, Freiburg, Federal Republic of Germany

Gilles Riveau   Attaché de Recherche at the Centre National de la Recherche Scientifique, Service d'Immunothérapie Expérimentale, Institut Pasteur, Paris, France

Max H. Schreier, M.D.   Basel Institute for Immunology, Basel, Switzerland

---

Present affiliations:

*Staff Scientist, Immunex Corporation, Seattle, Washington

† Director, Forschungsinstitut Borstel, Institut für Experimentelle Biologie und Medizin, Borstel, Federal Republic of Germany

Frank H. Valone, M.D.   Instructor in Medicine, Department of
Medical Oncology, Sidney Farber Cancer Institute, Boston,
Massachusetts

James D. Watson, Ph.D.*   Department of Microbiology, University
of California, Irvine, Irvine, California

David R. Webb, Ph.D.   Associate Member, Department of Cell
Biology, Roche Institute of Molecular Biology, Nutley, New Jersey

Otto Westphal, Prof. Dr. rer. nat.   Director, Max-Planck-Institut
für Immunbiologie, Freiburg, Federal Republic of Germany

Kenneth J. Wieder, Ph.D.†   Senior Scientist, Department of Molecular Genetics, Roche Institute of Molecular Biology, Nutley, New
Jersey

Present affiliations:

*Department of Pathology, Auckland University School of Medicine,
Auckland, New Zealand

†Department of Immunology, Du Pont-Ne Mours, Glenolden,
Pennsylvania

Contents

Immunopharmacology and the Regulation of Leukocyte Function

1

Antigen Induction of Specific and Nonspecific Signals in the Humoral Immune Response

MAX H. SCHREIER and SALVATORE CAMMISULI* Basel Institute for Immunology,† Basel, Switzerland

I. Introduction

According to the concept of clonal selection (1,2), B lymphocytes synthesize and express on their surface genetically determined recognition structures, the immunoglobulin molecules. The prediction was that interaction of antigen with these surface-expressed receptors would lead to selective proliferation and maturation of lymphocytes within the total repertoire of 10^5 to 10^6 different specificities, whereby the antibody secreted by the progeny of stimulated cells would retain its original specificity.

This simple concept of antigen-specific induction of a humoral immune response became more complex when it was found that the specific interaction of antigen with surface-immunoglobulin-bearing B lymphocytes was not a sufficient signal to induce an antibody response. For the majority of antigens, the participation of T lymphocytes (3-6) and of a third, nonspecific cell type, the macrophage (7) (accessory cell, adherent cell), turned out to be a stringent requirement for the induction of a specific antibody response. These cellular interactions are not only mediated by specific antigen but are also restricted by structures encoded in the major histocompatibility complex (8,9). Helper T cells can only exert their function in B cell induction if they are compatible in the I region with the B cells and/or macrophages (10,11).

In vitro studies over the last 10 years indicated that T cells can be replaced by soluble products which are found in the supernatants

---

*Present affiliation: Preclinical Research, Sandoz Ltd., Basel, Switzerland

†Founded and supported by Hoffmann-La Roche and Co., Limited Company, CH-4002 Basel, Switzerland.

of mixed lymphocyte cultures (allogeneic effect factors; 12,13) or antigen- or mitogen-stimulated T cells (14,15). No consensus could, however, be reached about the cellular origin of these factors, their antigen specificity, and their H-2 restricted or unrestricted mode of action, nor is there full agreement whether the same rules hold for all types of antigen.

In the last several years the number of possibilities for interpreting the sequence and mode of cellular interactions in the antibody response was further increased by reports about T cell subpopulations which either enhance or suppress the antibody response (16-18). Helper T cell subpopulations with synergistic effects and with isotype and idiotype specificity have been described (19-26). Moreover, it was shown that T cell help is counteracted by the concomitant induction of specific and nonspecific suppressor T cells (16,27,28). This increasing number of T cell subpopulations and soluble mediators with all their potential mechanisms of interactions makes the integration of all the described phenomena confusing for the outsider and leaves the investigator with much freedom to interpret experimental results.

Therefore, our own approach to deal with this complex problem aimed primarily at the establishment of experimental systems in which the number of variables was greatly reduced and controlled. To this end we have applied, wherever possible, culture conditions which allow discrimination between antigen-induced and nonspecific effects exerted by medium components or spontaneously released cell products during in vitro culture (29-31). We have used pure or highly enriched populations of specific helper T cells (31,32), and we have attempted to dissect the system by studying interactions between T cells and B cells and T cells and macrophages separately (31,33-39).

Many of these studies have been carried out with IgM antibody responses directed against heterologous erythrocytes. These particulate antigens have been shown to have less stringent requirements for B cell induction as compared with soluble antigens (40,41). In this review we will try, therefore, to trace the common features and basic differences between these antigen classes on the basis of our own experiments without reviewing the overwhelming literature in this controversial field. At this stage of rapid development, based on cloned cells, better defined biologically active mediators, and improved culture technology, we find it challenging to state the issues in their simplest form and to make the basis for present and future contradictory claims more translucent.

II. Experimental Systems: Critical Features
and Limitations

The study of interactions between lymphocyte subsets and accessory cells at the cellular or molecular level requires appropriate cell culture

techniques. When mixtures of lymphoid cells as present in spleen or
lymph nodes are placed in culture, the behavior and interaction of
these cells depend, more than in any other cell biological system, on
the culture conditions employed by the experimenter (42). Constituents
of the cell culture medium, as required for survival and growth of cells
in vitro, may exert a variety of effects on T cells, B cells, and macrophages during the culture period (28,43). Serum components and cellular products from disintegrating cells may exert stimulatory and inhibitory effects which under physiological conditions are only induced
by specific antigen (29,30). The magnitude of these complex effects
depends on the batch and concentration of serum, the cell density,
and previous immunological experience of the cell donor, which differs
for individual experiments. Therefore, within different experimental
systems as used in different laboratories, the same signal may be revealed as specific or nonspecific, may be identified as an absolute
requirement, or may escape detection altogether. The interpretation of
results which are obtained from in vitro studies, as well as the choice
of suitable culture systems for studying a given problem, requires,
therefore, some basic understanding of the critical features and
limitations inherent in in vitro techniques (30).

A. The Primary Antibody Response In Vitro

Cell culture systems which promote a primary in vitro antibody response of dispersed spleen cells in vitro have been described by
Mishell and Dutton (44,45) and Marbrook (46) and have been widely
used since with minor modifications. Dissociated spleen cells of unprimed mice, cultured together with particulate antigens [i.e., heterologous erythrocytes like sheep red blood cells (SRC) or horse red
blood cells (HRC)] give rise to a specific IgM response with similar
kinetics as observed in the intact animal upon immunization with the
same antigen. For the induction of a significant antibody response, it
is mandatory to fulfill at least two criteria. The cell concentration must
be high ($5{-}10 \times 10^6$/ml), and the culture medium has to be supplemented with selected batches of fetal bovine serum (29,30,42,45).
Depending on the actual cell density, the mouse strain, the health
status of the animal, and the batch-number and concentration of fetal
bovine serum (FBS) employed, the number of plaque-forming cells
(PFC) which arise after 4-5 days of culture may vary between very few
and several hundred thousand. This quantitative variation is not
found in the intact animal, where 1 mouse spleen (about 10^8 cells)
yields, quite consistently, 10^5 specific antibody-forming cells 4-5 days
after immunization with a "saturating" dose of SRC (47). Extensive
studies have traced, at least in part, the reasons for this variability
inherent in Mishell-Dutton culture systems and have provided explanations why high cell density and selected serum supplements are

required for the induction of a primary in vitro antibody response (29,30).

These studies have revealed that both high cell density and stimulatory serum are required to induce sufficient helper activity. Evidence for this notion came from simple titration experiments, where increasing numbers of normal spleen cells were cultured with antigen in culture media which were supplemented with either stimulatory or nonstimulatory FBS (Fig. 1). Irrespective of the serum supplement, no PFC arise if less than 2×10^6 spleen cells are present in a 1 ml culture, although, as shown below, 10^6 spleen cells contain at least 100 B cell precursors which recognize the antigen SRC and could, under different experimental conditions, give rise to 10^4 to 10^5 PFC after a 5-day culture period (30). As also shown in Figure 1, not even 5×10^6 spleen cells give rise to a measurable antibody response if the stimulatory effect of serum is absent. Since in vivo activated T cells (but not primed B cells) can overcome this stringent requirement for stimulatory FBS, we have concluded that the critical effect of serum was primarily exerted on T cells rather than on B cells (29).

Analysis of the effects of serum on the T cell compartment has revealed a rather complex picture. Both nonspecific helper and suppressor T cells arise antigen-independently, to a variable extent, during in vitro culture (28). T cells, reisolated from spleen cell cultures at various times of the culture period, exert similar effects on newly established antigen-induced spleen cell cultures as described by Dutton (48,49) for mitogen-induced T cells. Small numbers of T cells can almost completely abolish a primary antibody response to SRC if added at the onset of a normal spleen cell culture. Addition of these same cells reveals potent helper activity if added to T cell-depleted spleen cells together with SRC (28). These findings suggest that nonspecific helper and suppressor T cells are induced antigen-independently during in vitro culture of lymphoid cells. Their effect cannot be reliably discerned from antigen-induced specific helper and suppressor T cells. The relative proportions of helper and suppressor T cells in individual spleen cell pools and their variable degree of induction by medium components at high spleen cell density can fully account for the wide quantitative and qualitative variations inherent in Mishell-Dutton systems.

B. *Antigen-specific Induction of Unprimed B Cells In Vitro*

The analysis of the Mishell-Dutton system as outlined in the previous section and documented in more detail elsewhere (29,30,42) suggested the design of a culture system for antigen-specific induction of unprimed B cells with particulate antigens. Since the high cell density and the stimulatory effect of FBS are primarily required to provide sufficient T cell help, much lower cell densities and nonstimulatory

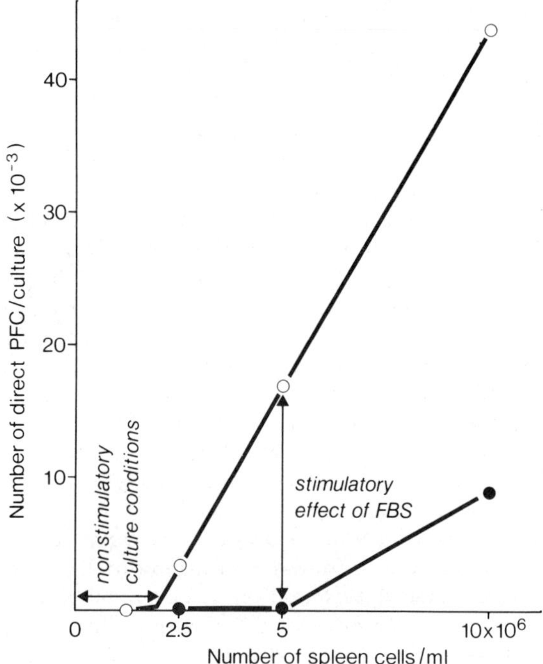

FIG. 1 Relationship between cell density requirement and serum supplement in Mishell-Dutton cultures (45). 1.25 to 10 × 10^6 normal C57BL/6J were cultured together with 5 × 10^6 SRC in 1 ml MEM supplemented with 5% stimulatory (o——o) or nonstimulatory (●——●) FBS, and the number of IgM-PFC per culture were enumerated 4 days after initiation of the cultures. The combination of low cell density and nonstimulatory FBS is termed "nonstimulatory culture conditions" (29).

serum or better defined serum supplements can be used if a reliable source of specific helper T cells is present in the culture system. Under these experimental conditions the induction of nonspecific T cell help is avoided and the dominant effects of suppression appear to be negligible (29,30).

By replacing serum with the combination of albumin, transferrin, and a mixture of lipids (50,51), and by working at lower cell density, it was possible to assure nonstimulatory culture conditions (29). As a consequence, coculture of unprimed T cells, B cells, and macrophages together with the particulate antigens SRC or HRC does not give rise to background antibody formation. However, if antigen-activated (T') T cells are added to the culture, extensive antibody formation is induced. On a per B cell basis, this antibody formation is about 100

times higher as compared with high cell density cultures. Such a
system reveals a high degree of specificity. T'$_{SRC}$ provide help for an
antibody response directed against SRC but not against HRC, and
vice versa (29-31).

This culture system is suited to limiting dilution analysis of B
cells provided that all cultures contain 1-2 × 10^5 in vivo activated
helper T cells and antigen. Contamination of the T cell compartment
with B cells can be eliminated by x-irradiation of the in vivo activated
helper T cells so that all PFC arise from an exogenous B cell source.
If more than about 20,000 surface-Ig-positive cells are added to large
numbers of such cultures (about 40 cultures per given B cell input),
all cultures will contain PFC after a 5-day culture period. At lower B
cell input the fraction of cultures which do not contain a B cell
precursor will increase, and the frequency of B cell precursors can
therefore be calculated from the zero term of the Poisson distribution.
Since 37% of all cultures remain negative at an input of about 3000
surface-Ig-positive cells, the frequency of B cell precursors which
recognize the antigen SRC is close to 1 in 3000 (29,30).

This experimental design reveals the same B cell precursor frequencies as mitogenic induction of B cells under conditions of limiting
dilution (52,53) and allows clone size determinations. The number of
antibody-forming cells which arise from one B cell precursor after 5
days of culture can vary between close to 10^2 and 10^3 (30). It is most
relevant that under these experimental conditions of limiting dilution,
B cell induction is essentially monoclonal. B cells which do not recognize a particulate antigen in these cultures are not induced to proliferate. This is due to the low cell density (5-10 × 10^3 nonirradiated
cells per 0.2 ml) and the lack of stimulatory effects which may be
exerted by serum. This feature of the system is a prerequisite for
defining differences between resting B cells and B cell blasts under
the influence of antigen-induced soluble mediators (see below) (33-37).

C. *T Cell-T Cell Interactions and Clones of Specific*
Helper T Cells

Spleen cells of irradiated, thymocyte-reconstituted, immunized mice,
as used for B cell induction at the single-cell level in the previous
section, provide a potent source of helper activity with specificity for
the particulate immunizing antigen. However, even upon optimal in
vivo priming, probably less than 1 in 1000 T cells is specific for the
priming antigen SRC or HRC. The fraction of helper T cells specific
for soluble antigens as obtained from draining lymph nodes, after local
injection of antigen, is most likely even lower. Such antigen-activated
T cells contain the whole repertoire of T cell specificities, a high fraction of alloreactive cells, and other T cell subpopulations together with
their precursors and accessory cells.

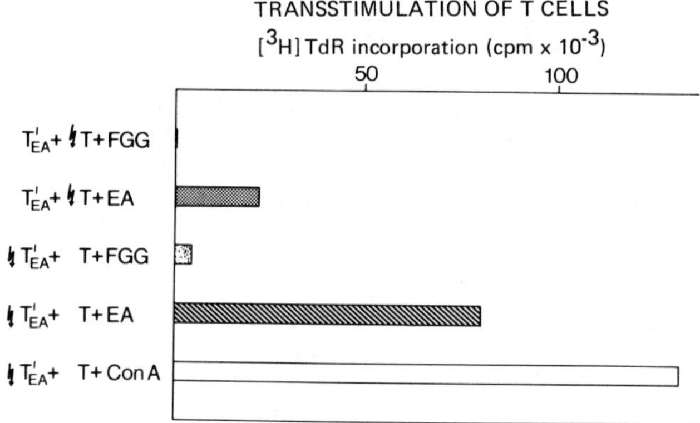

FIG. 2   "Transstimulation" of T cells (54). Antigen-specific induction of "polyclonal" T cell proliferation. 10^4 cloned helper T cells with
specificity for egg albumin (T'_{EA}, clone 7) were cultured together
with 1×10^6 nylon-wool-passed normal spleen cells in 0.2 ml IMDM-ATL
in Falcon II microtiter plates. The medium contained 50 μg/ml fowl
gammaglobulin (FGG), or chicken egg albumin (EA), or 1 μg/ml Concanavalin A. Irradiation of T cells (3300 R) is indicated by the symbol
↓. After 48 hr of culture, cell-proliferation was estimated with a 6-hr
thymidine pulse.

In vitro stimulation of in vivo primed T cell populations with
specific antigen leads to the activation of T cells with unrelated specificity as well (54). Such T cell-T cell interactions could be convincing-
ly shown when highly enriched populations of antigen-specific helper
T cells became available. Addition of specific antigen to a coculture of
small numbers of antigen-specific T cells and a large number of unprimed T cells leads to extensive T cell proliferation which cannot be
accounted for by selective proliferation of the antigen-specific T cells.
Moreover, it has been shown that x-irradiation of the antigen-specific
T cells does not abrogate the antigen-induced T cell proliferation
which, in terms of magnitude, is comparable to polyclonal T cell activation with the T cell mitogen Concanavalin A (ConA). An example of
this phenomenon, which Augustin et al. have termed transstimulation
(54), is documented in Figure 2. We have extended these findings with
cloned helper T cells (see below) specific for the soluble antigen egg
albumin (T'_{EA}). These cells can be induced to proliferate with the
homologous antigen egg albumin (EA), but not with an unrelated antigen [e.g., fowl gamma globulin (FGG)] in the presence of irradiated
syngeneic nylon-wool-passed spleen cells, containing T cells and adherent cells. If the T'_{EA} are prevented from proliferation by extensive
x-irradiation, specific antigen will still induce extensive proliferation

of the nonirradiated T cells in these cultures. Since these splenic T
cells originated from unprimed animals, virtually all the proliferating
cells are of unrelated specificity and do not recognize the inducing
signal egg albumin. The proliferation of these T cells is due to generation and accumulation of antigen-specifically induced T cell growth
factor (TCGF) and other soluble mediators which are generated upon
interaction of specific helper T cells, I-A compatible adherent cells,
and antigen (see Sec. III).

T cell growth factor, which is dealt with extensively in another
chapter in this volume, provided the key for establishing pure populations of T cells (55,56). Originally found in supernatants of allo-
antigen- or mitogen-stimulated lymphoid cells, this activity is now
understood to be an absolute requirement for both survival and proliferation of activated T cells (57). Supplementation of culture media
with this activity made it possible to maintain T cells in long term
culture and to expand single clones of functionally active T cells with
helper T cell characteristics. This technology provided pure helper T
cell populations which are free of adherent cells and allow us to overcome a great deal of the limitations and uncertainties inherent in
studies at the population level (31,32,39,58,59).

III. Antigen-Specific Induction of Nonspecific
   Soluble Mediators

It has long been observed that the induction of an antibody response
to a given antigen A in an in vitro culture system can facilitate
the antibody response against noncrossreacting antigen B which is
present in the same culture at the same time. Hartmann (60) was the
first to show that inclusion of HRC into cultures containing SRC-
primed T cells, B cells, and SRC led to the concomitant induction of
PFC directed against both antigens, although HRC alone gave rise
only to background PFC. This and similar findings from a great number
of laboratories can be and have been interpreted as antigen-specific
induction of nonspecific soluble mediators which help the antibody
response against the unrelated antigen. However, such findings cannot exclude either antigen-specific soluble mediators which may be
released from precursor T cells or limiting numbers of helper T cells
with unrelated specificity which may mature or expand under the
influence of either TCGF or another soluble mediator which is generated upon antigen-T cell-macrophage interaction. The extensive T
cell-T cell interactions in culture, as outlined in the previous section,
strongly emphasize this possibility. It is for this reason that the T
cell products contained in T cell-replacing factor (TRF) have been
interpreted as a family of antigen- or idiotype-specific factors which
contain the whole repertoire of T cell specificities (61). Such interpretation becomes untenable if clones of specific helper T cells are
applied.

A. The Bystander Effect In Vitro

By using low spleen cell density, nonstimulatory culture conditions, and pure populations of specific helper T cells, we could investigate whether a helper T cell specific for SRC (and selected against cross-reactivity with HRC) can provide T cell help for induction of an antibody response against HRC and vice versa.

Results shown in Table 1 indicate that helper T cells specific for HRC can indeed promote an anti-SRC response. Although T cells specific for horse red blood cells (T'_{HRC}) cannot provide help for an anti-SRC response if SRC are offered alone, they can promote an anti-SRC and an anti-HRC response to the same extent, provided that both particulate antigens are present at the same time (31).

This in vitro "bystander phenomenon" holds only for particulate antigens. If the second antigen is a soluble antigen, e.g., a hapten-carrier like phenyl arsonate conjugated to FGG (ARS-FGG), no anti-arsonate response can be induced with SRC-specific helper T cells, even if the B cell compartment has been primed in vivo with the hapten ARS on an unrelated carrier. However, if highly enriched long-term cultured helper T cells with specificity for the soluble carrier FGG that are able to induce an ARS-FGG response are used, addition of SRC to the cultures leads to the induction of a significant anti-SRC response as well (Table 2). In this case the induction of an anti-SRC response becomes strictly dependent on the antigen FGG. This response is not polyclonal under these experimental conditions, since the induction of a response against a third antigen HRC is only observed if this antigen is present during the culture period as well (Table 2).

The bystander phenomenon indicates that the antigen interferes in the antibody response at least twice: once at the level of the T cell and once at the level of the B cell. Since the induction of an anti-SRC response with T'_{HRC} is HRC dependent, it is reasonable to conclude that the antigen HRC is required to induce helper activity for the anti-SRC response. Moreover, this experimental protocol argues strongly against the involvement of antigen-specific factors in B cell induction with particulate antigen and suggests a basic difference in the requirement for B cell activation with particulate and soluble antigens.

B. Requirements for the Antigen-Specific Induction of Helper Activity

Original studies by Schimpl and Wecker (14) and Schimpl et al. (62) implied the T cell as the cellular source of a soluble helper factor(s). Adherent cells did not seem to be required for mitogenic induction of helper activity, nor did these cells themselves produce measurable amounts of it (62). This negative finding quite certainly reflects

TABLE 1 Specificity of Long-term Cultured and Cloned Helper T Cells and the Bystander Effect

T cells $(10^{3.5}/$ well)	Antigen added to culture[a]					
	SRC		HRC		SRC + HRC	
	IgM-PFC directed against[b]					
	SRC	HRC	SRC	HRC	SRC	HRC
T'_{HRC}	0	0	0	6240	5580	4260
T'_{SRC}	5613	0	0	0	6740	4394

[a]Cultures contained 2×10^5 congeneic nu/nu spleen cells, 5×10^5 SRC and/or HRC, and $10^{3.5}$ T'_{HRC} (clone 18-19) or $10^{3.5}$ T'_{SRC} (uncloned cell line, 14 weeks in culture) in a volume of 0.2 ml IMDM-ATL.

[b]The number of PFC directed against SRC and HRC was determined in individual culture wells after 120 hr of culture. Figures are the mean of 4 replicate cultures.

TABLE 2   Helper T Cells with Specificity for a Soluble Antigen Promote Antibody Response for Particulate Antigens, but not Vice Versa

Source of T cells[a]	Antigen present in culture	PFC directed against[b]		
		SRC	HRC	ARS (IgG)
T'_{HRC}	SRC	0	0	<10
	HRC	17	6080	<10
	SRC + HRC	8310	5255	<10
	HRC + ARS-FGG (0.04 µg/ml)	7	2173	<10
T'_{FGG}	SRC + HRC	56	14	—
	FGG (40 µg/ml)	6	—	<10
	SRC + FGG (40 µg/ml)	1538	0	<10
	SRC + ARS-FGG (0.04 µg/ml)	623	—	412
	SRC + HRC + FGG (40 µg/ml)	1675	615	—

[a] $10^{3.5}$ helper T cells with specificity for HRC [T'_{HRC}, clone 18-19, 10 months after cloning (49)] or with specificity for FGG [T'_{FGG}, uncloned line, after 6 months in culture (39)].

[b] After 5 days of culture, IgM-PFC directed against SRC and HRC and indirect anti-ARS-PFC were enumerated on SRC, HRC, and ARS-coupled SRC and/or ARS-coupled HRC in Cunningham's modification of the PFC assay (47).

Note: 2×10^5 T cell depleted ARS-KLH-primed spleen cells (3 months after priming) were cultured together with the indicated helper T cells and 5×10^5 SRC and/or HRC in 0.2 ml IMDM-ATL. The medium contained 0.04 µg ARS-FGG or 40 µg/ml FGG as indicated. Dashes indicate no data available.

inadequacies of depletion procedures, since improved methods of adherent cell removal revealed a stringent requirement for macrophages for mitogenic induction of soluble mediators.

Since pure populations of specific helper T cells are devoid of adherent cells and free of alloreactive T cells which may release helper activity by allogeneic stimulation, the requirement for antigen-specific induction of helper activity can be investigated.

To this end we have dissected the antibody response into two consecutive steps (31). In the first step, antigen and helper T cells are cultured alone or together with T cell-depleted spleen cells of various congenic mouse strains as a source of adherent cells. After a 48-hr culture period, the cell-free supernatants of these cultures are tested for soluble helper factors by adding them to T cell-depleted syngeneic spleen cells and a particulate antigen. The number of PFC, which arise in these cultures, is enumerated after a 5-day culture period. As shown in Table 3, significant helper activity arises only in cultures of C57BL/6 (H-2^b) helper T cells containing homologous antigen and adherent cells which share the same H-2 haplotype to the left of the I-B region. This type of experiment indicates that the induction of helper activity is both antigen specific and H-2 restricted. This experimental protocol does not allow for the conclusion as to whether T cells or adherent cells or both release the soluble helper factors.

Since the antigen-specific induction of helper activity requires I-A compatibility between helper T cells and adherent cells, it must be asked whether soluble helper factors, once induced in a syngeneic situation, are themselves H-2-restricted soluble mediators. If antigen-induced helper factors are added to unfractionated T cell-depleted spleen cells of various I-A compatible and incompatible congenic mouse strains, an anti-SRC response can be induced irrespective of the H-2 haplotype of the B cells (Table 4). This result suggests that I-A incompatible B cells can indeed respond to helper factors which were antigen-specifically induced in an I-A restricted T cell-macrophage interaction.

We have to stress, however, that this type of experimental protocol does not exclude I-A restricted soluble mediators, since the PFC may well have originated from a subpopulation of B cell blasts present in or induced by antitheta and complement treatment in the B cell source (33,34). Similarly, any H-2 restriction between B cells and macrophages would have gone unnoticed in this experimental protocol since all B cell sources contain I-A compatible adherent cells.

C. *Nature of Soluble Products Contained in Antigen-Activated T Cell Help*

The detailed functional definition and, even more, the biochemical characterization of biologically active mediators requires unambiguous

TABLE 3 Antigen-specific and H-2-restricted Induction of Helper Activity

Source of peritoneal cells[a]	H-2 Haplotype							Antigen present in culture	Number of IgM-PFC directed against SRC (day 5)[b]
				I					
	K	A	B	J	E	C	D		
None								SRC	8
C57BL/6J	b	b	b	b	b	b	b	HRC	14
C57BL/6J	b	b	b	b	b	b	b	SRC	4960
B10.A	k	k	k	k	k	d	d	SRC	12
B10.A(4R)	k	k	b	b	b	b	b	SRC	16
B10.A(5R)	b	b	b	k	k	d	d	SRC	3470
C57BL/10	b	b	b	b	b	b	b	SRC	2980

[a] α θ- and complement-treated normal peritoneal cells derived from the indicated congenic mouse strains.

[b] Number of direct PFC per culture after 5 days are indicated.

Note: 3×10^3 cloned helper T cells specific for SRC were cultured together with 10^4 peritoneal cells in 0.2 ml IMDM-ATL in the presence of 5×10^5 SRC or HRC. After 48 hr of culture, supernatants from 10 replicate cultures were harvested and sterilely filtered. 100 µliters of the 7 individual supernatants were added to cultures of C57BL/6J nu/nu spleen cells (2×10^5/0.1 ml) containing 5×10^5 SRC in Falcon II microtiter plates.

TABLE 4 Antigen-induced Helper Factors Promote an Anti-SRC Response Irrespective of H-2 Haplotype of Responder B-cell Population

Source of T cell-depleted spleen cells	Source of T cell help	
	"TRF" from rat[a]	Antigen-induced[b] helper activity
C57BL/6J	8290 ± 2111	6630 ± 512
B10.A	5540 ± 754	4190 ± 814
B10.A(4R)	5480 ± 2140	2640 ± 922
B10.A(5R)	2720 ± 615	2740 ± 393
C57BL/10	4882 ± 558	2533 ± 480

[a]TRF from ConA-induced rat spleen cultures was partially purified (64) and added in saturating amounts at time 0 of the culture period.

[b]Supernatants of cultures containing per 1 ml IMDM-ATL 5×10^4 cloned SRC specific helper T cells, 2.5×10^6 SRC, and 1×10^5 syngeneic T cell-depleted peritoneal cells were cultured for 48 hr. After removal of cells, by centrifugation and membrane filtration, this supernatant was diluted with one volume of fresh medium and was used for culture of the T cell-depleted spleen cells.

Note: 2×10^5 $\alpha\theta$- and complement-treated spleen cells of the indicated 5 congenic mouse strains were cultured together with 5×10^5 SRC in a final volume of 0.2 ml IMDM-ATL (29 30), supplemented with helper factors. Figures indicate the number of direct PFC directed against SRC after 120 hr of culture ±SEM. No PFC were detected in the absence of helper factors.

and reliable test systems. The TRF assay (14), i.e., coculture of T cell-depleted spleen cells with SRC and potential helper factors, is a test system of enormous complexity. Factors which are revealed as helper factors in this system could either act directly on B cells or B cell subpopulations or could exert their helper effect by acting primarily on residual T cells, on immature T cell precursors, or on various subpopulations of adherent cells. B cell induction, proliferation, and maturation may well be a secondary or tertiary event which can be achieved by a variety of pathways. Moreover, such mitogen- or antigen-induced factors may be obscured by, or act in concert with, mitogenic components or growth factors contained in serum in variable and limiting amounts. It is important to be aware of these shortcomings of the TRF assay since, in the majority of studies, quantitative considerations, based on precursor frequencies and clone size determinations, are ignored, and only a minor fraction of the potentially inducible B cell precursors are induced to respond and to expand clonally above a background or "spontaneously" arising PFC. It is for these reasons that efforts were made to study biologically active mediators in far less complex bioassays. Indeed, antigen-activated T cell help as obtained by specific stimulation of cloned T cells in the presence of I-A compatible adherent cells under serum-free culture conditions may provide a unique material to search for and define antigen-induced soluble products. Valid controls are provided by supernatants of cultures containing unrelated antigens or I-A incompatible adherent cells.

1. **T Cell Growth Factor** The close association of TRF and TCGF has been reported by a number of investigators (63,64) and the same partially purified material from ConA-induced supernatants is designated as TRF or TCGF, depending on the assay system. The close copurification of these activities by the criteria of size and charge by no means implies their identity. Schimpl and Wecker have recently succeeded in separating a TRF activity which is devoid of TCGF activity and has the functional characteristics of a B cell maturation factor from a TRF activity which promotes T cell growth as well (65). Similarly, Watson et al. could in part dissociate these activities by isoelectric focusing (64).

Since specific antigen induces growth of helper T cells in the presence of I-A compatible adherent cells, and since growth and survival of T cells is dependent on TCGF, it is to be expected that TCGF is antigen-specifically induced in this cellular interaction. TCGF activity in such culture supernatants has, therefore, been measured and quantitated on clones of killer or helper T cells, which provide an unambiguous probe for this activity (66).

These studies have revealed antigen-specific induction of TCGF activity in cultures containing cloned helper T cells and T cell-depleted I-A compatible peritoneal cells (32). The amount of TCGF which can be induced by antigen is up to 30-fold lower than the amount of TCGF induced with ConA (67). A comparison of TCGF activity, as measured on cloned killer T cells, and TRF activity, as determined by antibody formation in cultures of T cell-depleted spleen cells and particulate antigen, has not shown a correlation of these activities. Recent studies based on a large number of T cell clones with specificity for soluble antigens have revealed that culture supernatants of individual helper T cell clones may yield potent helper activity but no measurable TCGF activity, and vice versa (Schreier, Tees, and Nordin, work in progress).

2. Hematopoietic Growth Factors   Supernatants of cultures of lymphoid cells, stimulated with alloantigens or mitogens, have been shown to contain specific glycoprotein growth factors which promote colony formation by mammalian hematopoietic cells in vitro (68-70). The cellular mechanisms which lead to the release of granulocyte- or macrophage-colony-stimulating factors (G-CSF or M-CSF, respectively) for granulocytic or macrophage precursors (see Chapter 5), as well as for early committed erythroid cells (burst-promoting activity, BPA) have recently been studied with clonal populations of specific helper T cells (38). Both colony-stimulating factor (CSF) and BPA were found in cultures containing helper T cells and specific antigen, and the release of these activities depended strictly on the I-A region-restricted interaction with adherent cells from spleen or peritoneal cavity (38). Such an experimental protocol could prove useful in defining subpopulations of I-A positive cells which are involved in this factor release and to determine the nature of the I-A restricted interaction in a simple quantitative independent test system.

It is noteworthy that the antigen-specific and H-2-restricted induction could only be revealed at very low cell density and when the functional T cell compartment was represented by pure populations of specific helper T cells. Even in optimally primed spleen cells in vivo and under nonstimulatory culture conditions, the background levels of factor release were too high to reveal the stringent requirement of specific antigen in the induction of these glycoprotein growth factors.

Previous experiments by Watson and coworkers (71,72) had implicated G-CSF and M-CSF as the component of fetal calf serum critical in the induction of a primary in vitro antibody response. This claim was based on the observation that the addition of partially purified supernatants of the cell line JLSV5 to cultures of unprimed spleen cells and SRC led to the induction of a primary in vitro antibody response in the presence of nonstimulatory FBS. The activity which converted nonstimulatory into stimulatory FBS could not be separated from CSF over several purification steps (71). Although it has never been confirmed that CSF is involved in the induction of a primary antibody response to SRC in vitro, it is tempting to assume that CSF may have been the most readily determined mediator within a family of

copurifying activities which are present in these conditioned media or
in stimulatory sera.

3. Factors Affecting B Cell Growth and/or B Cell Maturation   Both in
vivo and in vitro studies have shown that the number of B cells proliferating (73) and the amount of antibody secreted (74) upon specific
antigenic stimulation are higher than can be accounted for by selective
proliferation and antibody secretion of B cells which recognize the
immunizing antigen. It is self-evident that in vitro analysis of this
question requires nonstimulatory culture conditions, since antigen-
independent blast-transformation of B cells by components of FBS will
partly or fully obscure the antigen-induced events, depending on the
batch and concentration of serum and the cell density employed.

Antigen-specific induction of B cells at low cell density and under
the experimental conditions as outlined in Section II.B has provided a
suitable test system. If unfractionated nu/nu spleen cells which are
almost exclusively composed of resting small B cells are added to cultures of activated spleen cells and homologous antigen, the number of
proliferating and specific antibody-secreting B cells is about the same
at the peak of the antibody response (29,30,34). A dramatically different picture arises if B cell blasts, purified from LPS-induced cultures of normal spleen, are used as a B cell source in these cultures
(33-37). In the presence of homologous antigen, an extensive B cell
proliferation is observed which cannot be accounted for by selective
proliferation of cells which recognize the antigen. Similarly, supernatants of cultures containing helper T cells, I-A compatible adherent
cells, and specific antigen will induce extensive proliferation of B cell
blasts but not of resting small B cells or low numbers of unfractionated
nu/nu spleen cells. These differences in behavior, as is obvious from
microscopic inspection of these cultures, can be documented with a
short term thymidine pulse as shown in Figure 3. A fivefold dilution of
antigen-induced helper activity induces [^{3}H]thymidine incorporation
of cultured B cell blasts which is comparable to LPS-induced cell proliferation. In contrast to B cell blasts, resting small B cells do not
proliferate significantly under the influence of antigen-activated T cell
help, while LPS exerts an extensive proliferative signal.

A detailed analysis of this phenomenon (33,34,36) revealed that the
proliferative response of B cell blasts under the influence of antigen-
specifically induced, soluble mediators is antigen-independent and
polyclonal, with 30-100% of B cell blasts being stimulated to proliferate.
This has been demonstrated by precursor frequency analysis, showing
that 1 in 1000-3000 proliferating B cell blasts lysed SRC, 1 in 1000
lysed HRC, and 1 in 100-300 lysed trinitrophenyl-conjugated sheep red
blood cells (TNP$_{30}$-SRC) (23). These frequencies are very similar to
those observed upon LPS activation (52,53). Although this activity
which promotes growth of B cell blasts is generated upon I-A restricted

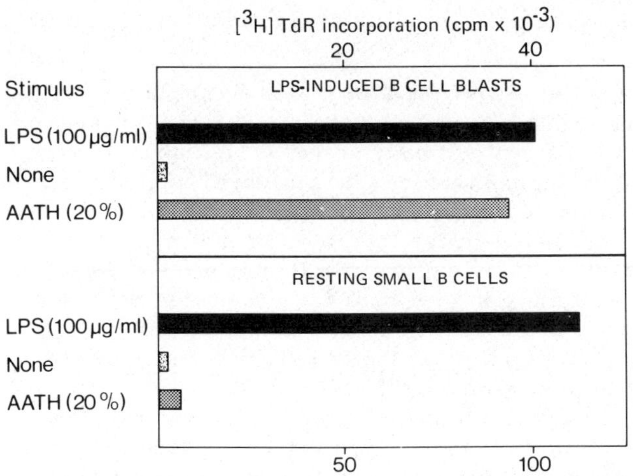

FIG. 3   Antigen induction of an activity which promoted proliferation
of B cell blasts but no resting small B cells. 2×10^4 LPS-induced
(48 hr) C57BL/6 B cell blasts or 5×10^4 resting small B cells were
cultured in 0.2 ml IMDM-ATL for 48 hr (33-37). The medium contained
100 µg/ml LPS, no further addition (None) or a 1:5 dilution of a 48
cell-free supernatant of a coculture of 5×10^4 SRC-specific helper T
cells, 10^6 congenic nu/nu spleen cells, and 2.5×10^6 SRC [designated
antigen-activated T cell help (AATH)] (33-37). After 48 hr of culture,
cell proliferation in B cell cultures was assessed with a 6-hr pulse of
[3H]thymidine.

T cell-macrophage interaction, its action is not H-2 restricted. B cell
blasts from any mouse strain, H-2 compatible or not, proliferate
antigen-independently and polyclonally in response to this B cell
growth factor (33,34). This finding mirrors the events in the T cell
compartment where T cell blasts, once activated, continue to proliferate under the control of TCGF, which is neither H-2 restricted nor
species specific (75,76).
    The adherent-cell dependence of B cell growth factor (BCGF)
production is obvious from Figure 4. If cloned helper T cells are
cultured together with homologous antigen, the 48-hr supernatant has
no effect on the growth of B cell blasts. If increasing numbers of syngeneic peritoneal cells are added to a constant number of helper T
cells and homologous erythrocytes, the activity of such culture supernatants in promoting proliferation of LPS-induced B cell blasts increases. There is a linear relationship between the number of normal
peritoneal (PE) cells present during antigen-specific induction and the
supernatant activity. This activity dilutes out linearly. The activity of

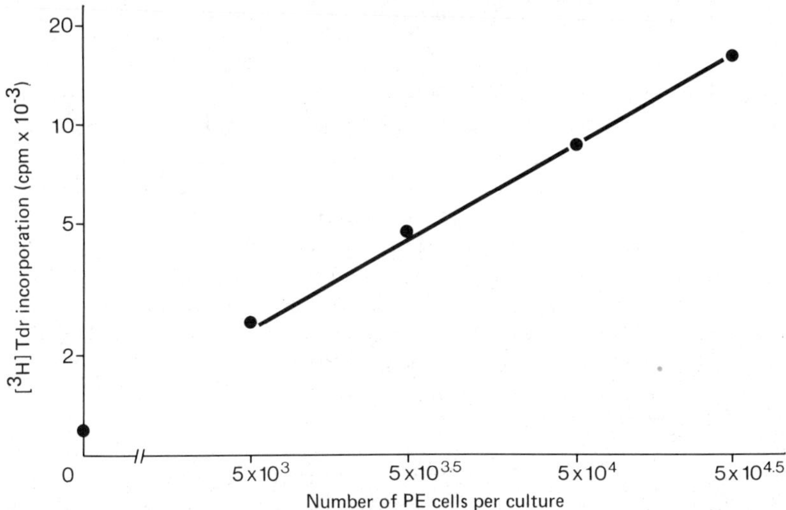

FIG. 4   Adherent-cell dependence of the antigen-specific induction of an activity which promotes proliferation of B cell blasts. HRC-specific cloned helper T cells ($5 \times 10^{3.5}$ cells/ml) were cultured for 48 hr together with 2.5×10^6 HRC/ml and increasing numbers of syngeneic peritoneal cells of congenic nu/nu mice as indicated on the abscissa. After removal of cells by membrane filtration, 2×10^4 LPS-induced B cell blasts (reisolated by velocity sedimentation) were cultured in 0.2 ml of a 1:2 dilution of the individual culture supernatants. Cell proliferation was measured after 48 hr by [³H]thymidine incorporation.

a 1:2 dilution of a supernatant generated in the presence of 10^4 PE cells is equivalent to the activity generated in the presence of 5×10^3 PE cells. This linear relationship allows for quantitation of PE cells under these experimental conditions.

IV.   Secondary Hapten-Carrier Responses

A.   *Hapten-Carrier Systems*

The majority of culture systems which are used for studying cellular interactions in the antibody response to soluble antigens are far more complex than the simplified experimental systems developed for particulate antigens (77) (Sec. II.B). Since significant primary responses cannot be induced, previous in vivo priming of both T and B cells is required. In vitro responses are carried out in FBS-supplemented media and often at rather high cell density. The IgM/IgG ratio may

vary widely, depending on antigen, culture conditions, and time after
onset of cultures. For a clear-cut interpretation of data, therefore, a
great number of variables have to be considered comparable to those
outlined for the Mishell-Dutton system in Section II.A. Previous in vivo
priming of B cells with hapten on an unrelated carrier introduces
another source of variability. Depending on the priming schedule, a
variable fraction of hapten-specific B cells may still be in an activated
state and, therefore, have an altered responsiveness to antigen-
induced signals. In contrast to particulate antigens, where mitogenic
induction (52,53) and T cell-dependent antigen-specific induction (29,
30) of B cells revealed comparable B cell precursor frequencies, there
is a considerable discrepancy in the efficiency of these two induction
mechanisms if this comparison is extended to soluble antigens. Limiting
dilution analysis revealed that close to 1 in 100 B cells can recognize
the hapten dinitrophenyl (DNP) or trinitrophenyl (TNP) (52). As yet
there are no consistent reports on the frequency of hapten-specific B
cell precursors which can be induced, with carrier-specific helper T
cells, to give rise to IgM and/or IgG-PFC. Quantitative analysis of the
majority of reported experiments—including our own—make it quite
obvious that only a minor fraction of B cells are antigen-specifically
induced to respond in vitro. Whether this inefficiency of in vitro
systems reflects inadequacies of the presently used culture systems
or a problem of cell interaction under in vitro conditions remains to
be clarified. As judged from our own experience, the supplementation
of culture medium with albumin, transferrin, and lipids does not
significantly increase the efficiency of secondary hapten-carrier systems and seems to favor IgM antibody formation. Limiting T cell help
or dominant T cell suppression does not fully explain the inefficiency
of hapten-carrier responses, since helper T cells at all stages of
enrichment have only in part improved the output of PFC on a per B
cell basis.

Since both particulate and soluble antigens are able to elicit
antigen-specific induction of soluble helper factors (Sec. III.A) which
are sufficient to promote an antibody response against particulate antigens, the difference between soluble and corpuscular antigens either
has been attributed to intrinsic properties of erythrocyte antigens
(see Sec. V) or has been explained by the existence of different B
cell subsets with different requirements for activation. At present, the
requirements for B cell induction with either soluble or particulate
antigens are not fully understood, and this central question is highly
controversial.

The implication of a B cell growth factor and the distinction between resting B cells and B cell blasts allows statement of the issue
with greater precision. On the basis of this it seems reasonable to
argue that the difference between soluble and particulate antigens
comes only to bear at the level of the resting small B cell. Once

activated, the B cell blast is able to proliferate and differentiate to specific antibody-secreting cells under the influence of nonspecific soluble factors which were induced by antigen-mediated and H-2 restricted interaction of the same helper T cell with adherent cells.

B. Experimental Models for B Cell Activation

Any model of B cell induction with soluble antigens has to account for the stringent requirement of hapten-carrier linkage, i.e., the fact that the activation of hapten-specific B cells by carrier-specific T cells requires bivalent binding of hapten and carrier (78,79). Experimentally, this stringent requirement for linked recognition can even be fulfilled by binding the antigen physically to the B cell surface, which suggests that the interaction of surface immunoglobulin and antigen is not mandatory for B cell activation (80-82).

The schematic illustration of such an experiment is given in Figure 5, where T cell-B cell interaction is brought about in the absence of antigen-surface Ig interactions (left panel of Fig. 5). The hapten p-azophenyl-β-D-lactoside (LAC) is bound to the surface of ARS-primed B cells via anti-H-2 antibodies, to which LAC had been covalently coupled. This hapten LAC is recognized by affinity-purified fowl-anti-LAC antibodies. Such B cells give rise to a significant anti-arsonate response upon coculture with FGG-primed T cells, since the FGG-anti-LAC-LAC-anti-H-2 bridge brings about cross-linking between FGG-primed T cells and ARS-primed B cells (80-82). Obviously, this activation modus leads to the activation of B cells of unrelated specificity as well and is, therefore, to a large extent, polyclonal.

In a similar type of experimental protocol there has been an attempt to focus ARS-specific B cells onto FGG-specific T cells via ARS-coupled anti-H-2 antibodies (right panel of Fig. 5). ARS-primed B cells, which recognize the hapten ARS on the T cell-bound haptenated antibody, are not induced to antibody formation during a 5-day culture period in the presence of the carrier FGG. This indicates that physical proximity between T and B cells is in itself insufficient as long as hapten and carrier are not linked. It is noteworthy that in both experimental protocols helper activity has been induced, as is obvious from a significantly enhanced anti-SRC response whenever SRC were added as bystander antigen.

Experiments of this type suggest that the mode of focusing antigen on the B cell membrane is not decisive. The physiological route via the Ig receptor has been bypassed by binding the antigen onto the B cell surface via anti-I-A or anti-H-2 antibodies or via the Fc receptor (80). Taken together, these experiments suggest that, for T-B cell cooperation, it is essential that T cells recognize the carrier molecule physically bound on the B cell surface.

Results obtained in these earlier experimental models have been confirmed recently in simpler experimental systems which made use of

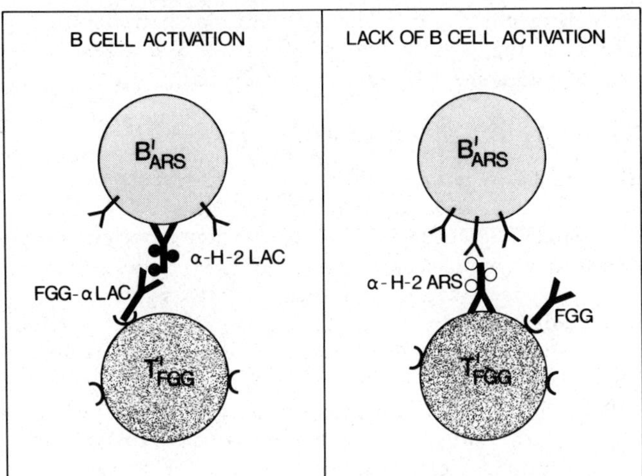

FIG. 5 Experimental model for B cell activation. T–B cell cooperation
occurs only if T cells recognize the carrier molecule physically bound
to the B cell surface. This is a schematic presentation of antibody-
mediated bridging of selected cells. For experimental details, see Refs.
80–82 and the text. Left panel: LAC-modified anti-H-2 antibodies are
used in conjunction with fowl-anti-LAC antibodies to bridge B cells
to T cells specific for fowl gamma globulin. Right panel: ARS-modified
anti-H-2 antibodies are used to bridge ARS-specific B cells to T cells
enriched for FGG specificity. The FGG antigen is present in culture.
In this case, no B cell activation is observed.

helper T cells selected for specificity to minor histocompatibility antigens as expressed on the B cell surface of congenic mice (83). The
interaction of T cells with these surface antigens leads to the activation of B cells. Similarly, polyclonal activation of hapten-coupled B
cells has been induced with T cells which were enriched for this
hapten specificity by long term in vitro culture in the presence of
haptenated syngeneic cells (84). The use of haptenated cells does,
however, not exclude the possibility that only surface immunoglobulin-
bound hapten mediates B cell activation.

C. *Effect of Soluble Mediators on the IgG Response*

The overwhelming evidence for a stringent requirement for hapten-
carrier linkage is occasionally contradicted by reports which claim
that hapten-specific B cell responses can be induced with carrier alone
in the presence of hapten coupled to an unrelated carrier (85,86).

Although such responses may be mediated in part by hapten-specific
T cells present in undefined in vivo primed T cell populations and may
be amplified by transstimulation (54), these results are obtained with
B cells which were primed in vivo shortly before (87). In this case,
the decisive induction step may have been carried out in vivo. Such
hapten-specific IgG-PFC can be induced by carrier alone, and it has
been shown that they arise from low density intermediate B cell types
which have been derived from resting cells by previous cell division
(87). It is noteworthy, however, that these hapten-specific B cell
responses are not explained by polyclonal activation of B cell blasts,
since the IgG-anti-hapten response was dependent on hapten linked
to an unrelated carrier and could be inhibited by an excess of free
hapten (85).

   Using hapten-primed B cells which were in a resting state, the
majority of investigators have found a stringent requirement for
hapten-carrier linkage. Under these experimental conditions, supernatants of cultures containing specific helper T cells, homologous
antigen, and adherent cells should not be able to induce a hapten-
specific response while promoting a response against erythrocyte-
antigen and antigen-independent growth of B cell blasts.

   We have tested the effect of such antigen-induced supernatants on
the secondary in vitro antibody response to the soluble antigen
phenylarsonate conjugated to keyhole limpet hemocyanin (ARS-KLH),
which is known essentially to give rise to an IgG response. As shown
in Table 5, such antigen-induced supernatant activity did not promote
an anti-ARS response in T cell-depleted ARS-KLH-primed lymph node
cells. However, it enhanced about 4-10-fold the response in untreated
ARS-KLH-primed lymph node cells which contained KLH-specific
helper T cells. Only few background PFC arose in the presence of
ARS-FGG (Table 5). Similarly, in cultures containing ARS-FGG and T
cell-depleted ARS-KLH-primed spleen cells, the effect of soluble helper
factors could only be detected if small numbers of FGG-specific T cells
(irradiated or nonirradiated) were present in the culture at the same
time.

   The enhancing activity revealed in the ARS-KLH or ARS-FGG
response correlated well with the B cell growth factor activity present
in antigen-activated T cell help (Fig. 6). The latter has been quantitated by its growth-promoting effect on purified LPS-induced B cell
blasts and has been generated by coculturing a constant number of
HRC-specific cloned helper T cells together with homologous antigen
in the absence or presence of variable numbers of T cell-depleted
syngeneic peritoneal cells (see Sec. III.C.3).

   These results indicate that clones of specific helper T cells,
which themselves help an IgM response both in vivo and in vitro,
promote the clonal expansion of B cells of different isotypes and
specificity for soluble antigen. The induction of this growth-promoting

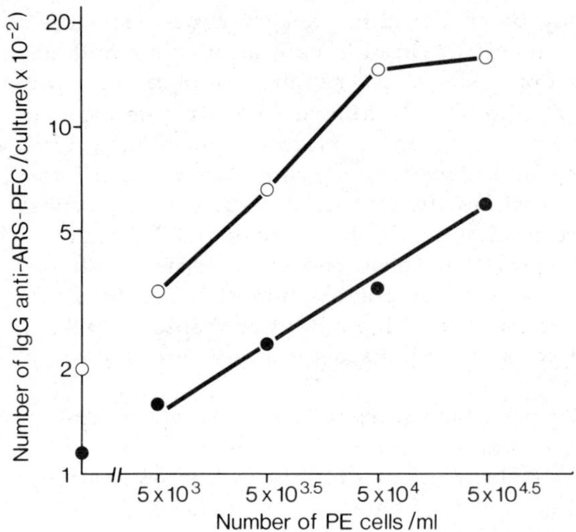

FIG. 6   Stimulation of a secondary hapten-carrier (IgG) response with supernatants of cultures of helper T cells which promote an IgM response. 2×10^5 ARS-KLH-primed BALB/c spleen cells (H-2^d) were cultured in the presence of 0.04 µg ARS-KLH in a 1:2 dilution of cell-free culture supernatants derived from 48-hr cultures of $5 \times 10^{3.5}$ HRC-specific cloned helper T cells, (H-2^b), 2.5×10^6 HRC, and various numbers of congenic peritoneal cells. Number of IgG-PFC directed against ARS was enumerated 5 days (●——●) and 6 days (o——o) after initiation of cultures. The effect of the very same supernatants on proliferation of B cell blasts is shown in Figure 4.

activity is antigen specific and requires the presence of syngeneic adherent cells. A likely explanation is that carrier-specific helper T cells are required to convert ARS-specific resting small B cells into a state where they are susceptible to B cell growth factor. However, we are aware that alternative explanations cannot be fully excluded and that a further dissection of these various steps is required.

D. *Regulatory Effects Exerted by Nonspecific Soluble Mediators*

In addition to a specific antibody response, in vivo immunization with a T cell-dependent antigen leads to an increase of Ig-secreting cells of unrelated specificity and of all antibody classes (74). We have, therefore, studied the effect of the soluble mediators, generated upon interaction of cloned helper T cells specific for SRC or HRC, homologous antigen, and adherent cells, on the nonspecific Ig-secreting cells in a secondary in vitro antibody response under conventional culture conditions.

TABLE 5 Antigen-induced Helper Activity Enhances the Secondary Antihapten Response Only in the Presence of Carrier-primed T Cells

Treatment of ARS-KLH primed lymph node cells (2×10^5/culture)	Antigen present in culture [a]	Source of supernatant[b]	IgG-PFC/culture directed against ARS
Anti-thy-1 + C'	ARS-KLH	T'_{HRC} + SRC	12
	ARS-KLH	T'_{HRC} + HRC	52
	ARS-FGG	T'_{HRC} + HRC	14
c'-treated only	ARS-KLH	Fresh medium	80
	ARS-KLH	T'_{HRC} + SRC	62
	ARS-KLH	T'_{HRC} + HRC	768
	ARS-FGG	T'_{HRC} + HRC	10

[a]The culture medium contained 0.04 µg ARS-KLH or ARS-FGG.

[b]Antigen-induced helper activity and control supernatants were generated by a 48-hr coculture of 5×10^3 cloned T'_{HRC} and 5×10^4 syngeneic peritoneal cells (C57BL/6J) per milliliter in the presence of 2.5×10^6 SRC or HRC per milliliter as indicated. The supernatant was depleted of cells by centrifugation and membrane filtration.

Note: ARS-KLH-primed BALB/c lymph node cells (2 months after priming; 2×10^5 cells/culture) were cultured in 200 µliter culture medium containing 50% supernatant of $T'_{HRC'}$, peritoneal cells, and SRC or HRC. After 120 hr of culture, IgG anti-ARS PFC were enumerated. Figures indicate mean number of PFC of 4 replicate cultures.

Addition of supernatants from such cultures to ARS-KLH-primed BALB/c lymph node cells alters the isotypic composition of non-specific Ig-secreting cells. The IgG/IgM ratio increases owing to an enhancement of IgG plaque-forming cells and to a suppression of IgM PFC, and the same effect is observed in the presence and absence of ARS-KLH in these cultures. There is a linear relationship between the number of adherent cells present during antigen-specific induction of the supernatant activity and the IgG/IgM ratio (Fig. 7). This effect is correlated with the activity of these supernatants in promoting proliferation of lipopolysaccharide (LPS) induced B cell blasts (see Fig. 4 and Sec. III.C.3).

There seems to be a threshold concentration of this supernatant activity above which growth of IgM B cell blasts is suppressed while the same concentration still promotes growth of IgG B cell blasts. At even higher concentrations the growth of IgG B cell blasts is inhibited as well. According to this notion, the IgG/IgM ratio depends on this differential sensitivity. In order to establish a relationship to

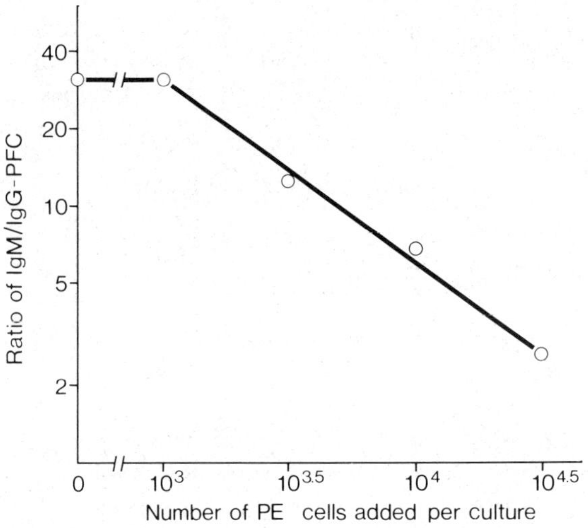

FIG. 7   The effect of antigen-induced helper factors on the ratio of IgM and IgG secreting splenic B cells in culture. 5×10^5 T cell-depleted ARS-KLH-primed BALB/c spleen cells were cultured in a 1:2 dilution of 48-hr culture supernatants of HRC-specific helper T cells, HRC, and various numbers of congenic PE cells (see legend to Figure 4). This medium was supplemented with 10% FBS and 0.04 µg ARS-FGG 1 ml. After 5 days of culture, the total number of IgM- and IgG-secreting cells, irrespective of specificity, was enumerated by the protein A-SRBC plaque assay (88).

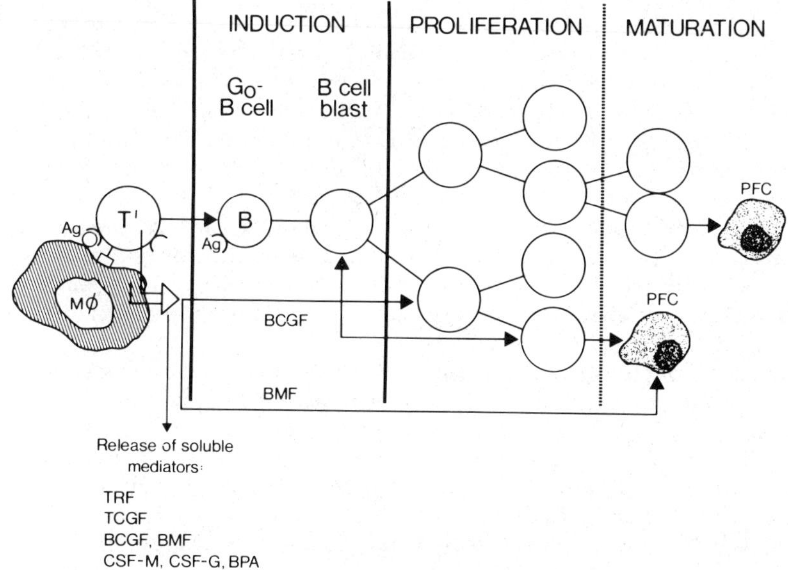

FIG. 8   Model for the induction of a humoral immune response. See text for explanation.

B cell growth factor, it is necessary to purify the factor responsible for this activity. Such antigen-induced soluble mediators may play an important role in the feedback suppression of an ongoing immune response and could be involved in the phenomenon of antigen competition.

V. Summary and Conclusions

Our partial synopsis of the complex sequence of events, which are initiated by specific antigen and which finally lead to specific antibody secretion, can be integrated in a simple, albeit not unchallenged, model for the induction of a humoral immune response. This concept, as outlined schematically in Figure 8, is compatible with a great number of experimental results, including our own, and allows us to pinpoint the open questions and state the points of major controversies.

From studies with cloned helper T cell populations we conclude that the same antigen-specific helper T cell can mediate B cell induction and provide a number of biologically active nonspecific mediators, which are generated upon antigen-mediated interaction with I-A compatible adherent cells. The list of such factors is certainly incomplete, and the cell of origin cannot be ascertained with this type of experimental protocol. One of these soluble factors, tentatively called B cell growth factor, promoted proliferation of activated B cells, irrespective of the mechanism which triggered the B cell to enter the cell cycle. After a BCGF-mediated proliferation phase which may vary considerably, depending on the experimental conditions, proliferating B cells mature to antibody-secreting cells under the influence of a B cell maturation factor (BMF), which is also generated by antigen-mediated, I-A restricted T cell-macrophage interactions. As indicated by the dotted line in Figure 8, there is at present no experimental system which allows for a reliable dissociation of proliferation and maturation signals exerted on proliferating cells.

Since both particulate and soluble antigens induce the release of the same soluble nonspecific mediators as required for proliferation and maturation of all B cell blasts, the difference between the two antigen classes comes only to bear at the level of B cell induction. The basis for such differences may be found in the phylogeny of the immune system, where the response to particulate antigens, like bacteria, may have preceded the response to the more "sophisticated" response to soluble antigens (89).

In the framework of this concept, the definition of the signals, which are required for converting a resting B cell into a growth factor-susceptible B cell blast is as yet the main subject of controversy. For soluble antigens the decisive induction event could result from direct I-A restricted and antigen-mediated T cell-B cell contact, or could be mediated by I-region-restricted and/or antigen-specific factors, for which there exists extensive experimental evidence [for reviews, see Feldman and Kontiainen (18) and Tada and Okumura (17)]. Such factors could act directly on B cells or may be presented on the macrophage surface together with antigen (90-94).

For particulate antigens, a T cell-B cell contact is obviously not necessary, since B cell induction can be achieved in the total absence of T cells. Our finding that clones of helper T cells with specificity for soluble antigens can provide helper activity for an antibody response to heterologous erythrocytes certainly does not point to the involvement of antigen-specific mediators in the induction of the immune response to particulate antigens. Some authors have reported I-region-restricted factors in the induction of an immune response to erythrocyte antigens (15,95). Such factors, as stated earlier (Sec. III.C.3) could readily be masked by the selective induction of B cell blasts.

The extensive work of Schimpl and Wecker and their colleagues (14,62,65,85,86,96-99) appears to be in conflict with our model in two major aspects. On the basis of autoradiographic studies, and as judged by results obtained upon delayed addition of helper factors, these authors claim that particulate antigens themselves are not only a

sufficient signal for B cell induction but are also a sufficient signal for
B cell proliferation. In this view, mitogen- or antigen-induced helper
activity comes only to bear late in the antibody response to particulate
antigens and provides essentially a maturation signal, as indicated by
the BMF arrow in Figure 8. Under the experimental conditions of these
investigators, the nonspecific induction and proliferation signals may
have been provided or induced by the stimulatory serum supplement
or may have been spontaneously released by spleen cells at the high
cell density of Mishell-Dutton culture systems (Sec. II).

Another major controversy is related to the question of whether
all the complex helper T cell functions are indeed mediated by the
same cell or by the combined action of two helper T cells (20-26, 41),
one (T1) triggering B cells to respond to soluble hapten-carrier
conjugates and the other (T2) providing nonspecific soluble mediators
(26). Although our experiments point to a single cell, a final answer
will require large numbers of individual helper clones and a detailed
analysis of their functional potential. Our present technology may
indeed select for helper clones which mediate both major functions.
Moreover, our in vitro hapten-carrier systems may reflect only the
behavior of a minor fraction of the totally inducible B cells.

The outlined experiments and the formulation of this simple concept provide a bridge between experimental approaches which were
concerned primarily with specific events, and were mostly derived
from hapten-carrier studies, and the extensive work on nonspecific
factors, which are, with few exceptions, studied with particulate
antigens.

A detailed understanding of the nature and sequence of specific
and nonspecific signals in the antibody response will require further
improvement of our culture technology and a further dissection of
experimental systems into unambiguously controlled individual steps.
This is in itself a prerequisite for the biochemical and functional
characterization of factors which mediate and regulate the antibody
response.

Acknowledgments

The authors wish to thank Ms. Reet Tees and P. De Riso for excellent
technical assistance, H. P. Stahlberger for the artwork, and Ms. P.
Kiss for typing the manuscript.

Abbreviations

AATH	antigen-activated T cell help
ARS	phenyl arsonate
ARS-FGG	phenyl arsonate conjugated to fowl gamma globulin

ARS-KLH	phenyl arsonate conjugated to keyhole limpet hemocyanin
B	bone-marrow derived
BCGF	B cell growth factor
BMF	B cell maturation factor
BPA	burst-promoting activity
ConA	Concanavalin A
DNP	dinitrophenyl
EA	egg albumin
FBS	fetal bovine serum
FGG	fowl gamma globulin
G-CSF	granulocyte-colony-stimulating factor
HRC	horse red blood cells
Ig	immunoglobulin
IMDM-ATL	Iscove's modification of Dulbecco's modified Eagles' medium, supplemented with albumin, transferrin, and lipids instead of FBS
KLH	keyhole limpet hemocyanin
LAC	p-azophenyl-β-D-lactoside
LPS	lipopolysaccharide of bacterial origin
M-CSF	macrophage-colony-stimulating factor
PE cells	normal peritoneal cells
PFC	plaque-forming cells
SRC	sheep red blood cells
T	thymus-derived
T'_{EA}	helper T cells specific for chicken egg albumin
T'_{HRC}	T cells specific for horse red blood cells
TCGF	T cell growth factor
TNP	trinitrophenyl
TNP_{30}-SRC	trinitrophenyl-conjugated sheep red blood cells
TRF	T cell-replacing factor

References

1. N. K. Jerne, The natural selection theory of antibody formation. *Proc. Natl. Acad. Sci. U.S.A. 41*:849 (1955).

2. F. M. Burnet, The clonal selection theory of immunity. Vanderbilt University Press, Nashville, Tenn., 1959.

3. H. N. Claman, E. A. Chaperon, and R. F. Triplett, Thymus-marrow cell combinations: Synergism in antibody production. *Proc. Soc. Exp. Biol. Med. 122*:1167 (1966).

4. J. F. A. P. Miller and G. F. Mitchell, The thymus and the precursors of antigen reactive cells. *Nature (Lond.) 216*:569 (1967).

5. E. L. Chan, R. I. Mishell, and G. F. Mitchell, Cell interaction in an immune response in vitro: Requirement for theta-carrying cells. *Science 170*:1212 (1970).

6.   M. C. Raff, Role of thymus-derived lymphocytes in the secondary humoral immune response in mice. *Nature 226*:1257 (1970).

7.   D. E. Mosier and L. W. Coppleson, A three-cell interaction required for the induction of the primary immune response in vitro. *Proc. Natl. Acad. Sci. U.S.A. 61*:542 (1968).

8.   B. Kindred and D. C. Shreffler, H-2 dependence of cooperation between T and B cells in vivo. *J. Immunol. 109*:940 (1972).

9.   D. H. Katz, T. Hamaoka, M. E. Dorf, B. Benacerraf, Cell interactions between histoincompatible T and B lymphocytes. III. Demonstration that the H-2 gene complex determines successful physiologic lymphocyte interactions. *Proc. Natl. Acad. Sci. U.S.A. 70*:2642 (1973).

10.   A. S. Rosenthal and E. M. Shevach, Function of macrophage in antigen recognition of guinea pig T lymphocytes. I. Requirement for histocompatible macrophages and lymphocytes. *J. Exp. Med. 138*:1194 (1973).

11.   P. Erb and M. Feldmann, The role of macrophage in the generation of T-helper cells. II. The genetic control of the macrophage-T-cell interaction for helper cell induction with soluble antigens. *J. Exp. Med. 142*:460 (1975).

12.   D. H. Katz, W. E. Paul, E. A. Goidl, and B. Benacerraf, Carrier function in anti-hapten antibody responses. III. Stimulation of antibody synthesis and facilitation of hapten-specific secondary antibody responses by graft-versus-host reactions. *J. Exp. Med. 133*:169 (1971).

13.   R. W. Dutton, R. Falkoff, J. A. Hirst, M. Hoffmann, J. W. Kappler, J. R. Kettman, J. F. Lesley and D. Vann, Is there evidence for a non-antigen specific diffusible chemical mediator from the thymus-derived cell in the initiation of the immune response? *Progress in Immunology* (B. Amos, ed.), Academic, New York, 1971, p. 355.

14.   A. Schimpl and E. Wecker, Replacement of T cell function by a T cell product. *Nature (Lond.) 237*:15 (1972).

15.   D. H. Katz, The allogeneic effect on immune responses. in *Lymphocyte Differentiation, Recognition, and Regulation* (F. J. Dixon and H. G. Kunkel, eds.), Academic, New York, 1977, p. 482.

16.   R. K. Gershon, T cell control of antibody production. in *Contemporary Topics in Immunobiology*, vol. 3, (M. D. Cooper and N. L. Warner, eds.), Plenum, New York, 1974, p. 10.

17.   T. Tada and K. Okumura, The role of antigen-specific T cell factors in the immune response. *Adv. Immunol. 28*:1 (1979).

18.   M. Feldmann and S. Kontiainen, The role of antigen-specific T cell factors in the immune response. in *Lymphokines*, vol. 2 (E. Pick, ed.), Academic, New York, 1981, p. 87.

19. H. Waldmann, Conditions determining the generation and expression of T helper cells. *Immunol. Rev.* *35*:121 (1977).

20. R. Woodland and H. Cantor, Idiotype-specific T helper cells are required to induce idiotype-positive B memory cells to secrete antibody. *Ear. J. Immunol.* *8*:600 (1978).

21. D. Hetzelberg and K. Eichmann, Recognition of idiotypes in lymphocyte interactions. I. Idiotypic selectivity in the cooperation between T and B lymphocytes. *Eur. J. Immunol.* *8*:846 (1978).

22. T. Tada, T. Takemori, K. Okumura, M. Nonaka, and T. Tokuhisa, Two distinct types of helper T cells involved in the secondary antibody response: Independent and synergistic effects of Ia^- and Ia^+ helper T cells. *J. Exp. Med.* *147*:466 (1978).

23. C. A. Janeway, Jr., D. L. Bert, and F. Shen, Cell cooperation during in vivo anti-hapten antibody responses. V. Two synergistic $Ly-1^+23^-$ helper T cells with distinctive specificities. *Eur. J. Immunol.* *10*:231 (1980).

24. R. M. Gorczynsky, B. Khomasunya, M. Kennedy, S. MacRae, and A. J. Cunningham, Individual-specific (idiotypic) T-B cell interactions regulating the production of anti-2,4,6 trinitrophenyl antibody. II. Development of idiotype-specific helper and suppressor T cells within mice making an immune response. *Eur. J. Immunol.* *10*:78 (1980).

25. T. Kishimoto and K. Ishizaka, Regulation of antibody response in vitro. VI. Carrier specific helper T cells for IgG and IgE antibody response. *J. Immunol.* *111*:720 (1973).

26. P. Marrack, J. E. Swiekosz, and J. W. Kappler, Functions of two helper T cells distinguished by anti-Ia antisera. in *Regulatory T Lymphocytes* (B. Pernis and H. J. Vogel, eds.), Academic, New York, 1980, p. 221.

27. E. L. Chan and C. Henry, Coexistence of helper and suppressor activities in carrier-primed spleen cells. *J. Immunol.* *117*:1132 (1976).

28. M. H. Schreier and I. Lefkovits, Induction of suppression and help during in vitro immunization of mouse spleen cells. *Immunology 36*:743 (1979).

29. M. H. Schreier, B cell precursors specific to sheep erythrocytes. Estimation of frequency in a specific helper assay. *J. Exp. Med. 148*:1612 (1978).

30. M. H. Schreier, The antibody response in vitro: Dissection of a complex system. *Lymphokines 2*:35 (1981).

31. M. H. Schreier and R. Tees, Clonal induction of helper T cells: Conversion of specific signals into nonspecific signals. *Int. Arch. Allergy Appl. Immunol. 61*:227 (1980).

32. M. H. Schreier, N. N. Iscove, R. Tees, L. Aarden, and H. von Boehmer, Clones of killer and helper T cells: Growth require-

ments, specificity and retention of function in long-term culture. *Immunol. Rev.* *51*:315 (1980).

33. M. H. Schreier, J. Andersson, W. Lernhardt, and F. Melchers, Antigen-specific T helper cells stimulate H-2 compatible and incompatible B cell blasts polyclonally. *J. Exp. Med.* *151*:194 (1980).

34. J. Andersson, M. H. Schreier, and F. Melchers, T cell dependent B cell stimulation is H-2 restricted and antigen-dependent only at the resting B cell level. *Proc. Natl. Acad. Sci. U.S.A.* *77*:1612 (1980).

35. F. Melchers, J. Andersson, W. Lernhardt, and M. H. Schreier, Functional studies on receptor complexes of B lymphocytes involved in regulation of growth and maturation. in *The Lymphocyte Cell Surface* (P. B. Garland and M. J. Crumpton, eds.), Biochemical Society, London, 1980, p. 75.

36. F. Melchers, J. Andersson, W. Lernhardt, and M. H. Schreier, H-2 unrestricted polyclonal maturation without replication of small B cells induced by antigen-activated T cell help factors. *Eur. J. Immunol.* *10*:679 (1980).

37. F. Melchers, J. Andersson, W. Lernhardt, and M. H. Schreier, Roles of surface-bound immunoglobulin molecules in regulating the replication and maturation to immunoglobulin secretion of B lymphocytes. *Immunol. Rev.* *52*:89 (1980).

38. M. H. Schreier and N. N. Iscove, Haematopoietic growth factors are released in cultures of H-2 restricted helper T cells, accessory cells and specific antigen. *Nature (Lond.) 287*:288 (1980).

39. S. Cammisuli and M. H. Schreier, Individual clones of carrier specific T cells help idiotypically and isotypically heterogeneous anti-hapten B cell responses. *Immunology 43*:581 (1981).

40. H. Waldmann, A. Munro, and P. Hunter, Properties of educated T cells. The ability of educated T cells to facilitate the immune response to non-crossreacting antigens in vitro. *Eur. J. Immunol.* *3*:167 (1973).

41. P. Marrack and J. W. Kappler, Antigen-specific and non-specific mediators of T cell/B cell cooperation. I. Evidence for their production by different T cells. *J. Immunol.* *114*:1116 (1975).

42. M. H. Schreier and A. A. Nordin, An evaluation of the immune response in vitro. in *B and T Cells in Immune Recognition* (F. Loor and G. E. Roelants, eds.), John Wiley, Chichester, 1977, p. 127.

43. S. M. Shiigi and R. I. Mishell, Sera and the in vitro induction of immune responses. I. Bacterial contamination and the generation of good fetal bovine sera. *J. Immunol.* *115*:741 (1975).

44. R. I. Mishell and R. W. Dutton, Immunization of normal mouse spleen cell suspensions in vitro. *Science 163*:1004 (1966).

45. R. I. Mishell and R. W. Dutton, Immunization of dissociated spleen cell cultures from normal mice. *J. Exp. Med. 126*:423 (1967).

46. J. Marbrook, Primary immune response in cultures of spleen cells. *Lancet 2*:1279 (1967).

47. N. K. Jerne, C. Henry, A. A. Nordin, H. Fuji, A. M. C. Koros, and I. Lefkovits, Plaque forming cells: Methodology and theory. *Transplant. Rev. 18*:130 (1974).

48. R. W. Dutton, Inhibitory and stimulatory effects of Concanavalin A on the response of mouse spleen cell suspensions to antigen. I. Characterization of the inhibitory cell activity. *J. Exp. Med. 136*:1445 (1972).

49. R. W. Dutton, Inhibitory and stimulatory effects of Concanavalin A on the response of mouse spleen cell suspensions to antigen. II. Evidence for separate stimulatory and inhibitory cells. *J. Exp. Med. 138*:1496 (1973).

50. L. J. Guilbert and N. N. Iscove, Partial replacement of serum by selenite, transferrin, albumin and lecithin in hemopoietic cell cultures. *Nature (Lond.) 263*:594 (1976).

51. N. N. Iscove and F. Melchers, Complete replacement of serum by albumin, transferrin and soybean lipid in cultures of lipopolysaccharide reactive B lymphocytes. *J. Exp. Med. 147*:923 (1978).

52. J. Andersson, A. Coutinho, and F. Melchers, Frequencies of mitogen-reactive B-cells in the mouse. II. Frequencies of B-cells producing antibodies which lyse sheep or horse erythrocytes, and trinitrophenylated or nitroiodophenylated sheep erythrocytes. *J. Exp. Med. 145*:1520 (1977).

53. J. Andersson, A. Coutinho, W. Lernhardt, and F. Melchers, Clonal growth and maturation to immunoglobulin secretion in vitro of every growth-inducible B-lymphocyte. *Cell 10*:27 (1977).

54. A. A. Augustin, M. H. Julius, and H. Cosenza, Antigen-specific stimulation and trans-stimulation of T cells in long-term culture. *Eur. J. Immunol. 9*:665 (1979).

55. D. A. Morgan, F. W. Ruscetti, and R. C. Gallo, Selective in vitro growth of T lymphocytes from normal human bone marrow. *Science 193*:1007 (1976).

56. S. Gillis and K. A. Smith, Long-term culture of tumor specific cytotoxic T cells. *Nature (Lond.) 268*:154 (1977).

57. K. A. Smith, S. Gillis, P. E. Baker, D. McKenzie, and F. W. Ruscetti, T cell growth factor mediated T cell proliferation. *Ann. N.Y. Acad. Sci. 332*:423 (1979).

58. R. Tees and M. H. Schreier, Selective reconstitution of nude mice with long-term cultured and cloned specific helper T cells. *Nature (Lond.) 283*:780 (1980).

59. A. T. J. Bianchi, H. Hooijkaas, R. Benner, R. Tees, A. A. Nordin, and M. H. Schreier, Clones of helper T cells mediate antigen-specific, H-2-restricted, delayed-type hypersensitivity. *Nature (Lond.) 290*:62 (1981).

60. K. U. Hartmann, Induction of a hemolysin response in vitro. Interaction of cells of bone marrow origin and thymic origin. *J. Exp. Med. 132*:1267 (1970).

61. R. R. Bernabe, C. Martinez-Alonso, and A. Coutinho, The specificity of "nonspecific" concanavalin A-induced helper factors. *Eur. J. Immunol. 9*:546 (1979).

62. A. Schimpl, Th. Hunig, and E. Wecker, Separate induction of proliferation and maturation of B cells. in *Progress in Immunology*, vol. 2 (L. Brent and J. Holborow, eds.), North-Holland, Amsterdam, 1974, p. 135.

63. J. Shaw, V. Monticone, G. Mills, and V. Paetkau, Effects of co-stimulator on immune responses in vitro. *J. Immunol. 120*: 1974 (1978).

64. J. Watson, S. Gillis, J. Marbrook, D. Mochizuki, and K. A. Smith, Biochemical and biological characterization of lymphocyte regulatory molecules. I. Purification of a class of murine lymphokines. *J. Exp. Med. 150*:849 (1979).

65. A. Schimpl, L. Hubner, C. A. Wong, and E. Wecker, Distinction between T helper cell replacing factor (TRF) and T cell growth factor (TCGF). *Behring Inst. Mitt. 67*:221 (1980).

66. S. Gillis, M. M. Ferm, W. Ou, and K. A. Smith, T cell growth factor: Parameters of production and a quantitative microassay for activity. *J. Immunol. 120*:2027 (1978).

67. M. H. Schreier, T cell growth factor (Interleukin 2) as a tool in establishing functionally active lines and clones of specific helper T cells. *Behring Inst. Mitt. 67*:184 (1980).

68. J. W. Parker and D. Metcalf, Production of colony-stimulating factors in mitogen-stimulated lymphocyte cultures. *J. Immunol. 122*:502 (1974).

69. G. R. Johnson and D. Metcalf, Pure and mixed erythroid colony formation in vitro stimulated by spleen conditioned medium with no detectable erythropoietin. *Proc. Natl. Acad. Sci. U.S.A. 74*:3879 (1977).

70. N. N. Iscove, Erythropoietin-independent stimulation of early erythropoiesis in adult marrow cultures by conditioned media from lectin-stimulated mouse spleen cells. in *Hematopoietic Cell Differentiation* (D. Golde, M. J. Cline, D. Metcalf, and F. Fox, eds.), Academic, New York, 1978, p. 37.

71. J. Watson and M. Thoman, A factor that can be used to regulate an in vitro primary immune response. *Proc. Natl. Acad. Sci. U.S.A. 69*:594 (1972).

72. J. Watson and R. Epstein, The role of humoral factors in the
     initiation of in vitro primary immune responses. I. Effect of
     deficient fetal bovine serum. *J. Immunol. 110*:31 (1973).
73. Y. Rosenberg and J. M. Chiller, Ability of antigen-specific
     helper cells to effect a class-restricted increase in total Ig-
     secreting cells in spleens after immunization with the antigen.
     J. Exp. Med. 150:517 (1979).
74. B. A. Askonas and J. H. Humphrey, Formation of specific
     antibodies and γ-globulin in vitro. A study of the synthetic
     ability of various tissues from rabbits immunized by different
     methods. *Biochemistry (New York) 68*:252 (1958).
75. K. A. Smith, S. Gillis, P. E. Baker, D. McKenzie, and F. W.
     Ruscetti, T cell growth factor mediated T cell proliferation.
     Ann. N.Y. Acad. Sci. 332:423 (1979).
76. A. Coutinho, E. L. Larsson, K. O. Gronvik, and J. Andersson,
     Studies on T lymphocyte activation. II. The target cells for
     concanavalin A-induced growth factors. *Eur. J. Immunol. 9*:
     587 (1979).
77. C. Henry, In vitro anti-hapten response to a lactoside-
     conjugated protein. *Cell. Immunol. 19*:117 (1975).
78. K. Rajewsky, V. Schirrmacher, S. Nase, and N. K. Jerne,
     The requirement of more than one antigenic determinant for
     immunogenicity. *J. Exp. Med. 129*:1131 (1969).
79. N. A. Mitchison, The carrier effect in the secondary response
     to hapten-protein conjugates. II. Cellular cooperation. *Eur. J.
     Immunol. 1*:18 (1971).
80. S. Cammisuli, C. Henry, and L. Wofsy, Role of membrane
     receptors in the induction of an in vitro secondary anti-hapten
     response. I. Differentiation of B memory cells to plasma cells is
     independent of antigen-immunoglobulin receptor interaction.
     Eur. J. Immunol. 8:656 (1978).
81. S. Cammisuli and C. Henry, Role of membrane receptors in the
     induction of an in vitro secondary anti-hapten response. II.
     Antigen-immunoglobulin receptor interaction is not required for
     B memory cell proliferation. *Eur. J. Immunol. 8*:662 (1978).
82. S. Cammisuli and H. Cosenza, Idiotypic profile of the response
     to phosphorylcholine induced in the absence of the homologous
     antigen. *Eur. J. Immunol. 10*:299 (1980).
83. A. Coutinho and A. A. Augustin, Major histocompatibility
     complex-restricted and unrestricted T helper cells recognizing
     minor histocompatibility antigens of B cell surfaces. *Eur. J.
     Immunol. 10*:535 (1980).
84. C. Martinez, A. A. Coutinho, R. R. Bernabe, A. Augustin,
     W. Haas, and H. Pohlit, Hapten-specific helper T cells. I.
     Collaboration with B cells to which the hapten has been directly
     coupled. *Eur. J. Immunol. 10*:403 (1980).

85. T. Hunig, A. Schimpl, and E. Wecker, Mechanism of T cell help in the immune response to soluble protein antigens. I. Evidence for in situ generation and action of T cell replacing factor during the anamnestic response to dinitrophenyl keyhole limpet hemocyanin in vitro. *J. Exp. Med. 145*:1216 (1977).

86. T. Hunig, A. Schimpl, and E. Wecker, Mechanism of T-cell help in the immune response to soluble protein antigens. II. Reconstitution of primary and secondary in vitro immune responses to dinitrophenyl-carrier conjugates by T-cell-replacing factor. *J. Exp. Med. 145*:1228 (1977).

87. J. R. North and B. A. Askonas, IgG response in vitro. I. The requirement for an intermediate responsive cell type. *Eur. J. Immunol. 6*:8 (1976).

88. E. Gronowicz, A. Coutinho, and F. Melchers, A plaque assay for all cells secreting Ig of a given type or class. *Eur. J. Immunol. 6*:588 (1976).

89. M. F. Burnet, Self and not-self. in *Cellular Immunology, Book One*. Melbourne University Press, 1969.

90. M. Feldmann and A. Basten, Specific collaboration between T and B lymphocytes across a cell impermeable membrane in vitro. *Nature (New Biol.) 237*:13 (1972).

91. M. Feldmann, Cell interactions in the immune response in vitro. II. Specific collaboration via complexes of antigen and thymus-derived cell immunoglobulin. *J. Exp. Med. 136*:737 (1972).

92. M. Feldmann and A. Basten, Cell interactions in the immune response in vitro. III. Specific collaboration across a cell impermeable membrane. *J. Exp. Med. 136*:49 (1972).

93. M. J. Taussig, T cell factor which can replace T cells in vivo. *Nature (Lond.) 248*:234 (1974).

94. M. Feldmann, A. Basten, A. Boylston, P. Erb, R. Gorczynski, M. Greaves, N. Hogg, D. Kilburn, S. Kontiainen, D. Parker, M. Pepys, and J. Schrader, Interactions between T and B lymphocytes and accessory cells in antibody production. in *Progress in Immunology II*, vol. 3 (L. Brent and J. Holborow, eds.), North-Holland, Amsterdam, 1974, p. 66.

95. T. L. Delovitch and H. O. McDevitt, In vitro analysis of allogeneic lymphocyte interaction. I. Characterization and cellular origin of an Ia-positive helper factor-allogeneic effect factor. *J. Exp. Med. 146*:1019 (1977).

96. A. Schimpl and E. Wecker, A third signal in B cell activation given by TRF. *Transplant. Rev. 23*:176 (1975).

97. A. Schimpl and E. Wecker, Lymphokines in nonspecific T cell-B cell cooperation. in *Biology of the Lymphokines* (S. Cohen, E. Pick, and J. J. Oppenheim, eds.), Academic, New York, 1979, p. 369.

98. T. Hunig, A. Schimpl, and E. Wecker, Autoradiographic
     studies on the proliferation of antibody-producing cells in vitro.
     J. Exp. Med. 139:754 (1974).
99. B. A. Askonas, A. Schimpl, and E. Wecker, The differentiation
     function of T cell replacing factor in nu/nu spleen cell cultures.
     Eur. J. Immunol. 4:164 (1974).

2

Purification of T Cell-Replacing Factors and T Cell-Growth Factors

JAMES D. WATSON,* DIANE MOCHIZUKI,† and MARK BARTON FRANK
University of California, Irvine, Irvine, California

STEVEN GILLIS   Fred Hutchinson Cancer Research Center, Seattle, Washington

I. Introduction

Antigen-sensitive lymphocytes are composed of two distinct cell populations which differ both in phenotype and function. The cells, found as resting cells in the peripheral lymphoid organs, have differentiated to a stage where they require a specific stimulus to drive them to their effector cell states, which represent the terminal stages in an extensive developmental sequence. Antigen-sensitive cells are triggered by the recognition of antigen in association with a cooperating system. The two types of specificity that are observed in the intercellular processes involved in lymphocyte activation include the antigen specificity of a given cell and the histocompatibility specificity involved in the cellular interactions.

The central problem in the analysis of functional responses of T lymphocytes lies in the characterization of recognition structures. The expression of T lymphocyte function requires both antigen-binding events and cellular interactions with other cell types. These two dissociable recognition specificities appear to be expressed in each cell and result in antigen binding (1-6) and in cellular recognition (7-15). Three major questions examine the involvement of the cooperating cell system in the activation of B and T cells (Fig. 1). First, what is the cell type that delivers the inducing signal to antigen-sensitive cells? Second, what is the chemical nature of the antigen-binding receptors and their relationship to histocompatibility recognition structures of T cells? Third, what is the signal that results following the binding of antigen to helper cells?

Present affiliations:
*Auckland University School of Medicine, Auckland, New Zealand
†Immunex Corporation, Seattle, Washington

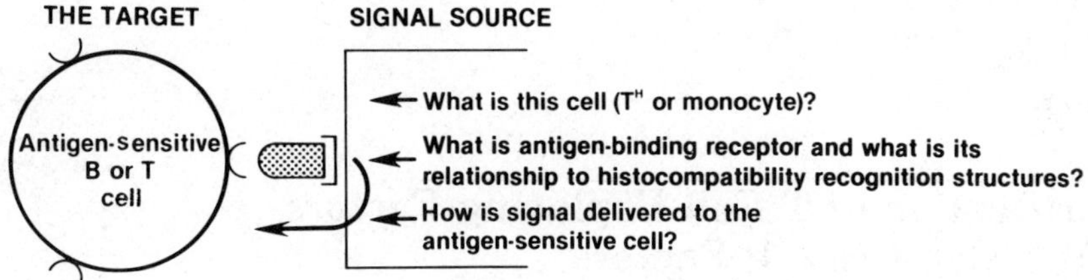

FIG. 1   Lymphocyte activation. A signal source involving helper
T cells and macrophages binds antigen and delivers a signal to
antigen-sensitive cells. The chemical mechanism of this intercellular
communication process is unknown.

A common approach to analyzing these problems is to delete one
cellular component of the cooperating system and attempt to determine how the function can be replaced. This approach has resulted
in the finding that lymphocyte culture supernatants contain a variety
of factors that stimulate lymphocyte maturation in T cell- or macro-
phage-depleted culture assay systems. Factors have been found in
murine, human, and rat lymphocyte culture supernatants which can
replace helper T cell function in the induction of in vitro antibody
production or cytotoxic T cell responses.

The induction of antibody synthesis involves an interaction of
helper T lymphocytes with macrophages in the activation of B cells.
There are numerous studies indicating that a direct interaction of T
helper cells and B cells may not occur. Since the antigenic determinant T cells recognize must be physically linked to the antigenic
determinant B cells recognize, one conclusion would be that T cells
cooperate with B cells via antigen-specific and nonspecific factors
that bind to macrophages and that B cells would interact via nonspecific factors.

A number of factors have been found to replace helper T cells in
the in vitro induction of antibody synthesis. Accordingly, these
factors fall into two classes, antigen-specific (16-19), or nonspecific (20-31), in their mode of action. While antigen-specific
factors are generally considered to be involved in the process of
binding antigen to cells, nonspecific factors may be involved as
mediators between different cell types.

II.   Lymphokine Assays

In this chapter we consider the purification of lymphokines, or
factors, that stimulate immune responses in lymphocyte cultures

depleted of T cells. In the past such factors have been commonly
referred to as T cell-replacing factors, or TRF. However, there are
a variety of ways that factors may stimulate immune responses in
T cell-depleted cultures, and these reflect the heterogeneity that is
now observed in TRF activity. For example, in a TRF assay a B cell
preparation depleted of functional T cells is incubated with heterologous erythrocyte antigens and the putative lymphokine, and a
primary IgM antibody is response measured 3-5 days later. Sources
of TRF activity are mixed lymphocyte supernatants (21,24,32),
primed mixed lymphocyte culture supernatants (18-20), supernatants
from spleen cell cultures with specific antigen or T cell mitogens
(16,17,27,30), and supernatants derived from activated macrophages
(33-35). At least four classes of different factors have been recognized which stimulate immune responses in such assays and have
been considered to have T cell-replacing activity.

A. Specific Factors

These factors can be separated into two categories: those factors
that are specific for the test antigen (16,17), and those factors that
appear specific for I-region-encoded antigens expressed on the
target B cells (18,19,32). It is highly likely that these factors
represent part, or all, of the antigen-binding receptor believed to be
synthesized by helper T cells (36,37). These factors may function,
after release by T cells and binding to a third party cell such as a
macrophage, to direct the signal required for the activation of the
antigen-sensitive target lymphocyte (Fig. 1).

B. Interleukin 1

It is likely that a number of factors defined in various assays are
really different manifestations of the factor which is now termed
interleukin 1 (IL-1). These include lymphocyte-activating factor
(LAF) (35), mitogen protein (38), helper peak 1 (HP-1) (39), T cell-
replacing factor III (TRF-III) (20), T cell-replacing factor$_{M\phi}$ (TRF$_M$)
(40), B cell-activating factor (BAF) (41), and B cell differentiation
factor (BDF) (42).

IL-1 has been shown to be produced by the murine macrophage
cell line P388D$_1$ which can be stimulated by a purified, phenol-
extracted K235 preparation of lipopolysaccharide (LPS), or phorbol-
myristic acetate (33). This seems to be the best evidence that IL-1 is
a macrophage product. The production of the factor by P388D$_1$ cells
can also be induced by T cells in the presence of mitogen, by
activated T cells, or by immune T cells if the immunizing antigen is
pulsed onto the cell line (33). These methods of induction are
analogous to the methods of induction of IL-1 activity (variously
termed MP, HP-1, LAF, TRF$_M$, TRF-III, BAF, and BDF) in more
complex systems (see Ref. 43).

C. *Interleukin 2*

Another group of T cell-replacing factors includes thymocyte-stimulating factor (TSF) (44), thymocyte mitogenic factor (TMF) (45), T cell growth factor (TCGF) (46-52), costimulator (53), killer cell helper factor (KHF) (54), and secondary cytotoxic T cell-inducing factor (55). This group of lymphokines all appear to express one common activity, namely the stimulation of continuous T cell growth in culture. This is the definitive assay for interleukin 2 (IL-2) (43), and such factors would appear to act by stimulating the maturation of functional helper T cells from immature precursor cells that remain in the assay system.

D. *A Late Acting TRF*

A late acting TRF, which appears to be distinct from the other three lymphokines in the expression of activity, is found in the supernatants of mitogen-activated T cell cultures and in antigen- or alloantigen-activated lymphocyte cultures (21,23,31). This activity appears to be more effective when added to the responding B cells at day 2 rather than with the antigen at the start of the culture period.

III.   Interleukin 2

In this section, we will focus on our work concerning the purification of murine and human IL-2. In the course of this work, we will discuss the appearance of other distinctive biological activities which may be due to the factors that fall into other classes of lymphokines.

A. *Expression of IL-2 Activity in Lymphocyte Cultures*

The definitive assay of IL-2 activity is the stimulation of T cell proliferation using cloned T cell lines that have been maintained in medium supplemented with IL-2. However, there are a number of lymphocyte culture systems which can be used to assay IL-2 activity during purification from culture supernatants (51,52). These include

1. T cell-growth assay. CTLL-2 cells, a continuous IL-2-dependent line of cytotoxic T cells, and HT-1, a continuous IL-2-dependent line of helper T cells, are used to perform T cell-growth assays as detailed elsewhere (51,52).
2. Mitogenic response assay. The induction of mitogenic responses to Concanavalin A (ConA) is measured in a micro-culture assay system utilizing adult murine thymocytes as detailed elsewhere (53).

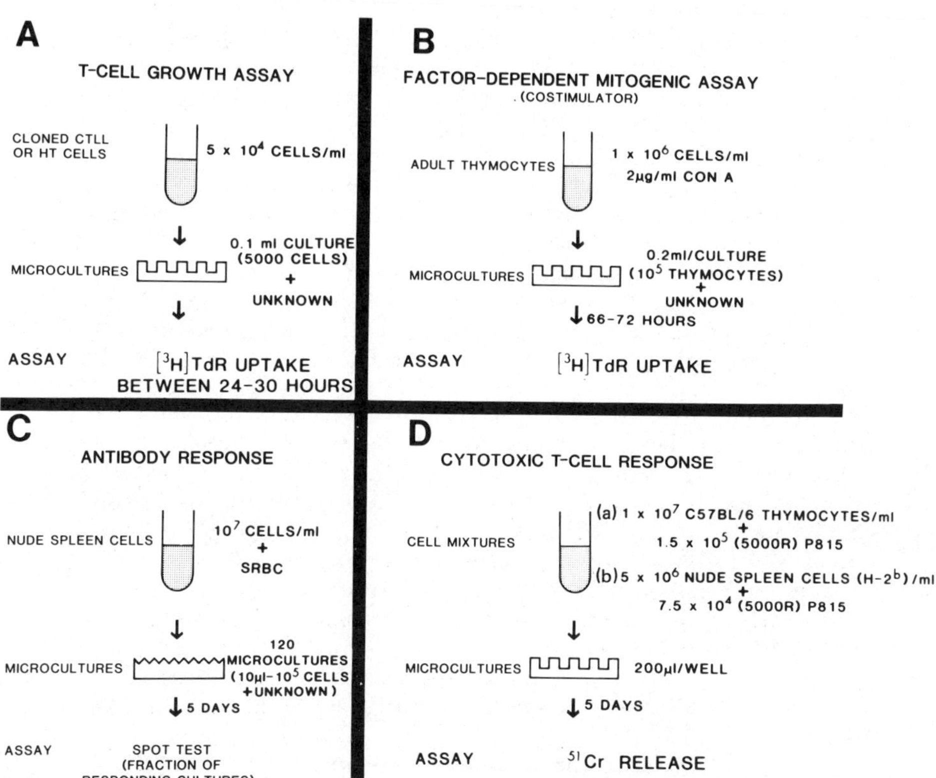

FIG. 2   Murine lymphocyte culture assays for interleukin 2 activities. A: T cell-growth assay utilizing cytotoxic (CTLL) or helper (HT) T cell lines of Gillis and Smith [47,48]. B: Costimulator assay system of Shaw et al. [53[. C: Antibody response assay using the microculture system of Lefkovits [22]. D: Cytotoxic T cell-response assays using thymocytes or nude spleen cells [51,52].

3. TRF activity and antibody synthesis. Antibody synthesis to heterologous erythrocyte antigens is measured in a microculture system using BALB/c.nu spleen cells (22).

4. Generation of CTL in thymocyte cultures. C57BL/6J (H-2^b) thymocytes are cultures in microwells with irradiated (5000 R) P815) (H-2^d) tumor cells. After 5 days of culture, microcultures are assayed for cytotoxic activity against ^{51}Cr-labeled P815 tumor cells (51,52).

The details of each assay have been summarized in Figure 2.

B. *Tumor Cell Sources*

It was apparent that there were two major difficulties in purifying
IL-2 from spleen culture supernatants. First, the low amount of
IL-2 obtained from activated murine, rat, or human sources made it
difficult to produce the quantities needed for molecular analysis.
Second, mitogen-activated lymphocyte culture supernatants contained
multiple lymphokine activities. Until a factor has been purified to
homogeneity, it remains difficult to definitively associate biological
activities with distinct molecular species.

We undertook the extensive screening of both human and murine
T cell leukemias for both constitutive and lectin-induced IL-2 production and have screened some 40 cell lines for IL-2 production. Of
the cell lines tested, only two parent tumor lines (one each in both
human and mouse systems) were found to produce high titer IL-2
upon mitogen-stimulation. As summarized in Table 1 (only a portion
of the cell lines tested is displayed), of the murine T cell lines tested,
1% phytohemagglutinin (PHA) stimulation of LBRM-33 cells resulted in
the generation of culture supernates which contained titers of IL-2
which sometimes range between 1,000 and 5,000 times the amount of
biologically active IL-2 which was routinely generated by identical
numbers (10^6 cells/ml) of optimally stimulated rat or mouse splenocytes. Similarly, PHA stimulation of the human leukemia T cell line
of JURKAT-FHCRC produced between 100 and 300 times the amount
of human IL-2 per milliliter normally generated by lectin-stimulated
human peripheral blood lymphocytes (PBL) or spleen cells (Table 1)
(56-58).

The LBRM cell line was originally derived from a radiation-
induced splenic lymphoma in B10.BR mice. LBRM cells express Thy-1,
Ly-1,2,3, Qa2-3, Qa3, Qa T4, and Ly-5 surface antigens. The expression of these T cell antigens on LBRM cells establish this line
as a T cell tumor (56,57).

The JURKAT cells were originally obtained from Dr. John Hansen,
Fred Hutchison Cancer Center, Seattle, and are a human leukemia T
cell line.

Because the experiments detailed in Table 1 monitored IL-2
activity on the basis of its capacity to sustain in vitro proliferation of
murine cells, it was not clear that PHA-stimulated JURKAT-FHCRC
cells produced significant amounts of human IL-2 activity. To
approach this problem, JURKAT-FHCRC and LBRM-33 cell PHA-
conditioned media were tested for relative capacities to induce proliferation of both murine CTLL and human antigen-specific T cells
harvested from long-term IL-2-dependent cultures. IL-2 microassays
using human CTLL (10^5 cells/ml) were also conducted. JURKAT-
FHCRC-derived IL-2 activity was capable of sustaining the in vitro
proliferation of both murine and human CTLL. LBRM-33-generated
conditioned medium proved effective only when tested on murine CTLL.

TABLE 1 Screening of Leukemia and Lymphoma Cells for IL-2 Production

Cell line		Units per milliliter of IL-2 activity present in 33-hr supernate following activation with	
	Medium	ConA (10 µg/ml)	PHA (1%)
Murine T cell tumors			
RBL-5	0.0	0.0	0.0
EL-4	0.0	0.0	0.0
L51784	0.0	0.0	0.0
S49	0.0	0.0	NT[a]
BW5147	0.0	0.0	NT
RDM 4	0.0	0.0	0.0
ASL-1	0.0	0.0	0.0
RLo-1	0.0	0.0	0.0
HRST 34	0.0	0.0	0.0
LBRM-33	0.0	26.0	517.0
LBRM-33 1A5	0.0	0.0	0.0
LBRM-33 4C1	0.0	0.1	4.3
LBRM-33 5A4	0.0	35.0	866.0
LBRM-33 4A2	0.0	42.0	1163.0
LBRM-33 6B1	0.0	32.0	927.0
Human T cell leukemias			
CEM-SK1	0.0	0.0	0.0
CEM-FHCRC	0.0	0.0	0.0
8402-FHCRC	0.0	0.0	0.0
HSB2-SK1	0.0	0.0	0.0
HSB2-FHCRC	0.0	0.0	0.0
MOLT-4-SK1	0.0	0.0	0.0
MOLT-4-FHCRC	0.0	0.0	0.0
Ke37-FHCRC	0.0	0.0	0.0
T-45-SK1	0.0	0.0	0.0
R-2-SK1	0.0	0.0.	0.0
PEER-SK1	0.0	0.0	0.0
HPB-ALL-SK1	0.0	0.0	0.0
JURKAT-FHCRC	0.0	93.7	225.0

[a]Not tested.

Tissue culture medium containing 1% PHA was incapable of inducing proliferation of either mouse or human activated T cells.

Experiments were also conducted to determine optimal cell and mitogen concentration for LBRM-33 and JURKAT-induced IL-2 production. In studies conducted with both cell lines, peak IL-2-containing supernates were harvested from 24-hr cultures (10^6 cells/ml) stimulated with either 1% PHA or 20 μg/ml ConA. LBRM-33 cells stimulated in such manner routinely generated conditioned medium containing greater than 1,000 U/ml IL-2 activity. Similarly prepared JURKAT supernates contained greater than 300 U/ml IL-2. It should be stressed that identical high titer IL-2-containing supernates could be produced by JURKAT or LBRM-33 cells under these conditions (10^6 cells/ml, 1% PHA stimulation) regardless of the presence of serum.

One of the most interesting facets of JURKAT or LBRM-33 cell IL-2 production was the consistent observation that peak production by 24-hr lectin-stimulated cultures was consistently accompanied by poor cell viability. Both LBRM-33 and JURKAT cells were greater than 95% trypan blue positive following 24 hr of 1% PHA stimulation. At present, it is difficult to distinguish whether JURKAT and LBRM-33 cells die as a result of IL-2 production, or whether IL-2 is released as a result of mitogen toxicity. Attempts to isolate active IL-2 from supernates of nonstimulated cells (via sonication or heat treatment) have been unsuccessful. The observation that increasing concentrations of IL-2 were found over a 16-hr period in supernates of stimulated tumor cells also argues against the hypothesis that mitogen activation simply stimulates cell death and concomitant release of preformed IL-2. Regardless of the mechanisms behind mitogen-stimulated LBRM-33 and JURKAT cell death, tumor-cell-line-derived serum-free, IL-2-rich supernates should prove to be of significant value for biochemical characterization and bulk purification of this lymphocyte regulatory molecule (56-58).

C. *Purification of Murine IL-2*

LBRM-33 cells are seeded at 5×10^4 cells/ml in 550 cm roller bottles in medium supplemented with 5% fetal calf serum (FCS) and grown to a density of $2-5 \times 10^6$ cells/ml. Cells are harvested by centrifugation and incubated in serum-free medium containing 1% PHA for 16-20 hr at 37°C. Cells are then removed by centrifugation (2000 *g* for 5 min). Our current studies indicate that these supernatants contain 500-5000 units IL-2 activity per milliliter. We have calculated that 1 unit is equivalent to approximately 100×10^{-12} g protein. Thus, 20 liters of LBRM supernatant is estimated to contain a total IL-2 quantity of 2×10^7 units, and a crude estimate is that this corresponds to about 2 mg IL-2.

1. **Ammonium Sulfate Precipitation**   The cell-free crude IL-2 supernatants are brought to 80% saturation with ammonium sulfate,
$(NH_4)_2SO_4$, by gentle stirring until dissolved at 4°C. The solution
is kept at 4°C for a minimum of 12 hr. Precipitated IL-2 is then
collected by centrifugation at 10,000 g for 20 min. The precipitate is
resuspended into the desired volume of the appropriate sterile
buffer. The resuspended IL-2 preparation is then dialyzed against
100 volumes of the appropriate buffer at 4°C.

2. **DEAE-Sephacel Ion-Exchange Chromatography at 4°C with
Sterile Buffers**   DEAE-Sephacel is obtained from Pharmacia Fine
Chemicals, Inc., Uppsala, Sweden. DEAE-Sephacel columns (1.5 ×
15 cm) are equilibrated in 50 mM NaCl buffered with either phosphate
(pH 7.6), or HEPES (ultrol grade, Calbiochem, La Jolla, California)
at pH 7.2. From 25 to 50 ml of the concentrated IL-2 preparation are
applied to the column. IL-2 is eluted with a salt gradient (140 ml) of
50 to 500 mM NaCl phosphate buffer (pH 7.6 or 7.2). The ionic
strength of the eluted fractions is determined using a conductivity
meter (type CDM, The London Company, Cleveland, Ohio). Column
fractions in the range of 0.1-0.2 M NaCl containing IL-2 activity are
pooled and then subjected to gel filtration.

3. **Gel-Filtration Chromatography at 4°C with Sterile Buffers**
Sephadex G-100 is obtained from Pharmacia Fine Chemicals, Uppsala,
Sweden. AcA54 is obtained from LKB, Bromma, Sweden. IL-2 is
fractionated on 2 × 90 cm gel filtration columns equilibrated in 0.9%
NaCl. The IL-2 preparation (≤10% bed volume) is applied to the
column and IL-2 is eluted with 0.9% NaCl into 7 ml fractions. The
protein content of the column fractions collected is monitored with the
aid of an LKB uvicord II calibrated for absorbance at 280 nm (LKB,
Bromma, Sweden). The column is calibrated with the following
molecular weight standards: bovine serum albumin (68,000 mol wt),
ovalbumin (43,000 mol wt), soybean trypsin inhibitor (21,500 mol wt),
and cytochrome c (12,500 mol wt). The column fractions containing
IL-2 activity are pooled and dialyzed against 1% glycine solutions.

4. **Preparative IEF**   Preparative flat bed IEF of IL-2 preparations
are performed in horizontal layers of Sephadez in an LKB multiphore
IEF apparatus [Schalch and Braun (59)] (LKB, Bromma, Sweden).
IL-2 preparations to be focused are dialyzed against 50-100 volumes
of 1% glycine. The IL-2 sample is made into a final concentration of
1% glycine, 2% ampholytes (pH 3-10 or 2.5-6, LKB) in 100 ml. The
IL-2 sample is added to 4 g ultrodex (specially treated Sephadex
G75, LKB), and the gel suspension is spread in a gel tray. The gel
is gently dried to the appropriate crack point of the ultrodex preparation with a blower. The tray is then transferred to a cooling plate
(5°C) and electrophoresed 20-26 hr under a constant current of 7 mA.

During electrophoresis the voltage increases from 100 to 1000 V.
After the gel reaches equilibrium at 1000 V, the gel is sectioned into
30 portions. Approximately 2% of each section is placed into 3 ml
sterile distilled water in polystyrene test tubes. The pH of the set of
tubes containing the water and gel is determined. The gel in each
section is transferred sterilely into a small 1×5 cm column. IL-2 is
eluted into a second set of test tubes with 3-5 ml of a sterile balanced
saline solution (BSS). In some instances, each fraction is dialyzed
against BSS (containing 1 µg/ml polyethylene glycol 6000) to remove
ampholytes which inhibit the biological assays.

5. **Polyacrylamide Gel Electrophoresis**   Partially purified IL-2 is fractionated by polyacrylamide gel electrophoresis (PAGE) using a modification of the Laemmli-modified Davis procedure (60). Using the modified Laemmli system, 0.1- or 0.2-cm-thick 16×12 cm slab gels with an
11.6% or 13% acrylamide 10-cm separation gel and 5% acrylamide 2-cm
stacking gel are used to fractionate IL-2. The stock acrylamide solution is 30% acrylamide by weight and 0.8% N,N'-bis-methylene acrylamide (BIS) by weight. The final concentrations in the separation gels
are 0.375 M Tris-HCl (pH 8.8), 0.045% N,N,N',N'-tetramethylethyl-
enediamine (TEMED) by volume, and 0.013% ammonium persulfate. The
stacking gels are 0.125 M Tris-HCl (pH 6.8), 0.1% TEMED, and 0.5%
ammonium persulfate. The electrode buffer contains 0.025 M Tris,
0.102 M glycine, and 0.03% sodium dodecyl sulfate (SDS). The samples
contain the final concentrations 10 mM Tris-HCl (pH 8.0), 1 mM ethyl-
enediamine tetra-acetic acid (EDTA), 0.1% SDS, 0.005% bromophenol
blue as the dye, and 10% glycerol. The molecular weight of IL-2 is
determined relative to the following molecular weight standards: bovine serum albumin (BSA) (68,000 daltons), ovalbumin (43,000 daltons), carbonic anhydrase (31,000 daltons), and soybean trypsin inhibitor (SBTI, 21,500 daltons). The samples are electrophoresed at
$4°C$ with a constant current of 10-15 mA per gel until the dye front
reaches the bottom of the gel.

6. **Sample Preparation for SDS-PAGE**   IL-2 is dialyzed against 50
mM ammonium bicarbonate and aliquoted into appropriate volumes,
the NH_4HCO_3 is removed by lyophilization, and the aliquots are
stored at $-70°C$ for future use. The lyophilized IL-2 sample is prepared for PAGE by resuspension in the appropriate volume of sample
buffer. The sample is then incubated at 70°C for 5-10 min and im-
mediately applied to gels and electrophoresed.

7. **Staining and Destaining Gels Subsequent to PAGE**   Following
PAGE the gel is fixed and stained for 20-25 min with rocking at room
temperature in 0.25% Coomassie Blue R, 50% methanol, and 7.5%
acetic acid. The gel is then destained for 1-2 hr with rocking at room
temperature with multiple changes of 20% ethanol and 7.5% acetic acid.

When the gel is sufficiently destained to allow visualization of the protein bands, the gel is photographed using Polaroid type 55 film.

8. Electrophoretic Elution and a Second Cycle of PAGE   A typical stained slab gel after PAGE is shown in Figure 3. Despite the large number of purification steps, there are 9 clear bands between the carbonic anhydrase (31,000 mol wt) and soybean trypsin inhibitor (21,000 mol wt) markers. Each band is cut out, and the stained protein is electrophoretically eluted and concentrated in a final volume of 0.2 ml. This recovered material is then titrated in a T cell-growth assay. The recovery of IL-2 activity from each band is also shown in Figure 3. There are 2 stained bands that have a proportionately large amount of IL-2 activity, one in the size range of 25,000 daltons and the other at 21,000. Recovery of biological activity after electrophoresis, staining, and destaining of the slab gel and subsequent electrophoretic elution is generally about 20% of the starting activity before electrophoresis.

The 25K and 21K material recovered from several slab gels is separately pooled and subjected to a second SDS-PAGE step exactly as described above. The resulting stained gels are depicted in Figure 4. Only 1 stained band of activity is observed, and the only IL-2 activity detected in the gel is associated with the stained band. Again, recovery of biological activity is in the range of 20% of the starting activity.

9. Flow Chart of Recovery of IL-2 Activity   A flow chart depicting the purification at 5 steps is outlined in Table 2. From 10 liters of starting supernatant, we recovered a total of 50 µg IL-2 with a specific activity of 1×10^7 units/mg. The final recovery of activity is generally estimated at less than 1% of the starting IL-2 activity in the crude supernatant.

D. Purification of Human IL-2

The purification of human IL-2 from JURKAT culture supernatants has not encountered some of the difficulties found with murine IL-2. Human IL-2 is found in the molecular weight range of 12,000–15,000, using both AcA54 column chromatography and SDS-PAGE. Fewer contaminants are copurified from culture supernatants in this size range than in the 20,000–30,000 size range where murine IL-2 is located. The following steps have thus far been utilized to purify human IL-2 from JURKAT supernatants.

1. Ammonium Sulfate Precipitation   The cell-free crude IL-2 supernatants are brought to 80% saturation with $(NH_4)_2SO_4$, and the precipitate is collected as described above.

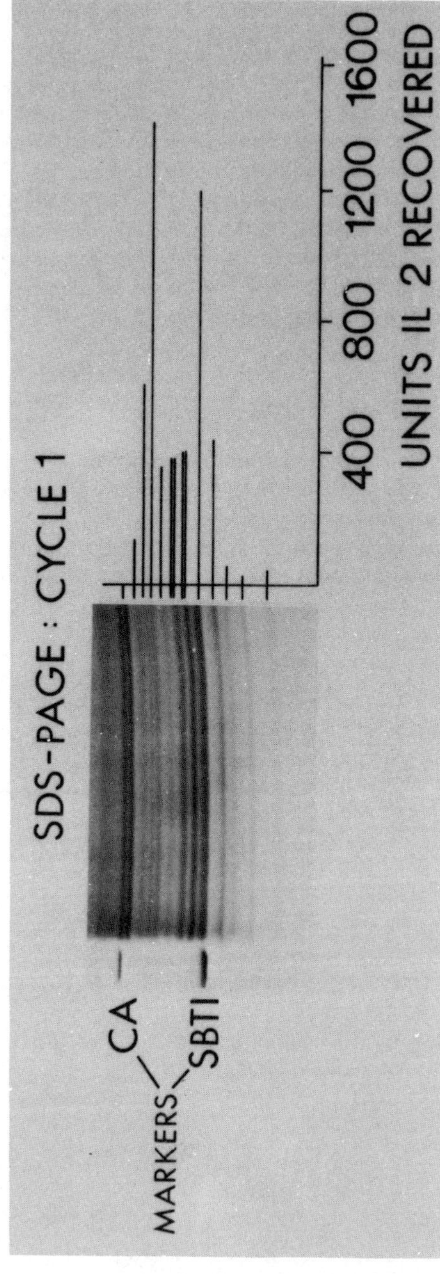

FIG. 3 SDS-PAGE: cycle 1 of LBRM IL-2. A typical stained slab gel after PAGE is shown. Despite the large number of purification steps, there are 9 clear bands between the carbonic anhydrase (31,000) and soybean trypsin inhibitor (21,000) markers. Each band is cut out, and the stained protein electrophoretically eluted and concentrated in a final volume of 0.2 ml. This recovered material is then titrated in a T cell-growth assay. The recovery of IL-2 activity from each band is also shown. There are two stained bands that have IL-2 activity, one in the size range of 25,000 daltons and the other at 21,000 daltons. Recovery of biological activity after electrophoresis, staining, and destaining of the slab gel and subsequent electrophoretic elution is generally about 20% of the starting activity.

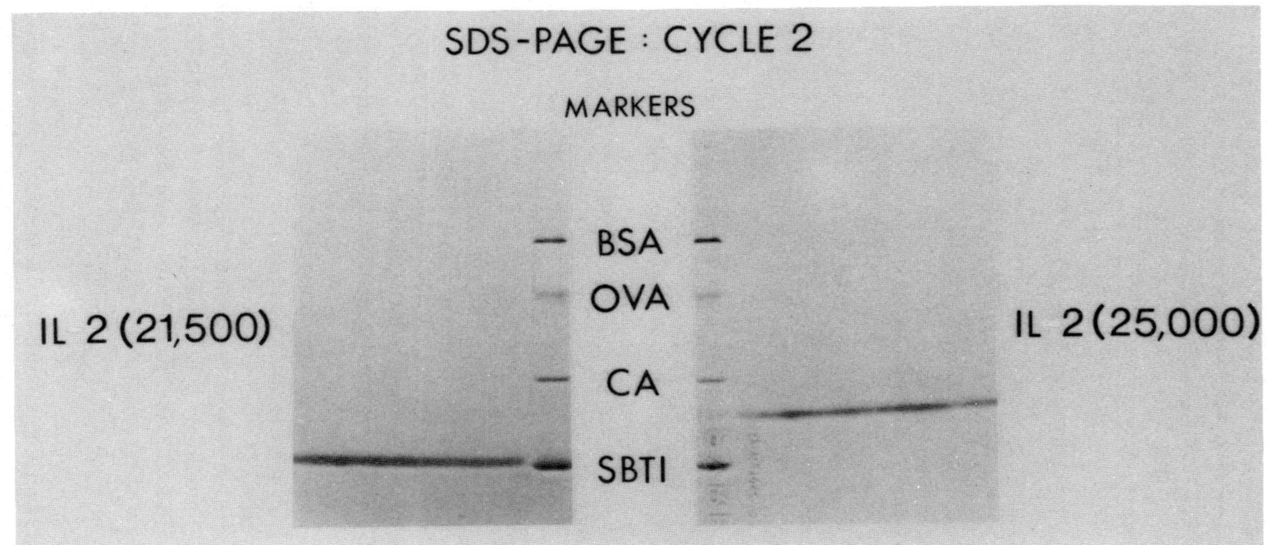

FIG. 4 SDS PAGE: cycle 2 of LBRM IL-2. The 25K and 21K material recovered from several slab gels is pooled and subjected to a second SDS-PAGE step exactly as described in Figure 3. The resulting stained gels are depicted in Figure 3. Only 1 stained band of activity is observed, and the only IL-2 activity detected in the gel is associated with the stained band. Again, recovery of biological activity is in the range of 20% of the starting activity.

TABLE 2 Recovery of IL-2 from PHA-stimulated LBRM
Cell Supernatants

Purification step	Total protein recovered (mg)	Total units	Specific activity (units/mg)
10 liters crude supernatant	52.8	1.63×10^{7}	3.1×10^{5}
DEAE Sephacel	22.0	1.30×10^{7}	5.9×10^{5}
Isoelectric focusing	7.5	6.0×10^{6}	8.0×10^{5}
AcA54 gel filtration	2.0	3.5×10^{6}	1.75×10^{6}
SDS-PAGE (25K + 21K bands)	0.05	5.0×10^{5}	1.0×10^{7}

2. DEAE-Sephacel Ion-Exchange Chromatography   The conditions
used are exactly as described above for LBRM-IL-2. However,
JURKAT IL-2 activity elutes in the range of 50 to 80 mM NaCl in HEPES
buffer (pH 7.2).

3. Gel-Filtration Chromatography   The IL-2 preparation is applied to
2 × 90 cm columns of AcA54 and equilibrated in 0.9% saline. JURKAT
IL-2 activity elutes in the size range of 12,000-15,000 daltons, relative
to marker proteins (cytochrome *c*, 12,500 mol wt; soybean trypsin
inhibitor, 22,000 mol wt; ovalbumin, 43,000 mol wt).

4. Polyacrylamide Gel Electrophoresis   AcA54 column fractions containing IL-2 activity are dialyzed against 0.1 M ammonium bicarbonate
and then lyophilized. Samples are then dissolved in a solution containing 10 mM Tris-HCl (pH 8.0), 1 mM EDTA, 0.1% SDS, 0.005%
bromophenol blue, and 10% glycerol. Samples are then heated to 70°C
for 10 min, cooled, and layered on a separation slab gel exactly as
described for LBRM-derived IL-2. Following electrophoresis, gels are
stained using Coomassie Blue R and destained, and then each band is
detected, cut out, and tested for IL-2 activity. Most of the IL-2
activity appears to be contained within a band of approximately 14,000
daltons.

5. Murine IL-2 Is a Single Polypeptide Chain   Treatment of purified
murine IL-2 with reducing agents prior to SDS-PAGE does not alter
its electrophoretic mobility. For murine IL-2, activity is recovered

after reducing treatment in 25K and 21K bands. It therefore appears
that murine IL-2 is a single polypeptide chain.

E. *Comparative Properties of IL-2 Derived from Normal and Malignant Cells*

We have found that LBRM-33-derived IL-2 is biochemically indistinguishable from conventionally prepared mouse-spleen-generated factor
(55). Mouse tumor cell-line-derived IL-2 appears to be localized in a
protein, isolatable by net charge into two electrophoretically distinct
species with isoelectric points of 4.3 and 4.9, respectively. Each
molecular species has the capacity to (1) enhance thymocyte mitogenesis, (2) sustain IL-2-dependent T cell-line proliferation, and (3)
induce CTL and PFC responses in thymocyte and nude spleen cell
populations, respectively (Fig. 5). Enzymatic analysis of conventionally generated murine spleen and LBRM-33-derived IL-2 activity
further confirms the identity of the two molecules. Regardless of the
source, murine IL-2 was found to be extremely sensitive to proteolytic enzyme treatment. Exposure to trypsin, subtilisin, and chymo-
trypsin completely destroyed both IL-2 activities. IL-2 activity purified from either LBRM-33 or murine spleen cells was remarkably stable
to chemical modification. Only treatment with 8 M urea or prolonged
exposure to high temperature (70°C for 30-60 min) resulted in a significant diminution of IL-2 activity. Of the 2 preparations tested, it
appeared that LBRM-33-generated IL-2 activity was consistently more
resistant to pH, urea, and heat treatment than splenic-derived material (55). JURKAT-derived IL-2 appears indistinguishable in size
but may differ in charge from IL-2 derived from normal human peripheral blood cells. These experiments are currently in progress.

   We would stress that one major difference exists between preparations of spleen and LBRM-derived IL-2 (Fig. 5). While IL-2 stimulates
antibody responses in nude spleen cultures, presumably via the clonal
expansion of helper T cell precursors, we have observed that in the
purification of murine spleen IL-2 there is another class of molecules
within the IL-2 fraction. This class of molecules may be true helper
T cell-replacing factors as detected by the ability to induce antibody
synthesis to heterologous erythrocyte antigens in nude spleen cultures,
and a total lack of T cell-growth factor activity. This material showed
considerable heterogeneity in charge ranging from pI values of 3.0-
4.2. LBRM cells do not secrete this class of lymphokine (56-58).

   The homologies between murine and human IL-2 in terms of biological activity are striking. Although the biological activities as determined in the assay systems outlined in Figure 2 utilizing murine cells
indicated that human IL-2 is identical to murine IL-2, their molecular
characteristics are considerably different. Human IL-2 appears as a
single molecular species of 15,000-17,000 daltons (as estimated from gel

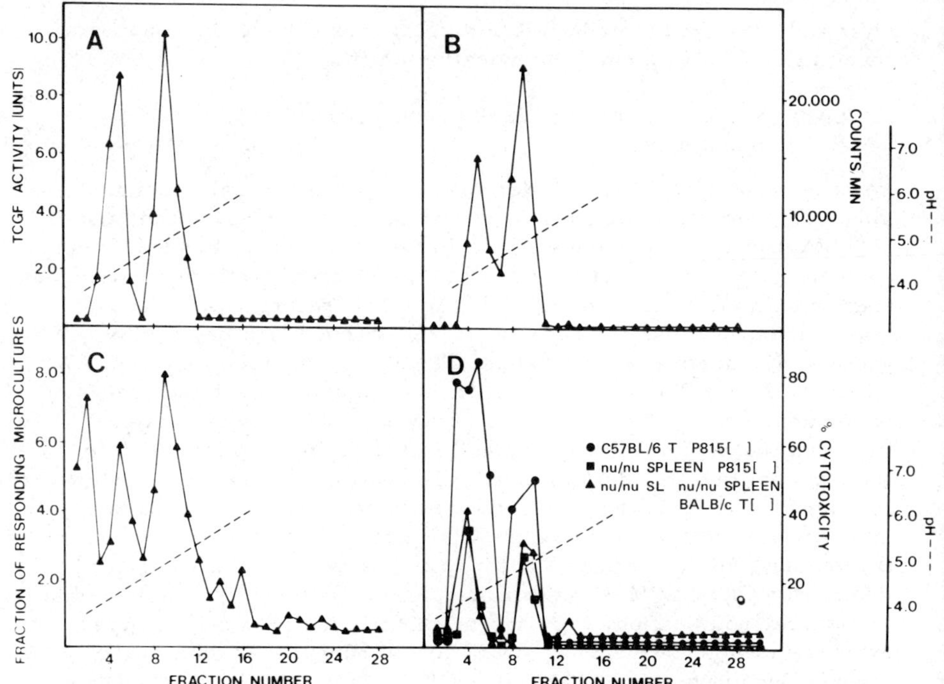

FIG. 5   Interleukin 2 activities from murine spleen-cell supernatants assayed following flat-bed isoelectric focusing (pH 3.5-10). A: T cell-growth assay. B: Ability to promote thymocyte mitogenesis. C: Ability to promote antierythrocyte antibody production in nude mouse spleen cell cultures. D: Ability to induce CTL responses in C57BL/6 thymocytes P815 MTLC (●), NIH nude spleen 815 (■), and NIH nude spleen by BALB/c thymocyte MLC (▲). The experiments are taken from Ref. 51.

filtration studies) and an isoelectric point of approximately 7.0. The observation that the activities of human IL-2 as assayed on murine lymphocytes, which (1) enhance mitogenesis to ConA and (2) amplify cytotoxic T cell and humoral antibody responses, under conditions considered to be limiting for helper activity, are inseparable from T cell growth-promoting activity following successive gel filtration, ion-exchange chromatography, and isoelectric focusing provides strong evidence that all biological activities are mediated by a single class of molecules.

IV. Conclusions

A. *Mode of Action of Interleukin 2*

Activated T cells, but not resting T cells, readily absorb IL-2. When combined with the proliferative effects of IL-2 on cloned cytotoxic and helper T cell lines, these observations imply that IL-2 interacts directly with T cells. However, the striking feature of IL-2 activity in the induction of antibody synthesis or CTL responses is that there is a strict requirement for antigen to observe cellular responses. We have suggested that, following interaction with antigen and mitogen, T cells or their precursors in thymocyte or nude spleen cultures respond by expressing receptors for IL-2. We have also suggested that the subsequent clonal expansion of T cells from each of the effector classes (helpers, killers, or suppressors) requires only the presence of IL-2. These suggestions are supported by the experimental finding that a brief treatment of thymocytes with ConA renders them responsive to IL-2 (61,62).

Such a mode of action has a number of implications. First, it is clear that the T cell mitogens ConA and PHA are not themselves mitogenic. They render T cells responsive to other humoral stimuli that result in cell proliferation. Second, in primary lymphocyte cultures, it is important to distinguish between IL-2 producer and responder cells. With regard to the generation of thymocyte reactivity, helper T cells (Ly-1$^+$) and adherent cells have been shown to be required for both the polyclonal sensitization of murine T cells by ConA or PHA and the generation of cytotoxic T cells from thymocyte cultures (52, 61). The T cells stimulated to proliferate and mature to effector cells are in fact antigen-sensitive T cells from killer, suppressor, and helper subclasses. ConA activation may have two roles, the first being to mimic the primary signal normally provided by an antigen, and the second being to stimulate the production of a proliferative factor, which appears to be identical to that which we have designated IL-2. Third, IL-2 can be used to express effector T cell activity in nude spleen cultures (52,53). Both antigen and IL-2 are required to generate both helper and cytotoxic effector T cells from nude mouse splenocytes; thus, pre-T cells must be present in the spleens of nude mice. Since T cell antigen or mitogen alone cannot initiate the proliferation of nude mouse lymphocytes, it follows that addition of IL-2 to responder pre-T cell populations promotes proliferation to the point where meaningful cytotoxic or helper reactivity can be witnessed. Although it cannot be concluded that IL-2 is the normal stimulus that drives pre-T cells to maturity, the implication is that the helper T cell-replacing activity of IL-2 is due to its ability to generate new helper cells (Fig. 6). The induction of B cell responses occurs then via the normal induction mechanism.

                                                    Watson et al.

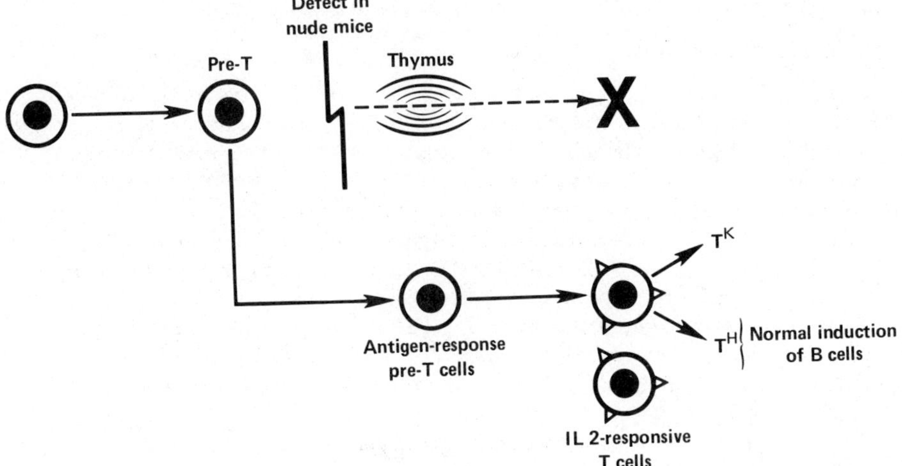

FIG. 6   The T cell-replacing activity of IL-2 in athymic (nude) mouse
spleen cultures. In nude spleen cultures, IL-2 may stimulate the clonal
proliferation of antigen-specific helper T cells. The subsequent induction of antibody synthesis observed may result from the normal interaction of helper T cells and macrophages with B cells.

We have used IL-2 as a reagent to select for and clonally expand
populations of antigen-specific helper T cells (50). IL-2 stimulates the
proliferation of antigen- or mitogen-activated T cells, but not non-
activated T cells. This finding has been utilized as a selection step in
the establishment of T cell lines in culture. Thymocytes are activated
to sheep red blood cell (SRBC) antigens in vivo and then cultured at
a density of 10^6 cells/ml. Cultures are supplemented with 10 units/ml
murine IL-2, 0.02% SRBC or horse red blood cells (HRBC), and irradiated syngeneic nude spleen cells as fillers at a final concentration
of 10^5 cells/ml. The success of this procedure depends upon removal
of ConA from IL-2 preparations, thereby avoiding polyclonal T cell
activation at the initiation of cell cultures. Thus, the T cells activated
to antigens in vivo would be stimulated to proliferation by IL-2. The
culture medium is replaced 3 times weekly by fresh medium supplemented with 10 units/ml IL-2. Each week, cells are recultured at a
density of 10^6 viable cells/ml with 10^5 irradiated filler cells. It is
readily apparent in these cell cultures that considerable proliferation
is occurring, and analysis of effector function reveals increases in
helper T cell activity (50). These findings imply that IL-2 will be an
extremely useful reagent for the selection and development of antigen-
specific T cell lines in culture.

B. Physiological Significance of Interleukin 2

It remains a difficult problem to associate a factor activity in an in vitro response assay with a physiological role in vivo. Studies on the purification of murine, rat, and human lymphokines with murine T cell-growth factor activity have revealed a class of hormonal-like molecules that exhibit a variety of biological activities in murine lymphocyte proliferative and differentiative assays. These assays appear to measure the clonal expansion of antigen- or mitogen-activated helper, suppressor, and cytotoxic T cells promoted by a single class of "hormones" which have many diverse effects in terms of the responses measured. The molecular analysis of these molecules from murine, rat, and human sources may reveal the existence of structure homologies in such molecules between species. However, it should be emphasized that the physiological significance of these molecules is unknown and that the hormonal activities they express may represent only one class of a diverse range of lymphocyte regulatory molecules. Interleukin 2 may represent one class of such regulatory molecules.

We have maintained in culture, for several years, murine T cell lines that retain their antigen-specific helper and cytotoxic effector activities and which remain absolutely IL-2 dependent for continued growth (Refs. 5,11,15, and 16). Whatever might be the physiological role of IL-2, it is of tremendous value as a tool to generate antigen-specific T cell lines.

Acknowledgments

Supported by a Research Career Development Award (AI-00182) and grant AI-13383 from the National Institute of Allergy and Infectious Diseases, and grant I-469 from the National Foundation to James Watson. Steven Gillis is a Special Fellow of the Leukemia Society of America, supported by grant 28419 from the National Cancer Institute, grant 1-725 from the National Foundation, and a grant from the National Leukemia Association, Inc.

References

1. N. Warner, *Adv. Immunol. 19*:67 (1974).
2. E. S. Vitetta and J. W. Uhr, *J. Exp. Med. 139*:1599 (1974).
3. A. Szenberg, J. J. Marchalonis and N. L. Warner, *Proc. Natl. Acad. Sci. 74*:2113 (1977).
4. D. Haustein, J. J. Marchalonis and A. W. Harris, *Biochemistry 14*:1826 (1975).
5. H. Binz and H. Wigzell, *J. Exp. Med. 142*:197 (1975).

6. H. Cosenza, M. H. Julis and A. A. Augustin, *Immunol. Rev.* *34*:3 (1977).

7. D. H. Katz, N. Chiorazzi, J. McDonald, and L. R. Katz, *J. Immunol.* *117*:1853 (1976).

8. R. M. Zinkernagel, G. N. Callahan, A. Althage, S. Cooper and J. Klein, *J. Exp. Med.* *147*:882 (1978).

9. P. Marrack and J. W. Kappler, *J. Exp. Med.* *147*:1596 (1978).

10. P. Marrack and J. W. Kappler, *J. Exp. Med.* *149*:780 (1979).

11. J. S. McDougal and S. P. Cort, *J. Immunol.* *120*:445 (1978).

12. W. E. Paul and B. Benacerraf, *Science* *195*:1293 (1977).

13. C. W. Pierce, J. A. Kapp and B. Benacerraf, *J. Exp. Med.* *144*:371 (1976).

14. C. W. Pierce and J. A. Kapp, in *Ir Genes and Ia Antigens* (H. O. McDevitt, ed.), Academic, New York, 1978.

15. R. H. Schwartz, A. Yano, and W. E. Paul, *Immunol. Rev.* *40*:153 (1978).

16. S. Howie and M. Feldman, *Eur. J. Immunol.* *7*:417 (1977).

17. M. J. Taussig, A. J. Munro, R. Campbell, C. S. David, N. A. Staines, *J. Exp. Med.* *143*:694 (1975).

18. D. Armeding and D. H. Katz, *J. Exp. Med.* *140*:19 (1974).

19. T. L. Delovitch and U. Sohn, *J. Immunol.* *1226*:1528 (1978).

20. J. Watson, *J. Immunol.* *111*:1301 (1973).

21. R. W. Dutton, R. Falkoff, J. A. Hirst, M. Hoffman, J. W. Kappler, J. R. Kettman, J. F. Lesley, and D. Vann, *Prog. Immunol.* *1*:355 (1971).

22. J. Watson, L. Aarden, and I. Lefkovitz, *J. Immunol.* *122*:209 (1979).

23. A. Schimpl and E. Wecker, *Nature (New Biol.)* *237*:15 (1972).

24. G. Doria, G. Agarossi, and S. Di Pietro, *J. Immunol.* *108*:268 (1972).

25. R. M. Gorczynski, R. G. Miller, and R. A. Phillips, *J. Immunol.* *108*:547 (1972).

26. S. Britton, *J. Immunol.* *1*:89 (1972).

27. O. Sjoberg, J. Andersson, and G. Moller, *J. Immunol.* *109*:1379 (1972).

28. L. Harwell, J. W. Kappler, and P. Marrack, *J. Immunol.* *116*:5 (1976).

29. I. Lefkovits, J. Quintans, A. Munro, and H. Waldmann, *Immunology* *28*:1149 (1975).

30. I. Lefkovits and H. Waldmann, *Immunology* *32*:915 (1977).

31. L. Hubner, G. Muller, A. Schimpl, and E. Wecker, *Immunochemistry* *15*:33 (1978).

32. J. S. McDougal, S. P. Cort, and D. S. Gordon, *J. Immunol.* *119*:1933 (1977).

33. S. B. Mizel, *J. Immunol.* *122*:2167 (1979).

34. L. B. Lachman and R. S. Metzgar, *J. Retic. Soc.* 27:621 (1980).
35. I. Gery and B. H. Waksman, *J. Exp. Med.* 136:143 (1972).
36. G. J. Prud'homme, U. Sohn, and T. L. Delovitch, *J. Exp. Med.* 149:137 (1978).
37. T. L. Delovitch, J. Watson, R. Battistella, J. F. Harris, J. Shaw, and V. Paetkau, *J. Exp. Med.* 153:107 (1981).
38. E. R. Unanue and J. M. Kiely, *J. Immunol.* 119:925 (1977).
39. W. J. Koopman, J. J. Farrar and J. Fuller-Bonar, *Cell Immunol.* 35:92 (1978).
40. M. K. Hoffman and J. Watson, *J. Immunol.* 122:1371 (1979).
41. D. D. Wood, *J. Immunol.* 123:2395 (1979).
42. M. K. Hoffman, S. Koening, R. S. Mittler, H. F. Dettgen, P. Ralph, C. Galanos, and U. Hammerling, *J. Immunol.* 122:497 (1979).
43. L. A. Aarden et al., *J. Immunol.* 123:2928 (1979).
44. D. M. Chen and G. Di Sabato, *Cell. Immunol.* 22:221 (1976).
45. J. J. Farrar, P. L. Simon, W. J. Koopman, and J. Fuller-Bonar, *J. Immunol.* 121:1353 (1978).
46. D. A. Morgan, F. W. Ruscetti and R. C. Gallo, *Science 193:* 1007 (1976).
47. S. Gillis and K. A. Smith, *J. Exp. Med.* 146:468 (1977).
48. S. Gillis, M. M. Ferm, W. Ou, and K. A. Smith, *J. Immunol.* 120:2027 (1978).
49. S. Gillis, P. E. Baker, F. W. Ruscetti, and K. A. Smith, *J. Exp. Med.* 148:1093 (1978).
50. J. Watson, *J. Exp. Med.* 150:1510 (1979).
51. J. Watson, S. Gillis, J. Marbrook, D. Mochizuki, and K. A. Smith, *J. Exp. Med.* 150:849 (1979).
52. S. Gillis, K. A. Smith, and J. Watson, *J. Immunol.* 124:1954 (1980).
53. J. Shaw, V. Monticone, and V. Paetkau, *J. Immunol.* 120:1974 (1978).
54. J. J. Farrar, P. L. Simon, W. J. Koopman, and J. Fuller-Bonar, *J. Immunol.* 121:1353 (1978).
55. H. Wagner and M. Rollinghoff, *J. Exp. Med.* 148:1523 (1978).
56. S. Gillis, M. Scheid, and J. Watson, *J. Immunol.* 125:2570 (1980).
57. D. Mochizuki, J. Watson, and S. Gillis, *J. Immunol.* 125:2579 (1980).
58. S. Gillis and J. Watson, *J. Exp. Med.* 152:1709 (1980).
59. W. Schalch and D. G. Braun, in *Research Methods in Immunology,* (I. Lefkovits and B. Pernis, eds.), Academic, New York, 1978.
60. U. K. Laemmli, *Nature (Lond.)* 227:680 (1970).
61. J. Watson and D. Mochizuki, *Immunol. Rev.* 51:355 (1980).
62. J. Watson, D. Mochizuki, and S. Gillis, in *ICN-UCLA Symposium on Control of Cell Division and Differentiation.* (D. Cunningham, E. Goldwasser, and J. Watson, eds.), Academic, New York, 1980).

3

Glucocorticoids, Stress, and the Immune Response

J. JOHN COHEN and LINDA S. CRNIC   University of Colorado
School of Medicine, Denver, Colorado

I.   Glucocorticoids, Stress, and the Immune Response

When considering the effects of glucocorticoids upon the immune and
inflammatory responses, it is helpful to remember that these effects
have been studied under three different sets of circumstances.
First, physiological effects, aspects of the immune system's function
which depend on normal levels of glucocorticoids and perhaps on
normal circadian rhythms, have been noted. Second, the patho-
physiological role of glucocorticoids has been studied in stressed
animals in which absolute levels of glucocorticoids in the blood have
been raised up to 20-fold and the circadian rhythm has been dis-
rupted. Third, glucocorticoids have been administered as drugs,
frequently in large doses and in long-acting forms. Under these
circumstances, of course, the desired result is immunosuppression
or reduction of inflammation. At these doses, effects upon the
immune system may be demonstrated which are not seen at the levels
obtained physiologically or even under stress. It is very important
for us to discover the cellular and molecular effects of glucocorticoids administered as drugs and to know to what extent these effects
also take place in the stressed animal. Furthermore, we need to know
how important glucocorticoids are in the normal functioning of immune responses, and to what extent this may influence experimental
and clinical studies in immunology. Finally, there is the very interesting question of whether or not stress produces an undesirable
immunosuppression, or, to put it another way, if the stress
response is harmful, why did it evolve?

II. Effects of Exogenous Glucocorticoids on the Immune Response

The profound effects of adrenal cortex extracts on the lymphatic system were discovered in the late 1930s (1,2), and this discovery stimulated so much research that a dozen years later investigators were pleading their inability to review the entire field (3-5). The growth of our knowledge about corticosteroids and their effects on immune and inflammatory responses has not lessened since the 1950s, and we also find ourselves unable to cover the new information comprehensively. Instead, we will deal briefly with certain areas which we feel promise to yield valuable insights into the effects of the glucocorticoids on lymphocyte function. These areas include glucocorticoid-sensitive and -resistant cells and processes, the mechanism of glucocorticoid-induced lymphocyte death, lymphocyte recirculation, the question of glucocorticoid-sensitive and -resistant species, and the role of endogenous glucocorticoids and their circadian rhythms in the normal functioning of the immune system. This last topic will naturally lead into a discussion of the results of disturbing endogenous glucocorticoid secretion, for example, by stress. The very interesting effects of glucocorticoids on the secretion of lymphokines and monokines will be considered in more detail in Chapters 4 and 11.

A. Glucocorticoid-Sensitive and -Resistant Cells and Processes

The earliest observations of exogenous glucocorticoid effects on the lymphatic system were profound "atrophy" of the thymus and lymph nodes. It is quite clear that many lymphocytes are, in fact, lysed by glucocorticoids (see Sec. II.B), and it was assumed that all immunosuppressive activity of these compounds was due to lympholysis. High doses of glucocorticoid were thought to be radiomimetic in that they killed all lymphocytes, with the fastest dividing being most sensitive.

Morphological evidence for glucocorticoid-sensitive and -resistant lymphocytes was obtained by Ishidate and Metcalf (6) and by Dougherty et al. (7). These workers showed that, in the thymus, the cortical lymphocytes are much more sensitive to pharmacological doses of glucocorticoids than are the lymphocytes of the medulla. The difference in sensitivity correlates with a difference in function; essentially all of the thymus's immunocompetent cells are contained within the corticosteroid-resistant fraction (8-13). This population does not exceed 5% of the total lymphocyte content. A related and overlapping subpopulation of cells in the thymus, ranging from 5 to 15%, can be identified by other means. These include a lack of the thymus lymphocyte (TL) surface antigen (14), agglutinability by the sialic acid-specific lobster lectin (P. A. Campbell, personal communication) but not by the galactose-specific peanut agglutinin (15), and concentrations of surface H-2 and Lyt antigens more like those of peripheral T cells than of the bulk of thymic lymphocytes (16). It is by no means clear that all these minor populations are the same, that they correspond to the cortico-steroid-resistant population, or that any of them consists exclusively of medullary lymphocytes. In fact, there is some evidence that, although most lymphocytes identified by surface antigen studies as similar to peripheral cells are, in fact, about to be exported [17], the glucocorticoid-resistant population is *not* exported, or at best is exported very slowly (18). This was demonstrated in mice that were given a chromosome-marked thymic implant. Long after the thymic cortex and peripheral T cells were mostly recipient type (indicating repopulation from bone marrow stem cells), the glucocorticoid-resistant portion of the implanted thymus remained of donor type: the cells had not been exported or replaced by cortex-derived precursors. The implication of this study is that movement from cortex to medulla, or maturation from glucocorticoid-sensitive to glucocorticoid-resistant, is not an obligatory step in the intrathymic maturation of T lymphocytes. Nabarra and Papiernik (19) have recent data which supports this idea.

There certainly are glucocorticoid-sensitive T cells in the periphery in mice, but their function has not been clearly elucidated. Determining the sensitivity of, for example, splenic T cells to glucocorticoids is complicated by the possibility of cell redistribution in addition to cell death (see Sec. II.C). Nevertheless, there is a dramatic fall in Thy-1$^+$ cells in the spleen following hydrocortisone administration (Fig. 1) which cannot be accounted for by an increase in Thy-1$^+$ cells in any other location, and therefore these cells are probably killed rather than redistributed. It seems reasonable to suppose that among the glucocorticoid-sensitive splenic population are many recent emigrants from the thymus retaining, at least for awhile, this "cortical" attribute. These cells may include precursors of other better-defined T cell populations, such as helpers and graft-versus-host inducers, which are quite glucocorticoid resistant (see below). Stutman (20) has described a "postthymic precursor" population which is glucocorticoid sensitive, spleen seeking, not recirculating, and of the Lyt-1$^+$2,3$^+$ phenotype; it probably constitutes most of the T lymphocytes in the spleen that are killed by glucocorticoids.

When spleen cells from a glucocorticoid-treated donor are transferred to an irradiated recipient, far less antibody is formed than if normal spleen cells had been transferred (21). The deficiency can be made up by addition of bone marrow but not of thymus, indicating that the glucocorticoid-treated spleen is depleted of B cells (13); this is supported by the data in Figure 1. However, in vitro, spleen cells from corticosteroid-treated donors, although deficient in antibody formation, can be reconstituted by T cells but not B cells (22,23). We do not know at present how to explain this interesting discrepancy.

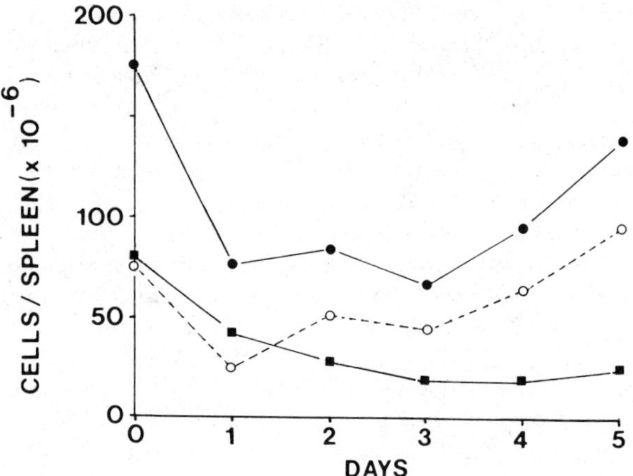

FIG. 1   Effect on spleen lymphocyte subpopulations of 2.5 mg of hydrocortisone acetate administered intraperitoneally to 11-week-old CBA/J male mice. ●——● = total lymphoid cells; ■——■ = B cells measured by immunofluorescence with rabbit antimouse IgM; O--- = T cells measured by immunofluorescence with anti-Thy 1.2, followed by rabbit antimouse Ig. Total lymphoid cell numbers were significantly (P = .05) lower than control on days 1-4, T cell numbers on days 1-3, and B cell numbers on days 1-5.

It illustrates some of the problems inherent in comparing in vitro with in vivo experimental systems: in one case the culture vessel is a plastic dish, but in the other it is a living, irradiated recipient. One has to take into account the cellular contribution of the recipient, especially antigen-presenting cells (probably macrophages). Mishell and colleagues (24) have shown that macrophages make a factor, GRMF (glucocorticoid response-modifying factor), which protects helper lymphocytes from the inhibiting effects of glucocorticoids. Perhaps the activation or recovery of helper T cells in the irradiated recipient is accelerated by GRMF produced by radio-resistant splenic macrophages, whereas in vitro there are insufficient macrophages to provide this effect. Evidence in favor of this hypothesis was obtained by Lee et al. (23), who found that the decreased antibody response of spleen cells from hydrocortisone-treated mice in vitro could be restored to normal by peritoneal exudate cells (mostly macrophages), or by 2-mercaptoethanol, which apparently stimulates macrophages. Also germane is the observation that macrophage secretion of enzymes of the activated state is suppressed by glucocorticoids (25). The conclusion that seems warranted is that helper T cells are probably not directly affected by reasonable doses

(10^{-6} M) of glucocorticoids in vitro, but their activation is diminished, probably through effects on accessory cells such as macrophages. A very reasonable possibility is that glucocorticoids inhibit synthesis of interleukin 1 (IL-1), the macrophage-produced factor that is essential for inducer T cell activation (26). This idea may be supported by the observations of Markham et al. (27) that a moderate dose (1 mg/ mouse) of a short-acting glucocorticoid, hydrocortisone sodium succinate, given 5 hr before priming helper T cells with antigen, completely inhibited such priming. Once primed, however, helper T cells were only marginally sensitive to glucocorticoid. It is likely that the drug given prior to priming suppressed the antigen presentation process.

Most studies show that, in vivo, cells of the helper, graft-versus-host inducer, and delayed hypersensitivity inducer phenotypes (all of which are Lyt-2⁻ and are very similar if not identical) are glucocorticoid resistant. The final immunological phenomena which are induced by these cells may be suppressed by glucocorticoids, but the lymphocytes themselves are spared. For example, the graft-versus-host reaction, as assessed by splenomegaly in the recipient, is suppressed almost completely, but the T cells which trigger the reaction are unaffected, as is their proliferation in vivo in response to allo-antigen (12,28). What *is* suppressed is the inflammatory response that would normally be called up by the activated T cells (28,29); apparently T cells make lymphokines in the presence of glucocorticoids, but inflammatory cells do not respond to them (30,31). A similar conclusion was reached in a study of contact hypersensitivity in mice (a form of delayed hypersensitivity) in which the inflammatory manifestations of hypersensitivity were abolished by hydrocortisone treatment during the sensitization phase; however, later challenge with the antigen showed that immunization (the expansion of T clones) had proceeded normally (32). Other groups also have come to the conclusion that the T cells that induce delayed or contact hyper-sensitivity are glucocorticoid resistant (33-35). A similar reasoning process indicates that the suppression of antibody synthesis by glucocorticoids may be due to inhibition of antigen-presenting cells or of B cells, or both; it is unlikely to be a result of direct toxicity or suppression of helper T cells.

The generation of cytotoxic or killer T cells involves a similarly complex set of cellular interactions. Antigen is presented by accessory cells, again probably macrophages, to helper or inducer cells. These cells help prekiller cells, which have interacted with antigen, to pro-liferate and express the full killer phenotype. This "help" is in the form of a mitogenic lymphokine, interleukin 2 (IL-2) (36). Recently, the effects of glucocorticoids have been examined within this context. It has been shown that the proliferation of killer cells is not affected to any great extent by glucocorticoids. On the other hand, the production of IL-2 by helper cells, upon which killer cell proliferation depends, is completely inhibited by dexamethasone (37-39). Once again, the locus of the drug's effect may be the helper/inducer cell itself, or, as we have discussed above, on the antigen-presenting IL-1-secreting accessory cell that is necessary for helper/inducer cell activation. Larsson (40) has preliminary results that suggest the latter to be the case: the suppression of T cell proliferation by dexamethasone can be overcome by the addition of a soluble macrophage product, presumably IL-1.

A separate class of T cell seems to have as its sole function the suppression of immune responses, which are thus under both positive and negative control. Suppressor T cells differ from inducer T cells in Lyt phenotype, being predominantly Lyt-2$^+$, and also in several metabolic properties. Here we must distinguish between the precursor cell--the suppressor cell that has not yet encountered antigen--and the activated suppressor cell several days after antigen exposure. For example, precursors of suppressor T cells are very sensitive to the alkylating agent cyclophosphamide, whereas activated suppressors and the other classes of T cells are relatively resistant. If cyclophosphamide is given several days before antigen, T cell-mediated responses--such as contact hypersensitivity--are enhanced, indicating the removal of a negative influence (41). A few studies in mice indicate that the suppressor cell precursor is also glucocorticoid sensitive (42-45), whereas the activated cell is resistant (44,45). The availability of a simple assay for human suppressor T cells (46) has allowed several groups to show that, in humans as well, suppressor T cell precursors are more sensitive to glucocorticoids (to which they were exposed in vitro) than are activated suppressors or other T cells (47-50).

The conclusion that must be drawn from the data presented above is that the observed effects of glucocorticoid treatment will be difficult to predict, depending as they do on at least the following variables: dose and chemical form of the drug, timing of treatment with respect to antigen administration, and complexity of the response—the degree to which accessory cells, helpers, suppressors, and inflammatory cells are involved. For example, in most immune mechanisms, antigen presentation by accessory cells is mandatory for the initiation of the response. This step seems to be relatively glucocorticoid sensitive, and so adequate levels of steroid at this time would be expected to suppress the response. Suppressor T cells are activated somewhat later than inducer cells, so that the presence of glucocorticoids early in the response would, by inactivating suppressor precursors, tend to increase the observed response. Since the drugs tend to inactivate B cells and inflammatory response cells, their administration in the later stages of the reaction will also tend to

be suppressive, although immunological memory (largely a property
of T cells) may be induced normally. It is not surprising that the
vast literature on the effects of glucocorticoids on the incidence of
disease in animals should show such a hodgepodge of results: in one
case the main resistance mechanism may involve antibody, in another
T cell-mediated immunity, in a third killer T cells; the antibody formation may be T dependent or T independent; the etiologic agent may
be a powerful activator of macrophages, producing glucocorticoid-
response-modifying factors; the drug administered may have been
long- or short-acting; and so on. In addition, this discussion has not
even considered the growing family of auxiliary, amplifier,
suppressor-inducer, suppressor-acceptor, and other regulatory cells
about whose function, not to mention glucocorticoid sensitivity, we
know almost nothing. It is essential that future studies concentrate on
the effects of glucocorticoids on defined cellular subpopulations and
interactions, so that a unified picture of the effects of these drugs
can be developed. Newer methods for identifying subpopulations by
surface markers are available in mice and humans, and the necessary
studies should be accomplished soon.

B.   The Mechanism of Glucocorticoid-induced Lymphocyte Death

Glucocorticoids have profound effects upon the structure and biochemical function of sensitive cells. Most of what we know in this
area comes from studies on thymocytes, most of which are exquisitely
sensitive to the lethal effects of these drugs. Unfortunately, thymocytes are not mature T or B cells, and it is probably wrong to extra-
polate from thymocytes to those mature, peripheralized lymphocytes
whose functions interest us more. Nevertheless, until glucocorticoid-
sensitive mature populations are isolated and studied, we can learn
some interesting things from the study of thymocytes.

   Biochemical changes in glucocorticoid treated thymocytes are extensive, and a review of them is beyond the scope of this paper; a
comprehensive monograph on the subject has recently appeared (51).
We will limit our discussion to the possible differences between
glucocorticoid-sensitive and -resistant thymocytes and to the mechanism
of cell death called apoptosis.

   Whatever the effects of glucocorticoids upon a cell, they are
generally considered to be the consequence of an interaction of the
hormone with cytoplasmic receptors. It should be pointed out,
however, that although this view has predominated since receptors
were first demonstrated in 1968 (52,53), it is possible that some
steroids can affect lymphocytes via other pathways, for example, by
acting as calcium ionophores (54). This is important to keep in mind
because a number of workers have failed to show a correlation between
numbers of cytoplasmic glucocorticoid receptors and susceptibility to

killing. There is an increase in receptor numbers when T cells are
stimulated by mitogens (55,56) or antigens (32,57), but in no case
were the activated cells found to be more susceptible to glucocorticoids as measured by macromolecular synthesis, glucose uptake, or
dye exclusion. Crabtree et al. (39) separated mitogen-activated T
cells into G_0 + G_1 and S + G_2 + M fractions and found a two- to
threefold increase in the number of receptors per cell in the latter.
Their observation, that cells increase their glucocorticoid receptor
content in S phase, is interesting, but one cannot conclude either
that cells in S or with high numbers of receptors are necessarily more
glucocorticoid sensitive or that extremely sensitive cells will be in
S + G_2 + M. In fact, cortical thymocytes have the same number of
glucocorticoid receptors per cell as medullary thymocytes (58), although they are easily killed by the steroids whereas medullary thymocytes are resistant (8-12). In addition, most cortical thymocytes
are in G_0 or G_1 (R. Chervenak, personal communication).

We are thus faced with the apparent paradox that a receptor-
mediated event cannot be correlated with the number of receptors
present to mediate it. Our knowledge of glucocorticoid receptor
economy is simply too sketchy at present to resolve this conflict.
Many other factors are involved: the ability of individual cell types to
metabolize the steroid (59), the ratio of active to inactive receptor
complexes in the cytoplasm, transport to the nucleus, and, probably,
the nature of the available sites at which the steroid-receptor complex
can effect an inducer- or derepressor-like action (for a review of receptors, see Refs. 60 and 61). Thus, cells with similar numbers of
receptors in a hormone-binding assay may have very different effective concentrations of receptors and very different derepression or
differentiation programs that are activated by glucocorticoid treatment.
One such program may be to die.

Wyllie has discussed extensively the difference between cell death
owing to toxic influences and that which seems to be physiologically
programmed (62). Examples of the latter include the resorption of the
tail during tadpole metamorphosis, or the cell death in a target organ
which follows ablation of the source of its trophic hormone. For this
sort of cell death the term apoptosis has been proposed. Probably the
most important difference between apoptosis and necrosis (the form
of cell death which follows injury) is that in necrosis there is a
collapse of the cell's homeostasis, with a termination of metabolism and
synthesis. In apoptosis, on the other hand, macromolecular synthesis
seems to be necessary for cell death to take place; the whole process
seems more "normal." Glucocorticoids, of course, are well known to
induce protein synthesis in a wide variety of cells (51), and it does
not seem unreasonable that, in susceptible cells, a "suicidal" protein
might be produced. Recently, Wyllie (63) has found in glucocorticoid-
treated thymocytes: small DNA fragments of size corresponding to a

few nucleosomes. It seems likely that the glucocorticoid induces
a new endonuclease which cuts DNA in the relatively unprotected
region between nucleosomes. This would lead to the collapse of
chromosomal structure characteristic of apoptosis, which was once
called, in fact, "shrinkage necrosis." We have found (M. Goncalves
and J. J. Cohen, unpublished) that the appearance of the DNA
breakdown products following exposure to glucocortocoid can be
eliminated by treatment with the protein synthesis inhibitor
cyclohexamide.

Thus it would appear that glucocorticoids can have three
possible effects on cells of the immune system. Either cells will be
unaffected or new protein synthesis will be induced. If there is new
protein synthesis, either it will survive, but in a metabolically
altered state, or it will die, depending on the program which that cell
type is designed to express. Within the immune system, cortical thymocytes, and possibly some suppressor T cells and B cells, are programmed to die. Much of what we observe clinically and experimentally to be the effects of glucocorticoids are due to alterations in the
metabolism of other cells, notably the inflammatory cells (neutrophils,
basophils, eosinophils, monocytes, and macrophages) (29,64,65).

C. Lymphocyte Recirculation

Glucocorticoid treatment causes a profound decrease in circulating
lymphocytes, monocytes, and eosionphils in all species tested. For
many years it was thought that this was due to cell death, but there
were hints, especially for eosinophils, that what was actually taking
place was a reversible sequestration of cells in the tissues (66,67).
When it was found that most mature T cells in the mouse were, in
fact, glucocorticoid resistant, the idea of sequestration of blood
lymphocytes, which are predominantly T cells, was examined. In 1972
one of us (J.J.C.) showed that ^{51}Cr-labeled T cells, injected intravenously into mice, could be found in the bone marrow of mice that
were hydrocortisone treated, but not in controls (68). This observation explained the decrease in recirculating lymphocytes that had
been reported earlier (69,70). Recirculating lymphocytes are those
that travel from blood via lymph nodes to the lymph, and then eventually back to the blood; they are the most mature T cells. We
originally assumed that the appearance of T cells in the bone marrow
after glucocorticoid treatment was just an index of a general sequestration of T cells in the tissues, but Zatz could not find increased T
cells in any tissue except bone marrow (71). Recent studies indicate
(D. Grier, unpublished) that the T cells which appear in bone
marrow after hydrocortisone treatment are numerically equal to those
which disappear from the blood. When T cells enter the marrow, T
cell activities can be observed which are normally very low or absent

in that tissue. Cole noticed this in 1960 (72): marrow from cortisone-
treated mice could induce graft-versus-host reactions, whereas control
marrow could not. We confirmed this (12) and also showed the appearance of helper T cells in the marrow of hydrocortisone-treated mice
(73). A rough time course study showed significant T cell entry at
2 days after hydrocortisone treatment, a peak at 5 days, and a
return to normal by about 9 days. In regard to this timing it should
be noted that the drug used was hydrocortisone acetate, a sparingly
soluble long-acting preparation. Other studies showed that mitogen-
responsive T cells also enter the marrow under the influence of glucocorticoids (21,74).

The sequestration of T cells in the marrow seems to be a wide-
spread phenomenon, having been documented in rats (75), guinea
pigs (76,77), and humans (78), although the evidence in rats and
humans is circumstantial. Two questions arise: Why and how are T
cells sequestered? Possible reasons why will be discussed in Sec. V;
how has not yet been elucidated. It is obvious that altered recirculation patterns could be due to an effect on the lymphocyte or on the
bone marrow endothelium. On the face of it, an effect on the lymphocyte seems less likely because the resulting redistribution is so specifically to the marrow. In preliminary experiments, D. Grier and
J. J. Cohen have found that the T cells which appear in marrow after
glucocorticoid treatment are not marrow-seeking when transferred to
a second, untreated recipient. Thus it is probable that glucocorticoids
induce a change in the bone marrow environment such that recirculating T lymphocytes are trapped within it for a period of time; the
effect is clearly reversible.

It should be obvious from this and the preceding sections that
the effects of glucocorticoids upon lymphocyte populations are complex. If, for example, spleen from a treated animal shows a reduced
helper T cell response to a particular antigen, one must consider
whether the effect was on the helper T cell itself, upon the antigen-
presenting cell, or upon the population of helper cells, some of which,
while unharmed, may have moved to another location. In fact,
Moorhead and Claman showed that T cells from the spleen can move to
the bone marrow after hydrocortisone treatment of mice (74,79).

D. Glucocorticoid-Sensitive and -Resistant Species?

It is repeatedly stated in the clinical literature that humans are glucocorticoid resistant, whereas mice, rats, and rabbits are glucocorticoid
sensitive (64,65,80,81). Because of this, investigators have been
cautioned that conclusions drawn from animal experiments should not
be extrapolated to humans. However, the data on which this distinction has been based do not, upon close examination, actually support
the contention. Thus Batra et al. (82) compared the survival of

peripheral blood lymphocytes from rat, rabbit, guinea pig, and man in vitro in the presence and absence of 10 μg/ml prednisolone sodium succinate. They found that survival in culture medium alone was very variable, being 26% at 2 days in the case of guinea pigs, and 40% at 3 days for mice, and 53% at 7 days for humans; therefore, their prednisolone data are from different incubation times. They showed that the excess death of lymphocytes was 49% (guinea pig), 96% (mice), and 23-40% (humans) at 2, 3, and 7 days, respectively. Another awkward point is that the medium was constant in all experiments and contained 20% rabbit serum. It is impossible to know if the conditions were optimal for survival of all species' lymphocytes, especially since normal sera often contain antibodies to cell surface structures of other species. In a similar study, Batra and Schrek (83) found that prednisolone caused 4% excess death of newborn rabbit thymocytes, 100% in mouse, and 77% in humans. This hardly supports the concept of rabbits as a glucocorticoid-sensitive species. However, the data are clouded by the fact that the human thymuses were studied 24-48 hr after excision. Finally, Shewell and Long (84) treated mice, rats, guinea pigs, rabbits, ferrets, and rhesus monkeys with 50 mg/kg, i.m. cortisone acetate daily for 10 days. They found muscle wasting in all animals except guinea pigs and monkeys, and all species had a fall in thymus weight. Rabbits, ferrets, guinea pigs, and monkeys all showed no decrease in spleen weights; mice and rats had a significant decrease. All species had decreased adrenal weights. They concluded that rats, mice, rabbits, and ferrets are cortisone sensitive, and monkey and guinea pigs are resistant.

These studies bring up some of the problems inherent in comparing any biologically active substance in different species. First, dosage is important: it may not always be proper to compare doses on a per kilogram basis. Of course, on the basis of dose per square meter of surface area, small animals like mice and rats receive much larger doses and might be expected to respond more profoundly. Second, the specific glucocorticoid employed must be taken into account. In humans, the predominant plasma glucocorticoid is hydrocortisone, whereas in rats and mice it is corticosterone. Thus it is not necessarily valid to compare effects of hydrocortisone in humans and mice; nonetheless, almost no studies have examined the potency of corticosterone in rodents (for a recent exception, see Ref. 85). In terms of causing thymus shrinkage, hydrocortisone is three times more potent than the natural corticosterone in mice (7). Synthetic glucocorticoids also differ widely, and unpredictably, in effect. Human peripheral blood mononuclear cells and thymocytes were found to be quite sensitive in vitro to hydrocortisone sodium succinate and methylprednisolone phosphate but were extremely resistant to dexamethasone phosphate (86). In this context it should also be noted that there are individual differences between people, and strain differences

between inbred mice, that may affect the outcome of glucocorticoid
therapy (87). A recent example of this is the Palmerston North mouse,
which, like the more familiar NZB/W, develops a spontaneous systemic
lupus erythematosus-like disease. Palmerston North mice do not im-
prove upon hydrocortisone treatment, unlike the NZB/W (88). If one
had studied only humans with lupus and Palmerston North mice, one
would conclude that humans are glucocorticoid sensitive and mice are
glucocorticoid resistant.

Perhaps the real clue to the persistent idea that mice and humans
differ in glucocorticoid sensitivity lies in the different doses and
forms of drugs used to treat the two species. Almost all studies done
in humans use soluble short-acting derivatives, frequently the
succinates. In mice, on the contrary, most studies have used cortisone or hydrocortisone acetate, an insoluble depot-effect form. Thus
it is not surprising that effects observed in rodents tend to be more
prolonged and profound. When 1 g prednisolone sodium phosphate was
given intravenously to human volunteers, a marked lymphopenia was
observed, in most cases within 1 hr. Some lymphocyte counts returned
to normal in 24 hr; all were normal at 48 hr (89). This rapid return
to normal is often compared with the relatively slow recovery of mice
treated with hydrocortisone acetate (for example, see Fig. 1) as
evidence of the relative glucocorticoid resistance of humans. However, if mice are treated with short-acting hydrocortisone sodium
succinate, there is almost no effect on spleen size or mitogen responses, even at doses approaching 400 mg/kg (90), and lymphocyte
counts are normal by 48 hr (unpublished observations). Note that in
the human study cited above, the dose of glucocorticoid was approximately 70 mg hydrocortisone equivalent per kilogram. Thus when dose
and pharmacodynamic properties are taken into account, there does
not seem to be any basis for the claim that humans and mice are
glucocorticoid resistant and sensitive. In fact, recent reviews of the
effects of glucocorticoids on the human immune response (65,81) show
that these are identical to those described in mice, whenever an adequate basis for comparison exists.

III. Effects of Endogenous Glucocorticoids and their Circadian Rhythms on the Immune Response

A. *Endogenous Glucocorticoids Modulate Immune Responses*

Normal plasma of almost all vertebrates contains glucocorticoids in the
range of 5×10^{-9} to 5×10^{-7} M. Because these agents regulate many
aspects of cellular metabolism in a wide variety of target cells, it
would not be surprising if normal lymphoid function were also regulated by them. Experiments to determine the extent of this effect can

be done in vitro and, for short periods of time, in vivo in adrenalectomized animals.

It has been claimed that, as is true of many culture systems,
antibody responses in vitro are absolutely dependent upon small
amounts of glucocorticoid. Ambrose (91,92), using a secondary
response model, showed that serum could be replaced by a mixture of
serine, vitamin B_{12}, insulin, and hydrocortisone in Eagle's medium.
Of these, only the requirement for hydrocortisone was absolute.
Optimal responses were achieved at 10^{-7} M. This observation has been
confirmed with human peripheral blood lymphocytes in vitro (93),
except that some serum was required. More recently, however, Iscove
has described a serum-free medium which does not contain glucocorticoids and yet seems to maintain many B (94) and T cell (95) activities
in culture for at least a week. Thus it is not clear to what extent
glucocorticoids are necessary for lymphoid function in vitro, although
their presence can increase several activities or growth rates. For
example, even when serum and other growth factors are optimal,
added hydrocortisone can double the number of pre-T cell colonies
grown from normal mouse bone marrow (96).

This difficulty in showing an absolute requirement for glucocorticoids in vitro is mirrored in in vivo experiments. In general, in
the relatively short time that adrenalectomized animals can be kept
healthy without steroid replacement, it has been found that immune
responses are *augmented*. By 4 days after adrenalectomy, spleen
size is significantly increased (97), as is thymus size, which can
reach twice normal at 12 days (98). It would appear that, at least in
the thymus, there are cells whose death is due to, or hastened by,
glucocorticoids. Shortman and Backson (98) showed that a large proportion (about 40%) of cells in normal thymus are "labile" in that they
die rapidly when placed in culture. After adrenalectomy this proportion falls to about 5%. It may be that labile cells represent cells about
to die due to in vivo glucocorticoid exposure. It would be interesting
to know if this represents the true steady-state situation or was due
to higher-than-normal glucocorticoid levels associated with stressful
animal handling. If the former, then glucocorticoids normally exert a
suppressive influence on the immune system, and their removal by
adrenalectomy would be expected to enhance responses. This has
been shown to be true for antibody formation (97,99,100) and T cell-
mediated graft-versus-host disease (101). Besedovsky et al. (102)
have suggested another role for glucocorticoids in the regulation of
immune responses. They have shown that serum corticosterone levels
are elevated 6 days following an injection of horse erythrocytes as
antigen into rats. This elevation is enough to be immunosuppressive,
and in fact a second antigen injected at that time evokes a smaller
antibody response than would have been expected had horse erythrocytes not been administered previously. This phenomenon is called

antigenic competition and is eliminated if the animals are first adrenalectomized. Besedovsky et al. (103) have further shown that when T cells are stimulated with the mitogen concanavalin A, they release a factor which, injected into rats, raises corticosterone levels three- to fourfold. This suggests a mechanism by which glucocorticoids might be involved in the regulation of normal immune responses: as T cells are stimulated by antigen, along with initiating a variety of immune responses, they release a factor which influences the hypothalamic-pituitary-adrenal axis in such a way as to increase the concentration of glucocorticoids, and the responses are suppressed and eventually terminated. In view of the large number of other suppressive mechanisms that have been demonstrated in immune responses, it would be very interesting to know the importance of this one.

In conclusion, it has been shown that glucocorticoids may play significant roles both in the maintenance of effective immune responses and in their control. Since glucocorticoid levels in plasma fluctuate over a considerable range in a diurnal fashion, it is of interest next to see what evidence there is for immune responses varying in a like manner.

B. *Circadian Rhythms of Glucocorticoids and Immune Phenomena*

All vertebrates higher than Agnatha have a circadian rhythm of glucocorticoid levels in the plasma. In general, the period is very close to 24 hr and is entrained on the light-dark cycle. Studies of circadian rhythms have not always clearly specified the duration of light and dark parts of the cycle, when they begin relative to clock time, or whether extraneous stimuli (such as cage cleaning, feeding, or outside noise) were carefully controlled. Because glucocorticoid levels are so responsive to stress (Sec. IV), it is also essential that no animal be bled more than once in an experiment, that other animals not be disturbed by the removal of cagemates, and that blood be obtained before stress can produce artificial elevations. Although the pattern varies among different species and strains, in general, glucocorticoid levels reach their peak around the time the animal wakes up or begins its active cycle. Thus humans have their highest cortisol levels at about 8 a.m. and their nadirs at 10 p.m. to midnight (104, 105); the difference may be as much as fivefold. In the guinea pig, the peak is reached at the end of the dark cycle, as in man (106); the difference between this peak and the nadir, at the end of the light cycle, is about twofold. Guinea pigs and humans are diurnal. In mice, which are nocturnal, the corticosterone peak comes at the end of the light cycle, when the animals become active (107-109). Corticosterone levels may fluctuate from 5-35 ng/ml in the morning (end of activity cycle) to over 200 ng/ml between 7 and 10 p.m. (107).

The circadian rhythm of glucocorticoids is superimposed on an ultradian rhythm. This was carefully studied in sheep, using indwelling venous cannulas to obtain frequent samples of blood (110). The sheep were given 3 weeks to adapt to the experimental environment. It was found that there were approximately 12 cycles of hydrocortisone secretion in 24 hr, in bursts lasting 30 min, 2 hr apart. The size of the bursts varied in a circadian manner (peak at about midnight, the dark phase of the cycle was from 6 p.m. to 6 a.m.). It should be noted that to do a study of this type required sampling blood at 10-min intervals (2-4 min intervals to analyze a single cycle) around the clock. The short mean transit time of hydrocortisone in the sheep's plasma (70 min) also helped in delineating the ultradian rhythm.

Although eosinophils in blood had been known for a long time to vary in a diurnal fashion, in 1965 Brown and Dougherty (111) showed that lymphocytes vary similarly. The peak was at late morning, the mouse's least active period, and the low point was at about 9 p.m., when the mouse was becoming most active. In C57B1 mice, the peak was about 18,000 lymphocytes/mm^3, and the nadir was about 6000. That this cycle was related to the corticosteroid cycle was shown by adrenalectomizing some subjects; the circadian lymphocyte rhythm was abolished, and the level stayed constant around the clock at about 20,000 lymphocytes/mm^3. This negative correlation between lymphocyte counts and glucocorticoid levels has been confirmed in mice, rats, and humans (112-114).

Given the circadian fluctuations in blood glucocorticoid levels and lymphocytes, it would not be surprising if similar fluctuations could be found in immune responses. Using a contact hypersensitivity model in rats, Pownall et al. (115) showed that the clock time at which previously immunized rats were skin tested was a very important determinant of the size of the reaction obtained. When the lights were on from 10 a.m. to 10 p.m., rats had lymphocyte counts of 4107 ± 304 at 10 a.m., and 2036 ± 165 at 10 p.m. Rats on this schedule were skin tested at 10 a.m. or 10 p.m., and swelling was measured 24 hr later. When testing was done at 10 a.m., when lymphocytes were high (and glucocorticoids, although not measured in this study, should be low), swelling averaged 160 μM; when testing was done at 10 p.m., swelling averaged only 40 μM. This study was very much enhanced by entraining another group of rats on a cycle with lights on from 10 p.m. to 10 a.m. (inverted); lymphocyte levels and contact hypersensitivity also became entrained. Circadian differences in other immune responses, both cellular and humoral, have been described (109,115-117). In humans the picture is less complete. Several studies have shown circadian variation in the ability of peripheral blood lymphocytes to respond to antigens and mitogens (114,118), but it is not so clear whether this reflects an inherent change in the responding lymphocytes or changes in subpopulations (119). When an immune response is tested, diurnal fluctuations are observed as well. Cove-Smith et al. (120) gave tuberculin tests to 180 volunteers at 3-hr intervals around the clock. Responses were maximal when the test was given at 7 a.m., and were minimal at 10 p.m. This cycle follows the usual curve of hydrocortisone *directly*; however, hydrocortisone was not actually determined in this study. If this pattern can be confirmed, it would mean that, in humans, immune responses are highest if elicited when glucocorticoids are high and blood lymphocytes are low; this is quite the opposite from the findings in animals. Skin thickness, circulation time, and the completeness of entrainment on a light-dark cycle all are different between small animals and humans and may all contribute to a difference in timing which is more one of detail than of fundamental mechanism.

It should be clear from this brief review that time of day is an important variable when immune function is assessed. Furthermore, it is obvious that controls and experimental groups should all be dealt with at the same time, or differences may appear which are not real, and real differences may disappear. Finally, for results to be reproducible from experiment to experiment and from laboratory to laboratory, good control of the light-dark cycle should be imposed, and the time of the experimental manipulations noted and kept constant.

IV. Effects of Endogenous Elevations in Glucocorticoids on Immunologic Phenomena

Given the effects of exogenous glucocorticoids on the immune system, (Sec. II) it is reasonable to ask whether the elevations in endogenous glucocorticoids produced by stressful stimulation influence the immune system. It is important first to define stress, to describe its effect on glucocorticoid secretion, and then to examine the evidence that immune system function and resistance to disease are altered by stress. In addition to contributing to our knowledge about the day-to-day variability in immune system function, we shall see that knowledge of stress-induced elevations in glucocorticoids has profound implications for laboratory practice.

A. Definition of Stress

Selye (121) originally defined stress as a nonspecific response to a variety of physically traumatic events. Included in his first stage of the stress response is elevations in glucocorticoids. It is now well established that glucocorticoid levels are, in addition, exquisitely responsive to psychological stimuli (122). It has been postulated, in fact, that the factor accounting for the common or nonspecific nature of the stress response is emotional arousal (123,124).

In almost all studies of stress in experimental animals, stress has been assumed, rather than proven, to have occurred. That is, experimenters have used manipulations which they assume are stressful but have not documented the stress response. This approach ignores one of the important features of the stress response, the interactive nature of its cause. Stress is produced by the interaction between environmental events and the animal's perception and evaluation of those events. Thus, what is stressful to one may not be to another, depending upon its resources to respond to the situation. These resources are probably a product of the animal's constitution, which is influenced by genetic and developmental events and its past experience with similar situations.

In the following review, we shall examine research in which the experimenters assumed that they have produced stress in ther experimental animals. We must be aware that this is an assumption and not a fact. We will therefore avoid the use of the term "stress" in all except summary statements, describing instead the experimental manipulations used upon the animals.

B. Control of Glucocorticoid Secretion

In rodents the acute glucocorticoid response to environmental stimulation is characterized by a very rapid rise (within 1-5 min) to levels many times higher than normal (125), which peak at about 30 min and can return to normal within an hour (126). Both the rate and extent of the rise depend upon when in the circadian rhythm of glucocorticoids the stimulation occurs (127-129). The response is also dependent upon the sex of the animal, with more dramatic responses shown by female rats (130) and male humans (131). Age is also important, with older animals producing lower responses (132).

Long-term elevations in glucocorticoids can be provoked by prolonged exposure to stimuli. Shipping mice has been shown to lead to high levels of corticosterone for 2 days, followed by a gradual return to normal after 13 days (133). Crowded caging can lead to prolonged elevations in adrenal weight (122).

A wide variety of stimuli can evoke elevations in glucocorticoids including, in rodents, 5 sec of handling or 3 min of exposure to a new environment (128,129). Reducing the frequency of reward of a rat working for food can increase corticosterone levels, whereas increasing the frequency of reward can reduce them (134). The response is so sensitive to environmental stimuli that, with few exceptions (135, 136), it has not been possible to produce a graded response. Hennessy and Levine (135) produced an approximately 7 µg/100 ml increase in corticosterone by putting C57BL/KA mice into a clean cage,

double that amount when the cage was empty of its usual bedding,
and more than three times that increase when the mouse was put into
a jar. Thus, only at very minimal levels of stimulation is the glucocorticoid response proportional to the amount of stimulation.

An important influence on glucocorticoid levels is social stimulation. Increasing the caging density of aggressive (C57BL/10J) but
not nonaggressive (*Peromyscus*) mice leads to adrenal hypertrophy
and adrenal ascorbic acid depletion (137). The psychological rather
than physical (e.g., wounds) causation of this response is shown by
the fact that mice exposed to trained fighter mice continue to show
glucocorticoid elevations even though time spent fighting decreased
with multiple exposures to the fighter (138). Further, exposure to a
fighter where actual contact is prevented can produce glucocorticoid
elevations in mice who have previously fought (138,139).

The previous example illustrates another important attribute of
the adrenocortical response: it is conditionable. That is, stimuli (in
the previous example, the sight and sound of a fighter mouse) which
have in the past accompanied events which elevate glucocorticoids
(fighting) can themselves come to evoke elevations in glucocorticoids
(reviewed in Ref. 140). Thus, glucocorticoid elevations can come to
occur in the absence of the original stimulus, and similarly, can be
made in anticipation of exposure to a stimulus.

Finally, daily exposure to a stimulus may not lead to habituation
of the response (123), although more frequent exposure may eventually do so (141,142).

It is obvious that both housing and care of laboratory animals as
well as routine laboratory procedures can have important influences
upon circulating glucocorticoid levels. There is, in fact, extensive
evidence that caging and handling conditions, as well as a variety of
experiences, can influence resistance to immunologically mediated
disease (for reviews, see Refs. 143-145). Thus, laboratory animals
cannot be treated as reagents to be taken from the shelf at the experimenter's convenience without regard to their circadian rhythms
(see Sec. III.B) and their psychological response to care and treatment. The following are important considerations when designing
immunologic experiments with laboratory rodents. First, they must be
allowed time after transport from the supplier to recover from the
effects of the journey, adapt to local environmental conditions, and
entrain to the light-dark cycle. Second, the light-dark cycle must be
consistent and well controlled. Most laboratory rodents are nocturnal
and thus sleep during the light portion of the day. They should not
be kept in noisy laboratories or well-traveled corridors where their
sleep is disturbed. Third, as follows from the discussion of circadian
rhythms in Sec. III.B, the time of day at which experiments are conducted must be controlled and preferably varied systematically for
greater generalizability of results. For example, control animals must

not be experimented upon in the morning, when their endogenous
glucocorticoids are at their minimum and their response to stimulation
large, while the experimental animals are used in the afternoon,
when their glucocorticoid levels are rising and their response to
stimulation less extreme. Fourth, caging density must be controlled
and crowding avoided, especially when using aggressive strains of
mice. Whenever there is more than one mouse in a cage, there is the
potential for differences in glucocorticoid levels owing to the establishment of dominance hierarchies. There is no good rule for caging
mice because isolation, which avoids the problem of dominance hierarchies, may be stressful or lead to altered response to stimulation
and altered susceptibility to disease (e.g., Refs. 146 and 147). Fifth,
when rodents are caged in groups, special care is needed to truly
randomly assign animals to experimental groups because the order in
which they are caught and taken from the cage is not random but is
related to their excitability and thus to their glucocorticoid response
to stimulation. Sixth, blood samples in which an acute rise in glucocorticoids must be avoided must be taken very rapidly after the first
disturbance of the cage (within 1-2 min), out of the sound and smell
of other animals. Seventh, conditioned rises in glucocorticoids may
precede procedures which are repeated several times, and their
effects must be taken into account, as must the effects of prior
traumatic manipulations such as blood sampling. Eighth, in the
absence of evidence to the contrary, age and sex differences in
hypothalamic-pituitary-adrenocortical system function must be
assumed to exist. Age and sex must be held constant or varied
systematically, and data gathered on one age or sex cannot be auto-
matically generalized to others. Finally, since past experience, and
especially rearing conditions, can influence both glucocorticoid responsiveness (148,149) and resistance to disease (reviewed in Ref.
146), past experience must be held constant.

C. Are Stress Effects on Immunologic Phenomena Mediated by Glucocorticoids?

There is an extensive literature on the effects of stress (defined as
the experimenter's manipulations) on cancer, autoimmunity, and
resistance to infectious disease. Although researchers have postulated
for more than 20 years that some of these effects may be mediated
through the pituitary-adrenocortical axis (e.g., Ref. 150), few have
addressed the question directly. To establish such a mechanism, one
would need to show that serum glucocorticoid and adrenal size changes
parallel changes in immunologic function, that exogenous glucocorticoid or adrenocorticotrophic hormone (ACTH) can mimic the effect of
stressful stimuli, and that adrenalectomy eliminates the effect. We
review here studies on immune function and resistance to disease which

address any of these types of evidence. This research is a small
subset of those studies which have examined "stress" effects on
disease. As noted in a previous section (II.A), glucocorticoids could
either enhance or decrease resistance to disease, depending upon the
particular disease and upon the timing of the glucocorticoid elevations. In this discussion we will not concern ourselves with the direction of the effects of glucocorticoids.

1. **Adrenal Weight Parallels Immunologic Effects**   There are few
enough studies in this category that no two address the same immunologic function. Several researchers have found that increases in
adrenal weight accompany changes in resistance to disease. The
adrenals of grouped C3H mice (absolute weights) were found to be
larger than those of isolated mice, and the grouped mice produced
lower antibody titers to bovine serum (151). Using C57BL/6 mice,
DeChambre and Gosse (152) found, in contrast, that isolated mice had
larger adrenals. Differences in the caging conditions or the strain
difference between mice may account for the disagreement between
these studies, although we can offer no specific hypotheses. The
larger adrenals of the isolated mice corresponded to increased ascites
fluid weights produced by Krebs-2 tumors. Independent of caging
condition, these same experimenters found a positive correlation between adrenal weight and ascites fluid weight, with the increase in
adrenal weight preceding the increase in fluid weight. They also
found that injection of ACTH prior to tumor cell injection mimicked the
effect of isolation. Teodoru and Schwartzman (153) found that seasonal
variation in adrenal reactivity to inoculatory trauma paralleled the
fluctuation in the incidence of paralysis in response to MEF_1 virus
in hamsters. Across a variety of environmental manipulations, the
percentage of animals with adrenal hypertrophy corresponded to the
percentage of paralytic poliomyelitis resulting from virus injection
observed in other animals under similar environmental conditions. On
the other hand, they found that chronic exposure to cold produced
chronic adrenal hypertrophy, although the incidence of paralysis
declined with increasing exposure to cold. They also found that injections of glucocorticoids reproduced the environmental effects.

Other investigators have shown a parallel, over several days,
among adrenal hypertropy, lowered leukocyte (mostly lymphocyte)
counts, decreased thymus and spleen weights during avoidance learning (in which the animal must learn to perform a response in order to
avoid electric shock to the feet), or confinement (154). Severe electric
shock has also been shown to decrease the numbers of tumors produced
by dimethylbenzanthracene (DMBA) while increasing relative adrenal
weights (155). In another study, the same group found that restraint
produced a decrease in the number of Huggins tumors which was not
accompanied by changes in adrenal weight, although the restrained

animals had lower adrenal ascorbic acid levels than did the controls
(156).

In the only study in which immune system function was measured
directly, adrenal hypertrophy accompanied the decrease in in vitro
antibody formation by spleen cells caused by accelerating mice in a
centrifuge or etherizing them prior to splenic explant (157).

Although the evidence on the correspondence between adrenal
hypertrophy and alterations in immunologic function is sparse, it is
consistent: in all cases either adrenal hypertropy or ascorbic acid
decrement have occurred when immunologic function changed. However, the temporal correspondence between the two events was not
always exact (153).

2. **Glucocorticoid Elevations Parallel Stress Effects**   Four studies
address the relationship between glucocorticoid levels and response to
immune system challenge. Mice had increasing adrenal weights and
increasing susceptibility to *H. nana* reinfection with increasing numbers of exposures per day to a cat (141). Plasma corticosterone did
not show a linear relationship to exposure number, being elevated at
all frequencies of exposure. Vervets exposed to multiple noxious
manipulations for several weeks showed glucocorticoid elevations
between the second and fourth week which corresponded to a delay
of about a week in the appearance of antibody to bovine serum albu-
men in Freund's complete adjuvant (158). Mice housed in isolation had
increased mortality to EMC virus and increased corticosterone at the
peak, but not the trough, of the daily corticosterone rhythm (159).
In this context the finding of Amkraut, Solomon, and Kraemer (160)
that overcrowded mice did not have glucocorticoid differences, although they did show an accelerated onset of adjuvant-induced
arthritis, must be interpreted carefully. In this study the glucocorticoid levels were measured at the trough of the daily rhythm, the
time at which Friedman et al. (159) did not find housing-induced elevations even though they did find them at the peak. Thus it is not
possible to interpret the Amkraut et al. study without evidence on
glucocorticoid levels at other times of day.

There were four other studies that examined glucocorticoid
parallels with immune system function more directly. Riley and
Spackman (133) found that shipping increased serum corticosterone
and decreased thymus weight and numbers of circulating T lymphocytes. The recovery of lymphocytes and thymus weight paralleled
the gradual return of the glucocorticoid levels to normal. Monjan and
Collector (161) found that the glucocorticoid response to noise over
several days paralleled the decrease in the response of splenic B
lymphocytes to lipopolysaccharide and the T lymphocyte response to
concanavalin A and ability to lyse P815 target cells. Although eventual
recovery of glucocorticoid levels corresponded to the recovery of B

and T cell function that occurred spontaneously during 20 days of
exposure to noise, there was no depression in glucocorticoids corresponding to a period of enhanced B and T cell function which occurred
after 20 days. They hypothesized that somatotrophic hormone was
responsible for the enhanced lymphocyte function, although no evidence is presented. Deficits in antibody response to in vitro immunization of mouse spleen explants has been shown to be related to the
glucocorticoid elevations produced by acceleration in a centrifuge,
etherization, and short-term exposure to crowded caging (142,162).
These effects were duplicated by injecting ACTH into intact but not
adrenalectomized animals.

These last four studies provide evidence that endogenous glucocorticoid levels can be responsible for alterations in lymphocyte circulation and function similar to those produced by exogenous glucocorticoids as described in Section II.C. The other studies indicate
that these effects may result in altered responses to disease. The
fact that glucocorticoid levels do not exactly parallel immunologic
changes in all cases indicates that we must consider other possible
mechanisms. These studies also point up the importance of measuring
glucocorticoids at more than one time of day, since selective changes
and alterations in the circadian rhythm are possible.

**3. Administration of Glucocorticoids or ACTH Mimics the Effects of
Stress**   Several of the studies mentioned in the previous sections
demonstrated that injections of glucocorticoids or ACTH could duplicate the effects of the experimental manipulations intended to produce
stress (142,152,153,162). In addition, Spry (70) used prednisolone
or ACTH to mimic the effect of surgery and ether anesthesia on
thoracic duct output of lymphocytes. As would be predicted, all of
these manipulations led to a rapid fall in circulating lymphocytes.
Glucocorticoids were also able to reproduce the effect of 18 hr of
restraint upon the ability of interferon-activated macrophages to kill
leukemia cells in vitro (163).

On the negative side, Amkraut and Solomon (164) could not reproduce the effect of exposure to electric shock on tumor size with
injections of ACTH.

The evidence in this and the previous sections makes it clear
that glucocorticoids may not account for all of the effects of stressful
manipulations on the immune system, but it is striking how much
agreement there is among studies which support some role for
glucocorticoids.

4. Adrenalectomy Eliminates the Effect of Stress   Adrenalectomy has
been shown to eliminate the increase in resistance to anaphylactic
shock produced by shuttle box avoidance learning (165), the protective effect of avoidance learning on splenic response to Rauscher
murine leukemia virus (166), and the leukopenia produced by

avoidance learning (167). On the other hand, adrenalectomy did not eliminate the effect of avoidance learning on the disappearance of vesicular stomatitis virus from the site of inoculation (168).

5. **Summary**   A series of studies by Gisler and colleagues (142,157, 162) has taken the most complete approach to determining the role of glucocorticoids in stress-induced alterations in in vitro measures of immunologic function. Using as their dependent variable antibody plaque-forming cells after in vitro immunization of spleen explants, they have shown depressions in response due to restraint, over-crowding, and acceleration. They have shown that corticosterone elevations parallel the effects of these manipulations, that they are duplicated by ACTH, and that ACTH treatment of adrenalectomized mice did not duplicate the effect. They have further explored both the immunological and psychological details of their paradigm. The plaque-forming capacity of spleen explants from immunized mice sub-jected to the stressful manipulations was restored by the addition of macrophages together with B lymphocytes, but not T lymphocytes. Using chromium-labeled cells they documented altered lymphocyte re-circulation with increased numbers of T and B cells in spleen and bone marrow. They found that frequent exposures to ether led to habitua-tion of the splenic depression and that diazepam decreased the effect of restraint. Finally, they showed that somatotrophic hormone can aid in the recovery from the effects of ACTH. They postulated that under normal circumstances, release of somatotrophic hormone con-current with ACTH serves to aid in the recovery from the effects of glucocorticoids. Although these hormones do seem to be released together in primates, the evidence for rodents shows that somato-trophic hormone release is decreased when glucocorticoids are re-leased (169), a fact which weakens this hypothesis.

The overwhelming majority of studies in which adrenal cortical function was explored support the role of glucocorticoids in mediating the effects of stress on resistance to disease and immune system function. As noted previously, exposure to stressors produces many other physiological effects, some of which would be expected to in-fluence immune system function. In addition, many of the studies measured resistance to disease rather than actual immune system function. In these studies, immune system effects can only be in-ferred, and other effects of glucocorticoids, including direct effects on the infectious organism (170), must be considered.

These studies clearly lack conclusive proof of the role of gluco-corticoids in the stress response of the immune system because none of them establish the multiple evidence necessary and few of them measure immune system function directly, focusing on tumors or in-fectious disease which may be influenced through a variety of modes. Several of the studies taken together do implicate the role of the glucocorticoids in the alteration of the circulation of lymphocytes produced by stress. Adrenalectomy eliminates the stress-induced leukopenia (167), adrenal hypertrophy parallels lowered leukocyte counts (154), increases in corticosterone parallel the absence of lymphocytes (133), whereas prednisolone and ACTH decrease thoracic duct output of lymphocytes (70).

V. Conclusion

When glucocorticoids are administered to humans or animals as drugs, their effects are profound and protean. This reflects the complexity of immune responses, which always have both positive and negative regulation. The ratio of positive to negative, or helper to suppressor, effects must be precisely regulated, and this regulation must be accurate qualitatively, quantitatively, and across time. Thus a disturbance in even a single element of the effector-control loop can have large effects on the ultimately observed immune response. If two or more elements are affected, it becomes nearly impossible to predict outcome. As in any complex system, there is a great need for a more complete understanding of the mechanisms of immune responses, so that modulation by drugs can be put in proper context. This will require, at first, a reductionist approach. The effects of glucocorticoids on antigen-presenting cells, helper T cells, B cells, etc., must be answered precisely, always keeping in mind that, in the immune system, the whole is very much more than the sum of the parts.

We have tried to emphasize that glucocorticoids are not only drugs; they are endogenous hormones and regulators whose concentrations in the blood vary with time and the physiological and psychological state of the subject. Considerable evidence indicates that these endogenous glucocorticoids are responsible for some of the effects of psychological stress on the immune system. In addition, we emphasize that animals are not test tubes to be taken off the shelf at the investigator's convenience without regard to their existence as living and feeling creatures. To do so reduces the generalizability of results obtained.

Finally, we still do not know the answer to the question that, if the response to stress is harmful, how was it retained in evolution? We should keep in mind that the response is primitive, occurring in most vertebrate groups, and may have evolved in response to acute, physical stress: injuries and attacks by predators. Is the function of elevated glucocorticoids to suppress possible autoimmune responses to injured tissues? If so, it is an uneasy trade-off, because responses to contaminants, toxins, etc., would also be suppressed. A great deal of work may be necessary before this fascinating problem is solved.

Acknowledgments

Preparation of this chapter was supported by NIH grants AI11661 to
J. J. C. and HD 08315 to L. S. C. L. S. C. is a member of the
Developmental Psychobiology Research Group of the Department of
Psychiatry, University of Colorado.

References

1. G. Charriere, J. Morel, and P. J. Gineste, *Compt. Rend. Soc. Biol. 126*:46 (1937).
2. D. J. Ingle, *Proc. Soc. Exp. Biol. Med. 38*:443 (1938).
3. T. F. Dougherty, *Physiol. Revs. 32*:379 (1952).
4. F. G. Germuth, Jr., *Pharmacol. Revs. 8*:1 (1956).
5. E. H. Kass and M. Finland, *Ann. Rev. Microbiol. 7*:361 (1953).
6. M. Ishidate and D. Metcalf, *Aust. J. Exp. Biol. Med. Sci. 41*: 637 (1963).
7. T. F. Dougherty, M. L. Berliner, G. L. Schneebeli, and D. L. Berliner, *Ann. N.Y. Acad. Sci. 113*:835 (1964).
8. N. L. Warner, *Aust. J. Exp. Biol. Med. Sci. 42*:401 (1964).
9. H. Blomgren and B. Andersson, *Clin. Exp. Immunol. 10*:297 (1972).
10. T. L. Vischer, *Immunology 23*:777 (1972).
11. H. Cantor and D. E. Mosier, *Transplant Proc. 4*:159 (1972).
12. J. J. Cohen, M. Fischbach, and H. N. Claman, *J. Immunol. 105*:1146 (1970).
13. J. J. Cohen and H. N. Claman, *J. Exp. Med. 133*:1026 (1971).
14. M. Schlesinger and V. K. Golokai, *Science 155*:1114 (1967).
15. Y. Reisner, M. Linker-Israeli, and N. Sharon, *Cell. Immunol. 25*:129 (1976).
16. H. Cantor and E. A. Boyse, *J. Exp. Med. 141*:1376 (1975).
17. R. Scollay, M. Kochen, E. Butcher, and I. Weissman, *Nature (Lond.) 276*:79 (1978).
18. E. V. Elliott, V. Wallis, and A. J. S. Davies, *Nature (New Biol.), 234*:77 (1971).
19. B. Nabarra and M. Papiernik, *Cell. Immunol. 51*:72 (1980).
20. O. Stutman, *Contemp. Topics Immunobiol. 7*:1 (1977).
21. M. A. Levine and H. N. Claman, *Science 167*:1515 (1970).
22. D. C. Vann, *Cell. Immunol. 11*:11 (1974).
23. K. C. Lee, R. E. Langman, V. H. Paetkau, and E. Diener, *Cell. Immunol. 17*:405 (1975).
24. R. I. Mishell, L. M. Bradley, Y. U. Chen, K. H. Grabstein, and S. M. Shiigi, in *Microbiology 1980*, American Society for Microbiology, 1980.
25. J. M. Norton and A. Munck, *J. Immunol. 125*:259 (1980).

26. J. J. Oppenheim, R. Moore, F. G'Melig-Meyling, A. Togawa, S. Wahl, B. J. Mathieson, S. Dougherty, and C. Carter, in *Macrophage Regulation of Immunity* (E. R. Unanue and A. S. Rosenthal, eds.), Academic, New York, 1980.

27. R. B. Markham, P. W. Stashak, B. Prescott, D. F. Amsbaugh, and P. J. Baker, *J. Immunol. 121*:829 (1978).

28. J. J. Cohen and H. N. Claman, *Nature (Lond.) 229*:274 (1971).

29. J. J. Cohen, *Ann. Allergy 29*:358 (1971).

30. W. L. Weston, H. N. Claman, and G. G. Krueger, *J. Immunol. 110*:880 (1973).

31. J. E. Balow and A. S. Rosenthal, *J. Exp. Med. 137*:1031 (1973).

32. A. Venetianer, P. Aranyl, Z. Bosze, and J. Fachet, *Scand. J. Immunol. 8*:355 (1978).

33. M. de Sousa and J. Fachet, *Clin. Exp. Immunol. 10*:673 (1972).

34. J. Fachet and D. M. V. Parrott, *Clin. Exp. Immunol. 10*:661 (1972).

35. A. S. Fauci, D. C. Dale, and J. E. Balow, *Ann. Int. Med. 84*:304 (1976).

36. S. Gillis and K. A. Smith, *Nature (Lond.) 268*:154 (1977).

37. S. Gillis, G. R. Crabtree, and K. A. Smith, *J. Immunol. 123*: 1624 (1979).

38. S. Gillis, G. R. Crabtree, and K. A. Smith, *J. Immunol. 123*: 1632 (1979).

39. G. R. Crabtree, A. Munck, and K. A. Smith, *J. Immunol. 125*:13 (1980).

40. E.-L. Larsson, *J. Immunol. 124*:2828 (1980).

41. L. Polak and J. L. Turk, *Nature (Lond.) 249*:654 (1974).

42. T. Hirano and A. A. Nordin, *J. Immunol. 116*:1115 (1976).

43. M. E. Weksler, D. Shell, and G. W. Siskind. *Cell. Immunol. 14*:98 (1974).

44. B. Schechter and M. Feldman, *J. Immunol. 119*:1563 (1977).

45. E. Clerici, B. Schechter, and M. Feldman, *Int. J. Cancer 25*: 349 (1980).

46. C. Hubert, G. Delespesse, and A. Govaerts, *Clin. Exp. Immunol. 26*:95 (1976).

47. G. J. Finlay, R. J. Booth, and J. Marbrook, *Aust. J. Exp. Biol. Med. Sci. 57*:597 (1979).

48. T. A. Waldemann, R. M. Blaese, S. Broder, and R. S. Krakower, *Ann. Int. Med. 88*:226 (1978).

49. B. F. Haynes and A. S. Fauci, *Cell. Immunol. 44*:157 (1979).

50. D. Sampson, C. Grotelueschen, and H. M. Kauffman Jr., *Transplantation 20*:362 (1975).

51. J. D. Baxter and G. G. Rousseau, eds., *Glucocorticoid Hormone Actions*, Springer-Verlag, Berlin, 1979.

52. A. Munck and T. Brink-Johnsen, *J. Biol. Chem. 243*:5556 (1968).

53. B. P. Schaumburg and E. Bojesen, *Biochem. Biophys. Acta. 170*:172 (1968).

54. F. Homo, F. Picard, S. Durant, D. Gagne, J. Simon, M. Dardenne, and D. Duval, *J. Steroid Biochem. 12*:433 (1980).

55. K. A. Smith, G. R. Crabtree, S. J. Kennedy, and A. Munck, *Nature (Lond.) 267*:523 (1977).

56. A. Munck, G. R. Crabtree, and K. A. Smith, in *Glucocorticoid Hormone Actions* (J. D. Baxter and G. G. Rousseau, eds.), Springer-Verlag, Berlin, 1979.

57. G. R. Crabtree, A. Munck, and K. A. Smith, *J. Immunol. 124*:2430 (1980).

58. F. Homo, D. Duval, J. Hatzfeld, and C. Evrard, *J. Steroid. Biochem. 13*:135 (1980).

59. A. Klein, H. Bessler, H. Hoogervorst-Spaller, H. Kaufmann, M. Djaldetti, and H. Joshua, *J. Steroid Biochem. 13*:517 (1980).

60. J. D. Baxter and J. W. Funder, *N. Engl. J. Med. 301*:1149 (1979).

61. G. G. Rousseau and J. D. Baxter, in *Glucocorticoid Hormone Actions* (J. D. Baxter and G. G. Rousseau, eds.), Springer-Verlag, Berlin, 1979.

62. A. H. Wyllie, J. F. R. Kerr, and A. R. Currie, *Int. Rev. Cytol. 68*:251 (1980).

63. A. H. Wyllie, *Nature (Lond.) 284*:555 (1980).

64. H. N. Claman, *J. All. Clin. Immunol. 55*:145 (1975).

65. A. S. Fauci, *J. Immunopharmacol 1*:1 (1978).

66. J. D. Romani, *Comp. Rend. Soc. Biol. 146*:1680 (1952).

67. V. Andersen, F. Bro-Rasmussen, and K. Hougaard, *Cell Tissue Kinet. 2*:139 (1969).

68. J. J. Cohen, in *Cell Interactions* (L. G. Silvestri, ed.), North-Holland, Amsterdam, 1972.

69. H. Schnappauf and V. Schnappauf, *Nouv. Rev. Franc. Hematol. 8*:555 (1968).

70. C. J. F. Spry, *Cell. Immunol. 4*:86 (1972).

71. M. M. Zatz, *Israel J. Med. Sci. 11*:1368 (1975).

72. L. J. Cole, in *Transactions of the IXth International Congress of Radiology*, Georg Thieme Verlag, Stuttgart, 1960.

73. J. J. Cohen, *J. Immunol. 108*:841 (1972).

74. J. W. Moorhead and H. N. Claman, *Cell. Immunol. 5*:74 (1972).

75. Z. Ben-Ishay, *Israel J. Med. Sci. 11*:978 (1975).

76. F. Brahim and G. Baradue, *J. Reticuloendothel. Soc. 25*:397 (1979).

77. A. S. Fauci, *Immunology 28*:669 (1975).

78. L. Borella and A. A. Green, *J. Immunol. 109*:927 (1972).

79. H. N. Claman and J. W. Moorhead, in *Cell Interactions* (L. G. Silvestri, ed.), North-Holland, Amsterdam, 1972.
80. H. N. Claman, *N. Engl. J. Med. 287*:388 (1972).
81. A. S. Fauci, in *Glucocorticoid Hormone Actions* (J. D. Baxter and G. G. Rousseau, eds.), Springer-Verlag, Berlin, 1979.
82. K. V. Batra, L. M. Elrod, and R. Schrek, *J. Pharmacol. Exp. Therapeut. 152*:525 (1966).
83. K. V. Batra and R. Schrek, *Proc. Soc. Exp. Biol. Med. 125*: 871 (1967).
84. J. Shewell and D. A. Long, *J. Hygiene 54*:452 (1956).
85. H. van Dijk, N. Bloksma, P. M. Rademaker, W. J. Schouten, and J. M. Willers, *Int. J. Immunopharmacol. 1*:285 (1979).
86. E. Dupont, G. Berkenboom, M. Leempoel, and P. Potvliege, *Transplantation 30*:387 (1980).
87. J. W. Hadden, *Int. J. Immunopharmacol. 1*:5 (1979).
88. S. E. Walker and B. Schnitzer, *Arth. Rheum. 23*:539 (1980).
89. A. J. Coburg, S. H. Gray, F. H. Katz, I. Penn, C. Halgrimson, and T. E. Starzl, *Surg. Gynecol. Obstet. 131*: 933 (1970).
90. M. J. Doenhoff and E. Leuchars, *Int. Arch. Allergy Appl. Immunol. 53*:505 (1977).
91. C. T. Ambrose, *J. Exp. Med. 119*:1027 (1964).
92. C. T. Ambrose, in *Hormones and The Immune Response* (G. E. W. Wolstenholme and J. Knight, eds.), J. & A. Churchill, London, 1970.
93. N. A. Sherman, R. S. Smith, and E. Middleton, Jr., *J. Allergy Clin. Immunol. 52*:13 (1973).
94. N. N. Iscove and F. Melchers, *J. Exp. Med. 147*:923 (1978).
95. N. N. Iscove, in *Hematopoietic Cell Differentiation*, (D. W. Golde, M. J. Cline, D. Metcalf, and C. F. Fox, eds.), Academic, New York, 1978.
96. B. A. Acuff and J. J. Cohen, *J. Supramol. Structure* (in *14*:215 (1980).
97. C. B. Streng and P. Nathan, *Immunology 24*:559 (1973).
98. K. Shortman and H. Backson, *Cell. Immunol. 12*:230 (1974).
99. D. F. B. Char and V. C. Kelley, *Proc. Soc. Exp. Biol. Med. 109*:599 (1962).
100. P. Crunkhorn and S. C. R. Meacock, *Immunology 20*:91 (1971).
101. L. R. Heim, R. A. Good, and C. Martinez, *Proc. Soc. Exp. Biol. Med. 122*:107 (1966).
102. H. O. Besedovsky, A. del Rey, and E. Sorkin, *Clin. Exp. Immunol. 37*:106 (1979).
103. H. O. Besedovsky, A. del Rey, and E. Sorkin, *J. Immunol. 126*:385 (1981).
104. G. W. Liddle, *Arch. Int. Med. 117*:739 (1966).

105. A. H. Vagnucci, *Am. J. Physiol. 236*:R268 (1979).
106. D. R. Garris, *Acta Endocrinol. 90*:692 (1979).
107. D. H. Spackman and V. Riley, *Science 200*:87 (1978).
108. J. E. Ottenweller, A. H. Meier, A. C. Russo, and M. E. Frenzke, *Acta Endocrinol. 91*:150 (1979).
109. M. H. Smolensky, A. Reinberg, and J. P. McGovern, eds., *Recent Advances in the Chronobiology of Allergy and Immunology*, Pergamon, Oxford, 1980.
110. W. J. Fulkerson and B. Y. Tang, *J. Endocrinol. 81*:135 (1979).
111. H. E. Brown and T. F. Dougherty, *Endocrinol. 58*:365 (1965).
112. T. Abo, T. Kawate, S. Hinuma, K. Itoh, W. Abo, J. Sato, and K. Kumagai, *Adv. Biosci. 28*:301 (1980).
113. R. Pownall, M. S. Knapp, I. C. Kowanko, D. Byme, H. Stockdale, and D. S. Minors, *Adv. Biosci. 28*:333 (1980).
114. J. Eskola, H. Frey, G. Molnar, and E. Soppi, *Clin. Exp. Immunol. 26*:253 (1976).
115. R. Pownall, P. A. Kabler, and M. S. Knapp, *Clin. Exp. Immunol. 36*:347 (1979).
116. J. P. McGovern, M. H. Smolensky, and A. Reinberg, eds., *Chronobiology in Allergy and Immunology*, Chas. C Thomas, Springfield, 1977.
117. R. F. Bargatze and D. H. Katz, *Fed. Proc. 39*:567 (1980).
118. H. B. Tavadia, K. A. Fleming, P. D. Hume, and H. W. Simpson, *Clin. Exp. Immunol. 22*:190 (1975).
119. B. F. Haynes and A. S. Fauci, *J. Clin. Invest. 61*:703 (1978).
120. J. R. Cove-Smith, P. Kabler, R. Pownall, and M. S. Knapp, *Br. Med. J. 2*:253 (1978).
121. H. Selye, *Nature (Lond.) 138*:32 (1936).
122. J. W. Mason, *Psychosom. Med. 30*:576 (1968).
123. J. W. Hennessy and S. Levine, in *Progress in Psychobiology and Physiological Psychology* (J. Sprague and A. Epstein, eds.), Academic, New York, 1979.
124. J. Weinberg and S. Levine, in *Coping and Health* (S. Levine and H. Ursin, eds.), Plenum, New York, 1980.
125. L. D. Keith, J. R. Winslow, and R. W. Reynolds, *Steroids 31*:523 (1978).
126. R. Ader, *Ann. N.Y. Acad. Sci. 159*:791 (1969).
127. R. Ader, S. B. Friedman, and L. J. Grota, *Anim. Behav. 15*:37 (1967).
128. G. M. Brown and J. B. Martin, *Psychosom. Med. 36*:241 (1974).
129. J. A. Seggie and G. M. Brown, *Canad. J. Physiol. Pharmacol. 53*:629 (1975).

130. R. Ader and S. M. Plaut, *Psychosom. Med. 30*:277 (1968).
131. M. Frankenhaeuser, *Neb. Symp. Motiv. 26*:123 (1979).
132. B. E. Eleftheriou, *Gerontologia 20*:224 (1974).
133. V. Riley and D. Spackman, *Fogarty Intl. Center Proc. 28*:
      319 (1977).
134. L. Goldman, G. D. Coover, and S. Levine, *Physiol. Behav.
      10*:209 (1973).
135. M. B. Hennessy and S. Levine, *Physiol. Behav. 21*:295
      (1978).
136. M. B. Hennessy, J. P. Heybach, J. Vernikos, and S. Levine,
      Physiol. Behav. 22:821 (1979).
137. F. H. Bronson and B. E. Eleftheriou, *Physiol. Zool. 36*:161
      (1963).
138. F. H. Bronson and B. E. Eleftheriou, *Physiol. Zool. 38*:406
      (1965).
139. F. H. Bronson and B. E. Eleftheriou, *Science 147*:627 (1965).
140. S. C. Woods and S. R. Burchfield, in *The Comprehensive
      Handbook of Behavioral Medicine* (J. M. Ferguson and C. B.
      Taylor, eds.), Spectrum, New York, 1980.
141. D. R. Hamilton, *J. Psychosom. Res. 18*:143 (1974).
142. R. H. Gisler, *Psychother. Psychosom. 23*:197 (1974).
143. R. C. LaBarba, *Psychosom. Med. 32*:259 (1970).
144. R. Ader, in *Perspectives in Behavioral Medicine* (S. Weiss,
      A. Hurd, and B. Fox, eds.), Academic, New York, 1981.
145. S. M. Plaut and S. B. Friedman, in *Psychoneuroimmunology*
      (R. Ader, ed.), Academic, New York, 1981.
146. R. Ader, in *Modern Trends in Psychosomatic Medicine 3*
      (O. W. Hill, ed.), Butterworths, London, 1976.
147. S. M. Plaut and L. J. Grota, *Neuroendocrinology 7*:348 (1971).
148. R. Ader, in *Hormonal Correlates of Behavior*, vol. 1 (B. E.
      Eleftheriou and R. L. Sprott, eds.), Plenum, New York, 1975.
149. J. W. Hennessy, R. Levin, and S. Levine, *J. Comp. Physiol.
      Psychol. 91*:770 (1977).
150. D. E. Davis and C. P. Read, *Proc. Soc. Exp. Biol. Med. 99*:
      269 (1958).
151. S. H. Vessey, *Proc. Soc. Exp. Biol. Med. 115*:252 (1964).
152. R. P. Dechambre and C. Gosse, *Cancer Res. 33*:140 (1973).
153. C. V. Teodoru and G. Schwartzman, *Proc. Soc. Exp. Biol.
      Med. 91*:181 (1956).
154. J. J. Marsh and A. F. Rasmussen, Jr., *Proc. Soc. Exp. Biol.
      Med. 104*:180 (1960).
155. B. H. Newberry, G. Frankie, P. A. Beatty, B. D. Maloney,
      and J. C. Gilchrist, *Psychosom. Med. 34*:295 (1972).
156. B. H. Newberry, J. Gildow, J. Wogan, and R. L. Reese,
      Psychosom. Med. 38:155 (1976).

157. R. H. Gisler, A. F. Bussard, J. C. Mazie, and R. Hess, *Cell Immunol.* 2:634 (1971).

158. C. W. Hill, W. E. Greer, and O. Felsenfeld, *Psychosom. Med.* 29:279 (1967).

159. S. B. Friedman, R. Ader, and L. A. Glasgow, *Psychosom. Med.* 32:285 (1970).

160. A. A. Amkraut, C. F. Solomon, and H. C. Kraemer, *Psychosom. Med.* 33:203 (1971).

161. A. A. Monjan and M. I. Collector, *Science 196*:307 (1977).

162. R. H. Gisler and L. Schenkel-Hullinger, *Cell. Immunol.* 2:646 (1971).

163. N. Pavlidis and M. Chirigos, *Psychosom. Med.* 42:47 (1980).

164. A. Amkraut and G. F. Solomon, *Cancer Res.* 32:1428 (1972).

165. P. E. Treadwell and A. F. Rasmussen, Jr., *J. Immunol.* 87:492 (1961).

166. M. M. Jensen, *Proc. Soc. Exp. Biol. Med.* 127:610 (1968).

167. M. M. Jensen, *J. Reticuloendothel. Soc.* 6:457 (1969).

168. A. Yamada, M. M. Jensen, and A. F. Rasmussen, Jr., *Proc. Soc. Exp. Biol. Med.* 116:677 (1964).

169. G. M. Brown, J. Seggie, and P. Ettigi, in *Cancer, Stress, and Death* (J. Tache, H. Selye, and S. B. Day, eds.), Plenum, New York, 1979.

170. H. E. Varmus, G. Ringold, and K. R. Yamamoto, in *Glucocorticoid Hormone Action* (J. D. Baxter and G. G. Rousseau, eds.), Springer-Verlag, Berlin, 1979.

4

Polymorphonuclear Leukocyte Chemotaxis: Lipid Chemotactic Factors

FRANK H. VALONE   Sidney Farber Cancer Institute, Boston, Massachusetts

I. Introduction

Lipid chemotactic factors for human polymorphonuclear (PMN) leukocytes were initially recognized as components of inflammatory exudates isolated after immunological challenge of the rat peritoneal cavity (1) and of filtrates from *Escherichia coli* (2) and *Corynebacterium parvum* (3) cultures. Subsequently, oxygenation products of the arachidonic acid cyclooxygenase and lipoxygenase pathways were shown to account for the bulk of the observed chemotactic activity, with hydroxyeicosatetraenoic acids (HETEs) (4,5), leukotriene B_4 (LTB$_4$) (6), 12-L-hydroxy-5,8,10-heptadecatrienoic acid (HHT) (7), and a partially characterized principle termed LCF$_r$ (1,8) being the predominant factors. While the diverse lipid chemotactic factors were initially identified by their capacity to elicit neutrophil and eosinophil chemotaxis, recent studies have led to the recognition of additional functional specificities for these principles as exogenous mediators and, under some circumstances, as intracellular messengers (Fig. 1). This chapter will review recent developments in our understanding of the functional properties of lipid chemotactic factors as well as preliminary attempts to delineate the contributions of these principles to in vivo inflammatory conditions.

II. Lipid Chemotactic Factors Derived from the Lipoxygenase and Cyclooxygenase Pathways

A. *Lipoxygenase Products*

Specific immunological perturbation of cell membranes leads to the mobilization of arachidonic acid and other fatty acids from membrane

"

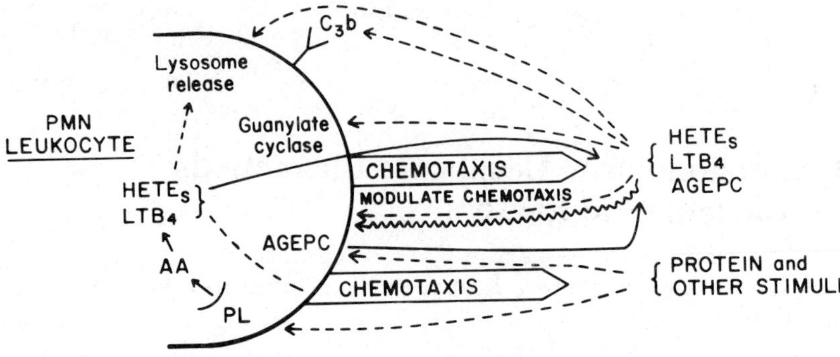

FIG. 1 Modulation of PMN leukocyte chemotaxis. ——→ = release;
----→ = enhancement; ∿∿→ = inhibition; PL = phospholipids; AA =
arachidonic acid; C_3b = C_3b receptor; AGEPC = alkyl-ether phospholipids.

phospholipids (9). Subsequent oxidation by either the lipoxygenase
(10) or cyclooxygenase (11) pathways leads to the appearance of unstable peroxide intermediates which are rapidly transformed to diverse factors that are capable of modulating leukocyte migration and
other functions and of modulating the actions of other immunological
effector cells and vascular permeability (12). The initial hydroperoxy-
eicosatetraenoic acid (OOHETE) products of the lipoxygenase pathway
are transformed largely to the corresponding monohydroxyeicosate-
traenoic acids which differ mainly in the position of the hydroxyl
group. The nature and quantities of the HETEs generated differ
for each cell studied, so that rabbit alveolar macrophages (13) and
human neutrophils, eosinophils, basophils, and monocytes (14,15)
generate predominantly 5-HETE and 11-HETE, whereas human lymphocytes generate 5-HETE and probably 12-HETE (16), human platelets
produce 12-L-HETE (10,17), and rat serosal mast cells produce 11-
HETE, 12-HETE, and 15-HETE (18). While stimulation of alveolar
macrophages with zymosan yields predominantly 5-HETE and 11-
HETE, analysis of cell homogenates revealed the capacity to generate
a range of mono-HETEs including 8-, 9-, 12-, and 15-HETE, as well
as 5- and 11-HETE (13). That these diverse HETEs are the products
of the alveolar macrophage lipoxygenase rather than of spontaneous
oxidation is demonstrated by experiments in which the addition of
the lipoxygenase inhibitor 5,8,11,14-eicosatetraynoic acid (ETYA)
diminished the generation of the different HETEs by more than 80%
(13).

Initial investigations demonstrated that platelet-derived 12-L-
HETE at concentrations of 0.3 to 24 µg/ml is chemotactic for human
neutrophils and eosinophils in vitro (4,5) and stimulates an early

accumulation of eosinophils and subsequent influx of neutrophils into
the guinea pig peritoneal cavity (19). Series of mono-HETE isomers
which differed in the position of the hydroxyl group were purified
subsequently from diverse cell sources and were shown to elicit neutrophil chemotactic responses of comparable magnitude with a rank
order of potency of 5-HETE > 8-HETE = 9-HETE > 11-HETE = 12-HETE
(13,20). Preincubation of PMN leukocytes with peak chemotactic concentrations of 12-L-HETE at 37°C for 30 min, followed by washing,
reduced the chemotactic responsiveness of the exposed leukocytes by
more than 90% when compared with leukocytes preincubated with
buffer (5). This phenomenon of chemotactic deactivation is characteristic of peptide (21), and of other lipid chemotactic factors (1), and
suggests a mechanism for trapping leukocytes at sites of inflammation.

In addition to yielding 5-HETE, 5-OOHETE is the unique intermediate in the generation of a family of complex lipids termed leukotrienes that contain additional polar substituents and three conjugated
double bonds (22,23). 5-OOHETE is converted to the highly reactive
5,6-epoxy-7,9,11,14-eicosatetraenoic acid, or leukotriene A (LTA$_4$)
(22), that reacts rapidly with water to form 5,12-dihydroxyeicosate-
traenoic acid (5,12-di-HETE), or leukotriene B$_4$ (24), and with
cysteine-containing peptides to form 5-hydroxy-6-sulfidoglutathionyl-
eicosatetraenoic acid, or leukotriene C$_4$ (LTC$_4$) (23,25,26). LTC$_4$ is
subsequently converted by γ-glutamyltranspeptidase to leukotrienes
D$_4$ and E$_4$ (27). That LTC$_4$, LTD$_4$, and possibly LTE$_4$ are functionally
critical constituents of the slow-reacting substance of anaphylaxis
(SRS-A) is suggested by comparable dependence for their generation
on the integrity of the lipoxygenase pathway, release by identical
stimuli in the same time period, and similar functional properties with
respect to smooth muscle contraction and alterations in vascular permeability (23,25,26,27). Of the lipoxygenase products that are stable
enough to permit purification of sufficient quantities for in vitro
studies, LTB$_4$ is the most potent chemotactic factor for human PMN
leukocytes (6,28). LTB$_4$ elicits a maximal chemotactic response at
30 ng/ml of approximately 50 PMN leukocytes per high power field
(hpf), which is comparable in magnitude to that evoked by 1000-2000
ng/ml of 5-HETE and 10,000-20,000 ng/ml of 11-HETE or 12-HETE
(6,28). In contrast, the structurally related LTC$_4$ and platelet-
derived tri-HETEs lack significant chemotactic potency. While LTB$_4$ is
the more potent chemotactic factor, the substantially greater quantities of 5-HETE released by most cells indicates that accurate quantitation of those factors present during inflammatory conditions is essential to delineating the contributions of these principles to disease
states.

The lipoxygenase products of arachidonic acid are more selective
in their leukocyte-directed effects than nonlipid factors such as C5a
and the formyl-methionyl peptides. For example, HETEs do not alter

leukocyte oxidative metabolism or adhesiveness to plastic petri dishes
(12,20,29). The expression of C3b receptors on neutrophil and eosinophil membranes is enhanced by the mono-HETEs and LTB_4, whereas
lesser effects are observed on the expression of IgG receptors (6,12,
28,29). Concentrations of LTB_4 as low as 30-100 ng/ml increase the
release of lysozyme and, to a lesser extent, β-glucuronidase from
human neutrophils in the presence of cytochalasin B. The maximal
release, however, was one-third or less of that achieved by optimal
concentrations of the chemotactic fragment of the fifth component of
complement (C5a) or of the formyl-methionyl peptides. Of the mono-
HETEs, only 5-HETE increases marginally the release of lysozyme
alone, and the levels required to achieve this effect exceed the optimal chemotactic concentrations. HETEs increase the level of guanosine
3':5' cyclic monophosphate (cyclic GMP), with a maximal one- to twofold increase at concentrations of 1/200 to 1/50 of those required for
a maximal chemotactic effect (30). Compared with their mono-HETE
products, the OOHETE precursors are both more potent and elevate
cyclic GMP levels for more prolonged periods. For example, 12-L-
OOHETE induces a twofold increase in cyclic GMP at 5 ng/ml as
compared with 50 ng/ml for 12-L-HETE, and the elevation is maintained for 30 min as compared with 10-20 min for 12-L-HETE.

B. Cyclooxygenase Products

Oxidation of arachidonic acid by the cyclooxygenase pathway yields
unstable endoperoxide intermediates which rapidly decay to more
stable compounds including thromboxane B_2, prostaglandins (PG) D_2,
E_2, and $F_{2\alpha}$, prostacyclin, and the 17-carbon compound 12-L-hydroxy-
5,8,10-heptadecatrienoic acid which is a potent chemotactic factor for
human PMN leukocytes (7,31). Although prostaglandins and thromboxanes have been considered capable of eliciting a PMN leukocyte
chemotactic response (32,33), much of the observed chemotactic activity may be attributed to oxidation products developing spontaneously during storage under aerobic conditions (2). Under some circumstances, however, prostaglandins D_2, E_2, and $F_{2\alpha}$, modulate PMN
leukocyte nondirected migration, termed chemokinesis (34). Immunological stimulation of rat peritoneal mononuclear leukocytes in vivo
and in vitro leads to the recovery of lipid chemotactic and chemo-
kinetic factors whose appearances are dependent upon the integrity
of the cyclooxygenase and lipoxygenase pathways, respectively (1,8).
That the chemotactic factor termed LCF_r is a unique principle is
demonstrated by its chromatographic resolution from defined cyclooxygenase products which are known to modulate leukocyte migration
(8) and from other lipid mediators generated simultaneously with
LCF_r, including a platelet-activating factor and a slow-reacting
substance (35). In recent studies, arachidonic acid oxygenation

products of rat peritoneal mononuclear cells were radiolabeled by pre-incubation of 10^8 cells with 2 µCi [^{3}H]arachidonic acid prior to stimulation with a calcium ionophore. LCF_r released into the supernatant phase was purified by sequential chromatography on neutral Amberlite, silicic acid, DE-52, silica gel thin-layer plates, and Zorbax C-18 reverse phase high performance liquid chromatography (HPLC), and the radioactivity and chemotactic activity recovered in the HPLC fractions were assessed. LCF_r eluted at 46 min, with 2% of the eluate eliciting a chemotactic response of 40 leukocytes per high power field. No net radioactivity was associated with LCF_r, whereas peaks of radioactivity were recovered at 36 and 52 min which corresponded to $PGF_{2\alpha}$ and 12-L-HETE, respectively. Thus, LCF_r appears to be a cyclooxygenase pathway product of a fatty acid other than arachidonic acid. Such nonarachidonic acid cyclooxygenase products have been described previously and include prostaglandins E_1 and $F_{1\alpha}$ which are derived from eicosatrienoic acid but which have little chemotactic activity (36).

Determination of the structure of LCF_r will require isolation of sufficient quantities of material for gas chromatography and mass spectroscopy. Preliminary structural information has been attained, however, by simple chemical modification of LCF_r employing techniques such as methylation of carboxyl groups with ethereal diazomethane and acetylation of hydroxyl and amino groups with acetic anhydride (8,19). Acetylation of LCF_r completely eliminated the chemotactic activity of this principle. Methylation, on the other hand, had no effect on the chemotactic activity of LCF_r, suggesting that a hydroxyl or amino group susceptible to acetylation is critical to the chemotactic activity of LCF_r, whereas any carboxyl group present plays a lesser role in the expression of chemotactic activity. Addition of acetylated LCF_r to chemotactic chambers completely blocks the chemotactic effect of an equal quantity of native LCF_r while having no effect on the chemotactic response to 10^{-7} M f-Met-Leu-Ala-Phe (8). That the diminished chemotactic response is due to competitive inhibition is suggested by the specificity of inhibition and by the reversal of inhibition by washing the exposed leukocytes. Employing identical chemical modification techniques, a critical role for a hydroxyl group in the chemotactic activity of LTB_4 is shown by loss of chemotactic activity after acetylation (6), whereas for the mono-HETEs the loss of chemotactic activity after methylation indicates a critical role for a carboxyl group (19). As was observed for LCF_r, the chemically inactivated LTB_4 and mono-HETEs reversibly blocked the chemotactic activity of the unmodified material, but not of other chemotactic factors. The demonstration of different functionally critical substituents and the competitive inhibition between inactivated and native chemotactic factors suggests the presence of unique membrane receptors for the different lipid chemotactic factors. Although such receptors

receptors have not been demonstrated directly, their presence is
suggested by the observation that exogenous radiolabeled 5-HETE
and 12-L-HETE remain associated with neutrophil membranes for up to
2 hr (12,29). While a minor portion of the added mono-HETEs becomes
incorporated into membrane phospholipids (37), the bulk of the material can be recovered as the free acids indistinguishable from the
authentic HETEs (12).

III. Effects of Alkyl-Ether Phosphorylcholine Mediators on Human Leukocyte Function

The recent demonstration that 1-O-alkyl-2-acetyl-sn-glycero-3-
phosphorylcholine possess platelet-activating activity (38) suggests
that 1-alkyl-ether phospholipids (AGEPC), which are present in only
trace quantities in most mammalian cells, might also modulate leukocyte function. The effects of 2-acetyl, 2-succinyl, 2-maleyl, and 2-
phthalyl analogues were examined in a variety of in vitro assays of
neutrophil function (39). The 2-acetyl, 2-succinyl, and 2-maleyl
analogues elicited maximal neutrophil chemotactic responses of approximately 30 neutrophils per hpf, with 50% of the maximal response
occurring at concentrations of 3×10^{-7} M, 10^{-6} M, and 10^{-6} M, respectively (39). The 2-phthalyl analogue was only marginally chemotactic, and none of the analogues significantly enhanced leukocyte
nondirected migration. The double bond of the 2-maleyl analogue resulted in increased chemotactic potency, and a free carboxyl group
endowed the 2-maleyl and 2-succinyl analogues with the capacity to
enhance neutrophil adherence, whereas only the 2-acetyl analogue
possessed lysosomal enzyme secretagogue activity.

The most striking leukocyte-directed effect of this class of lipids,
which also was dependent on the nature of the 2-acyl substituent, was
the modulation of chemotactic responses to homologous or other stimuli. When PMN leukocytes were preincubated with the analogues for
15 min at 37°C and washed twice in buffer, the chemotactic responses
to C5a, 10^{-5} M 2-acetyl analogue, and 10^{-6} M 2-maleyl analogue were
suppressed significantly by optimally chemotactic concentrations of
the 2-acetyl, 2-maleyl, and 2-phthalyl analogues, but not by the 2-
succinyl analogue. At concentrations of 10^{-10} M, which is well below
the chemotactic range, preincubation of leukocytes with the 2-succi-
nyl, 2-maleyl, and 2-phthalyl analogues, but not with the 2-acetyl
analogue, significantly enhanced the chemotactic response of the exposed leukocytes to other stimuli.

IV. Contribution of Endogenous Lipoxygenase Products to Polymorphonuclear Leukocyte Function

The presence of endogenous lipoxygenase products in PMN leukocyte membranes in approximately nanomolar quantities which are affected rapidly and transiently by changes in other membrane constituents and by exogenous stimuli suggests that endogenous HETEs serve a role in the expression of critical leukocyte functions. Human neutrophil membranes contain approximately 500–600 ng of 5-HETE, 300–2000 ng of 11-HETE, and 150–300 ng of LTB_4 per 10^8 neutrophils (40). The intracellular content of these mono-HETEs begins to rise within 15 min of the addition of a chemotactic stimulus, achieves peak elevations to 2- to 10-fold by 30 min, and returns to baseline by 60–120 min. Preincubation of neutrophils for 30–60 min with lipoxygenase inhibitors such as 10 μM ETYA or 5 μM nordihydroguaiaretic acid (NDGA), followed by washing in the presence of the inhibitors, diminishes the endogenous mono-HETE by greater than 50% and suppresses both random migration and chemotaxis to diverse stimuli (40). This effect is reversed by the addition of nanomolar quantities of 5-HETE even in the continued presence of the lipoxygenase inhibitors. The suppression of migration and depletion of endogenous mono-HETEs demonstrated similar time course and lipoxygenase inhibitor concentration dependence. In contrast, inhibitors of cyclooxygenase activity, such as indomethacin, enhanced leukocyte random migration and chemotaxis. The specificity of the functional consequences of depleting endogenous HETEs has been assessed in a range of neutrophil activities (12). The release of neutrophil lysosomal enzymes by optimally chemotactic concentration of C5a and formyl-methionyl peptides was suppressed to an extent which generally correlated with the degree of depletion of neutrophil mono-HETEs by NDGA or ETYA, whereas, indomethacin had no effect. In contrast, the expression of C3b receptors and the phagocytosis of EAC43b cells were inhibited significantly only by the maximal depletion of mono-HETEs achieved by preincubation with 10 μM NDGA. Thus, leukocyte random and chemotactic migration and lysosomal enzyme release appear to be critically dependent on the integrity of the lipoxygenase pathway, whereas phagocytosis and the expression of some membrane receptors are less dependent.

The capacity of platelet-activating factors of the 1-alkyl-ether phospholipid family to modulate leukocyte migration has been appreciated only recently (39), and the range of possible leukocyte-directed effects of these principles has not been explored fully. The structural similarity of AGEPC to membrane phospholipids and the observation that polymorphonuclear and mononuclear leukocytes release AGEPC (41) suggest that these principles may function as intracellular messengers in a manner analogous to the endogenous HETEs.

The human leukocyte AGEPC have not been structurally characterized,
however, and in preliminary studies the monocyte-derived material is
chromatographically distinct from the rabbit basophil AGEPC (2-
acetyl analogue) (unpublished data). Thus, delineation of a role for
endogenous AGEPC in leukocytes requires structure elucidation of the
endogenous material as well as development of specific inhibitors.

V. Contribution of Lipid Chemotactic Factors to In Vivo Inflammatory Reactions

The establishment of an in vivo role for the different lipid chemotactic
factors is dependent in part on the demonstration of functionally relevant concentrations of the products in inflamed tissues and biological
fluids and on the ability to suppress in parallel the levels of these
mediators and the intensity of the leukocytic infiltration with specific
inhibitors. LCF_r was recognized initially as the predominant chemotactic factor generated during immunological challenge of the rat peritoneal cavity (1). Similarly, challenge of the guinea pig peritoneal
cavity with 4-8 µg of 12-L-HETE led to an initial accumulation of eosinophils at 30 min and a subsequent influx of neutrophils at 5 hr
(19). Methylated 12-L-HETE which is chemotactically inactive had no
direct effect on the peritoneal leukocytes, but reduced the leukocyte
influx evoked by an equimolar amount of native 12-L-HETE. Psoriatic
skin is characterized by an intense neutrophilic infiltrate, and the
content of 12-L-HETE in psoriatic plaques is elevated as compared
with noninvolved skin in the same subjects (42). The synovial fluid
levels of LTB_4 and the synovial tissue levels of 5-HETE are elevated
in patients with rheumatoid arthritis when compared with levels observed in patients with noninflammatory arthropathies which lack a
prominent leukocytic infiltration (43). The concentrations of LTB_4
and of 5-HETE observed in rheumatoid synovial fluid are sufficiently
high to elicit maximal PMN leukocyte chemotactic responses. That
lipoxygenase products may be the predominant stimuli of the leukocyte
component of some inflammatory responses is supported by the finding
that the lipoxygenase inhibitor BW755C suppresses the PMN leukocyte
infiltration, but not the edema, in rat paws injected with carrageenin
(44). The development of more specific and less toxic lipoxygenase
inhibitors will be required in order to provide more definitive proof of
the proposed physiological role of the HETEs in inflammatory disease
states.

VI. Summary

The diverse activities of lipid chemotactic factors as extracellular and
intracellular mediators of leukocyte function in vitro suggest an

important contribution of these principles to the initiation and maintenance of the cellular component of in vivo inflammatory reactions
(Fig. 1). Immunological stimulation of a variety of cells, including
polymorphonuclear and mononuclear leukocytes, leads to the rapid
appearance of lipid chemotactic factors, including the lipoxygenase
products mono-HETEs and leukotriene B_4, the cyclooxygenase products
HHT and LCF_r, and 1-alkyl-ether phospholipids. In addition to evoking
leukocyte chemotaxis, the different chemotactic factors express a
variety of leukocyte-directed effects. AGEPC analogues are potent
modulators of the chemotactic response to other factors while having
only modest secretagogue and adherence-enhancing actions. Exogenous LTB_4 and mono-HETEs elevate leukocyte cyclic GMP, induce lysosomal enzyme release, enhance the expression of C3b receptors, and
enhance the leukocyte chemotactic response to other chemotactic factors. In addition to the extracellular functions of these lipoxygenase
pathway products, the integrity of the lipoxygenase pathway may be
a biochemical prerequisite for leukocyte migration, phagocytosis, and
lysosomal degranulation, since these functions are suppressed by
lipoxygenase inhibitors which deplete the leukocytes of their endogenous HETEs. In some cases these functions have been restored by
the addition of exogenous lipoxygenase products in the continued
presence of the lipoxygenase inhibitors. Mono-HETEs, LTB_4, and LCR_r
have been isolated from tissues and body fluids in association with a
leukocytic infiltrate during the in vivo inflammatory reactions characteristic of psoriasis, rheumatoid arthritis, and anaphylaxis, respectively. Further delineation of the roles of lipid chemotactic factors
in pathophysiologic processes requires accurate quantitation of those
principles present and the development of specific, nontoxic inhibitors
of their generation.

References

1. F. H. Valone and E. J. Goetzl, *J. Immunol.* *120*:102 (1978).
2. S. Sahu and W. S. Lynn, *Inflammation* 2:47 (1977).
3. R. J. Russell, R. J. McInroy, P. C. Wilkinson, and R. G.
   White, *Immunology 30*:935 (1976).
4. S. R. Turner, J. A. Tainer, and W. S. Lynn, *Nature (Lond.)*
   257:680 (1975).
5. E. J. Goetzl, J. M. Woods, and R. R. Gorman, *J. Clin. Invest.*
   59:179 (1977).
6. E. J. Goetzl and W. C. Pickett, *J. Immunol. 125*:1789 (1980).
7. E. J. Goetzl and R. R. Gorman, *J. Immunol. 120*:526 (1978).
8. F. H. Valone and E. J. Goetzl, *Immunology 41*:517 (1980).
9. M. Hamberg, J. Svensson, P. Hedqvist, K. Strandberg, and
   B. Samuelsson, in *Advances in Prostaglandin and Thromboxane*

Research (B. Samuelsson and R. Paoletti, eds.), Raven, New York, 1976, p. 8.

10. H. Nugteren, *Biochim. Biophys. Acta 380*:299 (1975).

11. M. J. Hamberg, J. Svensson, and B. Samuelsson, *Proc. Natl. Acad. Sci. U.S.A. 71*:3824 (1974).

12. E. J. Goetzl, D. W. Goldman, and F. H. Valone, in *The Biochemistry of the Acute Allergic Reaction*, Alan R. Liss, New York, in press.

13. F. H. Valone, M. Franklin, and E. J. Goetzl, *Cell. Immunol. 54*:390 (1980).

14. E. J. Goetzl and F. F. Sun, *J. Exp. Med. 150*:406 (1979).

15. E. J. Goetzl, P. F. Weller, and F. F. Sun, *J. Immunol. 124*: 926 (1980).

16. C. W. Parker, W. F. Stenson, M. G. Huber, and J. P. Kelley, *J. Immunol. 122*:1572 (1979).

17. M. Hamberg and B. Samuelsson, *Proc. Natl. Acad. Sci. U.S.A. 71*:3400 (1974).

18. L. J. Roberts, R. A. Lewis, J. A. Oates, and K. F. Austen, *Biochim. Biophys. Acta 575*:185 (1979).

19. E. J. Goetzl, F. H. Valone, V. N. Reinhold, and R. R. Gorman, *J. Clin. Invest. 63*:1181 (1979).

20. E. J. Goetzl, A. R. Brash, A. I. Tauber, J. A. Oates, and W. C. Hubbard, *Immunology 39*:141 (1980).

21. P. A. Ward and E. L. Becker, *J. Exp. Med. 127*:693 (1968).

22. P. Borgeat and B. Samuelsson, *Proc. Natl. Acad. Sci. U.S.A. 76*:3213 (1979).

23. R. C. Murphy, S. Hammarstrom, and B. Samuelsson, *Proc. Natl. Acad. Sci. U.S.A. 76*:4275 (1979).

24. P. Borgeat and B. Samuelsson, *J. Biol. Chem. 254*:2643 (1979).

25. H. R. Morris, G. W. Taylor, P. J. Piper, M. W. Sankoun, and J. R. Tippins, *Prostaglandins 19*:185 (1980).

26. C. W. Parker, M. M. Huber, M. K. Hoffman, and S. F. Flakenheim, *Prostaglandins, 18*:673 (1979).

27. L. Orning, S. Hammarstrom, and B. Samuelsson, *Proc. Natl. Acad. Sci. U.S.A. 77*:2014 (1980).

28. E. J. Goetzl, C. K. Derian, C. J. Owens, and F. H. Valone, in *Proceedings of the First International Conference on Immunopharmacology*, in press.

29. E. J. Goetzl, *Med. Clin. North Am.* (in press).

30. E. J. Goetzl, H. R. Hill, and R. R. Gorman, *Prostaglandins 19*:71 (1980).

31. B. Samuelsson, in *Advances in Prostaglandin and Thromboxane Research* (B. Samuelsson and R. Paoletti, eds.), Raven, New York, 1976, p. 1.

32. G. A. Higgs, E. McCall, and L. J. F. Youlton, *Br. J. Pharmacol. 53*:539 (1975).

33. J. R. Boot, W. Dawson, and E. A. Kitchen, *J. Physiol. (Lond.)* **257**:47P (1976).

34. E. J. Goetzl, P. F. Weller, and F. H. Valone, in *Advances in Inflammation Research* (G. Weissmann, B. Samuelsson, and R. Paoletti, eds.), Raven, New York, 1979, p. 157.

35. F. H. Valone, D. Whitmer, and E. J. Goetzl, *Immunology* **37**:841 (1979).

36. F. H. Valone, K. F. Austen, and E. J. Goetzl, *J. Clin. Invest.* **54**:1100 (1974).

37. W. F. Stenson and C. W. Parker, *J. Clin. Invest.* **64**:1457 (1979).

38. C. A. Demopoulos, R. N. Pinckard, and D. J. Hanahan, *J. Biol. Chem.* **253**:9355 (1979).

39. E. J. Goetzl, C. K. Derian, A. I. Tauber, and F. H. Valone, *Biochem. Biophys. Res. Commun.* **94**:881 (1980).

40. E. J. Goetzl, C. K. Derian, and F. H. Valone, *J. Reticuloendothel. Soc.* **28**:105S, 1980.

41. G. Z. Lotner, J. M. Lynch, S. J. Betz, and P. M. Henson, *J. Immunol.* **124**:676, 1980.

42. S. M. Hammarstrom, M. Hamberg, B. Samuelsson, E. A. Duell, M. Stawiski, and J. J. Voorhees, *Proc. Natl. Acad. Sci. U.S.A.* **72**:5130 (1975).

43. L. B. Klickstein, T. Shapleigh, and E. J. Goetzl, *Arthritis Rheum.* **23**:704 (1980).

44. G. A. Higgs, S. Moncada, and J. R. Vane, in *Advances in Inflammation Research* (G. Weissmann, B. Samuelsson, and R. Paoletti, eds.), Raven, New York, 1979, p. 278.

5

Regulation of Monocyte-Macrophage Differentiation

LOUIS M. PELUS* and MALCOLM A. S. MOORE   Sloan-Kettering Institute for Cancer Research, New York, New York

I.   Introduction

The importance of the macrophage in antitumor activity, microbial clearance, and the complex interactions of the cellular and humoral immune responses are now well recognized (1-6). Although the macrophage was initially thought only to play a role in body defense to microbes as a phagocytic scavenger, the recognition of the multiplicity of monocyte cell-derived factors and the myriad of regulatory interactions provided by and participated in by these cells indicate a more central role for macrophages in host defense. Thus, the monocyte-macrophage system today is believed to be central to body integrity, necessary to provide the diversity of immunological reactions, and important to the overall mobilization of host defense mechanisms.

In recent years it has become apparent that monocytoid cells are endowed with an abundant synthetic capacity and actively synthesize and release a multiplicity of factors into their pericellular environment. These factors have been shown to play important roles in immune cell function and regulation, in proliferatory response, particularly those involving clonal hematopoietic progenitor cell expansion, and in inflammatory reactions. Thus, the secretory activity of these cells plays a predominant role in their overall function. Indeed, the macrophage itself can be regulated by its own synthetic products. Among the diverse products of members of this cell lineage are two groups of factors which regulate the prolifera-

---

*Scholar of the Leukemia Society of America, Inc.

tion and differentiation of monocytoid cells themselves, namely, colony-stimulating factors, CSF (7-9), and the acidic lipids, the prostaglandins (10-12).

The importance of the monocyte-macrophage lineage in overall host defense mandates that homeostatic mechanisms exist to maintain adequate numbers of functionally mature cells, as well as provide for heightened production in response to specific demands. In vitro studies indicate that the proliferation of mature monocytic cells from their stem cells within bone marrow (13) and from more mature monocytoid cells in various peripheral tissues (14) is under the control of a specific macrophage growth factor, granulocyte-macrophage colony-stimulating factor, GM-CSF. The recognition that GM-CSF is produced by monocytes and macrophages and that tissues rich in macrophages are invariably good sources of GM-CSF (13) creates a problem, since the macrophages are themselves a result of elevated GM-CSF levels. This then is a positive feedback system and raises the question of what mechanisms act to counterbalance the positive stimulus. Unchecked, CSF production leads to monocyte-macrophage production, which leads to elevated CSF production, etc. However, studies have indicated that prostaglandin E (PGE), a major monocyte-macrophage biosynthetic product, profoundly inhibits monocyte-macrophage proliferation and differentiation in vitro (12). Just as GM-CSF promotes the continued replication of bone marrow myeloid stem cells and their progeny, PGE limits this effect by an opposing action on the responsiveness of the myeloid stem cell and its proliferative progeny to stimulation. Thus, monocyte-macrophage-derived products ultimately control the production of monocytoid cells.

This chapter will deal with the mechanisms whereby monocyte-macrophage-derived PGE and GM-CSF effect regulation of monocytoid-committed stem cell proliferation and monocyte-macrophage differentiation.

II. Assessment of Macrophage Proliferation and Differentiation

A. Methodology

The development of in vitro techniques which support the growth of hematopoietic progenitor cells has permitted the investigation of potential regulators and established a means to detect, quantitate, and categorize the proliferating stem cells. In vivo, the various hematopoietic populations are inextricably intermixed, and delineation of the regulatory mechanisms controlling hematopoiesis have proven extremely complex. Moreover, ethical reasons prevent their adequate study. Thus, the in vitro culture assays afford us the only means to study control mechanisms. Albeit, the overall significance of culture studies to in vivo mechanisms is not direct, their importance lies in the ability to (1) study cells only of a given lineage at one particular time, e.g., erythropoiesis, (2) to observe the clonal expansion from discrete single cells suspended in a semisolid matrix, and (3) to assess the proliferative capacity of specific stem cells. Furthermore, established diagnostic and prognostic values support their significance.

The in vitro proliferation and differentiation of monocytes and macrophages (as well as granulocytes) from their committed progenitor cell, the granulocyte-macrophage colony-forming cell, or colony-forming-unit granulocyte-macrophage (CFU-GM), and from the more mature unipotential monocyte-macrophage colony-forming cell (M-CFC) are dependent upon the continuous presence of specific stimulating factors, granulocyte-macrophage colony-stimulating factors. The proliferation of these lineage-restricted marrow or tissue progenitor cells can be quantitated in semisolid agar culture. Suspensions of murine or human bone marrow cells at a concentration of 7.5 to 10×10^4 cells in 1.0 ml of 0.3% agar medium containing the appropriate source of CSF are aliquoted into 35 mm petri dishes and incubated in a well-humidified atmosphere of 5% CO_2 in air. Alternatively, cell suspensions can be overlayed upon underlayers of GM-CSF-producing cells, such as human peripheral blood leukocytes and/or monocytes and murine peritoneal macrophages, suspended in 0.5% agar medium or adherent to the petri dish, and separated from the target overlay by a 1.0 ml layer of 0.5% agar medium. This bilayer culture system represents an in vitro hematopoietic environment in which direct cellular contact is prevented, yet permits the analysis of the effects of diffusible molecules upon progenitor cell proliferation. The direct proliferation of the more mature bone marrow or tissue unipotential M-CFC is assayed by incubating 1×10^4 thioglycollate-elicited murine peritoneal exudate cells (or cells from other anatomical sites) in 0.3% agar medium containing 10% fetal calf serum and 5% horse serum, in the presence of either GM-CSF or M-CSF or, alternatively, over feeder layers of resident peritoneal macrophages.

B. Colony-forming Cells

Various classes of progenitor cells are detected depending on the time of scoring of the cultures. Following 7 days of incubation, clones (clusters of 3-50 cells and colonies of >50 cells) composed exclusively of either neutrophils, eosinophils, monocytes-macrophages, or a mixture of neutrophils and macrophages can be quantitated. If M-CSF is used as the proliferative signal, all colonies will be composed exclusively of monocytes and macrophages. Similarly, the proliferative progeny of more immature GM-CFC can be detected after 14 days of incubation. The maturational state of these two classes of GM-CFC have been established following biophysical separation (15) and sensitivity to growth regulators (16,17).

The 7- and 14-day clones composed solely of monocytes and macrophages apparently derive from the proliferation of both bipotentially committed GM-CFC and unipotential bone marrow monocyte-macrophage stem cells. In this regard, paired daughter cell transfer studies have shown that GM-CSF levels can modulate some degree of pathway differentiation (18). These studies suggest that irreversible unilineage differentiation occurs, and likewise in some cases, perhaps within the first several divisions of the colony-forming cell, the level and specific subtype of CSF can alter differentiation.

The colony-forming cells just described are distinct from those bone marrow-derived M-CFC which can be detected in many tissues as well as in bone marrow. These colony-forming cells form colonies composed exclusively of monocytes and macrophages in the obligate presence of GM-CSF or M-CSF. These M-CFC are characterized by an initial 13-18-day lag period prior to initiation of colony formation. During this lag period, CSF is not required, which is in contrast to GM-CFC which require the continuous presence of CSF. These cells are further characterized in that their differentiation to monocytes and macrophages cannot be influenced by GM-CSF levels. The available data suggest that this macrophage-colony-forming cell is present in bone marrow, spleen, thymus, lymph node, peripheral blood, stimulated peritoneal and pleural cavities, and alveolar spaces. They are heterogeneous in many respects and may be site-specific subpopulations of progenitor cells (14).

C. Colony-stimulating Factors

As described, the proliferation and differentiation of granulocytes and macrophages from their committed progenitor cell is dependent upon a diffusible activity termed granulocyte-macrophage colony-stimulating factor. This factor is likely to be the major regulator of granulocyte and monocyte-macrophage formation in vivo (13). It can be detected in human and mouse serum (19,20) and extracted directly from various tissues (21). All murine GM-CSF are glycoproteins of 23,000 mol wt (21). Human active GM-CSF, isolated from human placental cells, is a glycoprotein of 30,000 mol wt as determined by gel filtration (22). In the mouse, a distinct subclass of colony-stimulating factor which only stimulates monocyte-macrophage colony formation, M-CSF, has been isolated from L cells and yolk sacs (23,24). Purified M-CSF from mouse L cells is a 70,000 mol wt glycoprotein composed of two disulphide-bound 35,000 mol wt subunits (23). Recently, the GM-CSF produced by the murine WEHI-3 myelomonocytic leukemia cell line has been shown to contain both granulocyte (G-CSF) and macrophage (M-CSF) specific subtypes (25). In addition, a low molecular weight G-CSF can be isolated from mouse-endotoxin lung-conditioned medium (26). Likewise, variants of human placental GM-CSF which preferentially stimulate day 7 versus day 14 colony formation have been identified (22). While it

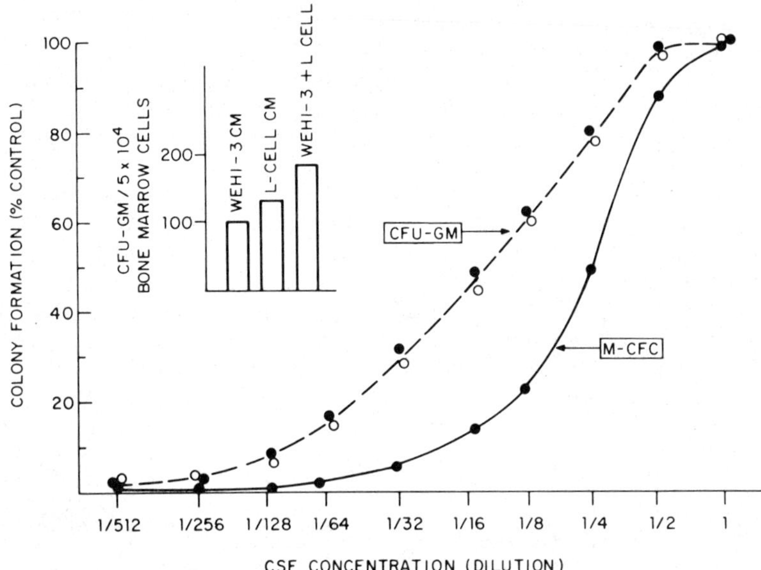

FIG. 1   The cloning capacity of bone marrow CFU-GM and peritoneal M-CFC stimulated by various concentrations of L-cell M-CSF (●) and WEHI-3 GM-CSF (○). Colony-forming capacity is expressed as a percentage of the maximum number of colonies obtained. Quadruplicate cultures were scored for each point.

may appear that considerable heterogeneity exists among materials having colony-stimulating activity, it is becoming apparent that micro-environmental or cellular factors are intimately involved in the regulation of every facet of hematopoietic differentiation. It is conceivable that in the near future, with continued biochemical analysis, factors for each proliferative and maturation step in the pathway of hematopoietic cell differentiation will be isolated and characterized.

The colony-stimulating factors are not simple inducing agents, their presence is required throughout the growth of the colony for promotion of survival, proliferation, and differentiation. Concentrations as low as 10^{-11} M are sufficient to induce stem cell proliferation. Colony-stimulating factor acts remarkably fast on target cells; RNA synthesis increases within 5 min, noncycling GM-CFC enter the cell cycle within 3 hr, the rate of proliferation of the GM-CFC and the progression to recognizable granulocyte-macrophage precursors and mature forms are accelerated by increasing concentrations of GM-CSF, and the mean cell cycle time is decreased.

In vitro, the relationship between colony-stimulating activity and colony number is represented by a sigmoidal curve (Fig. 1). For bone marrow, throughout the linear portion of the dose response curve, increases in GM-CSF and macrophage-specific M-CSF (provided by WEHI-3 and mouse L cell-conditioned medium, respectively) result in increased GM-CFC proliferation. Plateau colony formation occurs at half maximal stimulator levels and represents the maximum potentially clonable progenitor cells in the bone marrow suspension. It should be noted, however, that the addition of both GM-CSF and M-CSF to the marrow sample results in greater proliferation than either alone, indicating that the responding colony-forming cell populations both share and differ in responsiveness to CSF. The proliferation of the more mature tissue M-CFC likewise follows a sigmoidal dose response curve, although approximately fourfold higher CSF levels are required for equivalent half maximal proliferation. Thus, the net monocytoid proliferative response is dependent upon the type of CSF present, the number of given colony-forming cells capable of responding, and the intrinsic sensitivity of the colony-forming cells to stimulation.

III. Regulation of Monocyte-Macrophage Proliferation

As stated earlier, the major source of GM-CSF within the hematopoietic system has been identified as the monocyte and tissue macrophage (8,9,27,28). The release of GM-CSF by macrophages can be augmented by bacterial endotoxins, suggesting a mechanism whereby the presence of bacterial products can increase granulocyte and monocyte production by the bone marrow (28). Enhancement of monocyte-macrophage GM-CSF production by lymphokine also provides a mechanism for increasing macrophage production during certain immunological reactions. The role of GM-CSF in recruiting monocytes and macrophages from the GM-CFC compartment, as well as promoting local macrophage proliferation, indicates an operative positive feedback control based upon monocytoid cell GM-CSF production. In culture, mouse peritoneal macrophages release GM-CSF during the first 24 hr of incubation, after which no further GM-CSF production occurs unless the growth medium is changed. In contrast, daily medium replacement promotes incremental production of GM-CSF (29). This suggests that GM-CSF secretion can be modulated by GM-CSF in the external milieu or that some inhibitor of GM-CSF production or of the effect of GM-CSF on its target cell accumulates in the medium.

The recognition that prostaglandins are a major secretory product of monocytoid cells (11,30) and that the E series prostaglandins in particular are inhibitory in a variety of cell proliferatory assays (31, 32) suggests that monocyte-macrophage-derived PGE might represent a cosynthesized inhibitor serving to counterbalance the positive drive of GM-CSF. Simultaneous measurements of GM-CSF activity and PGE in

TABLE 1   Effects of Prostaglandin E on Murine-Macrophage Colony-Stimulating Factor Production

Addition to control	Mean CFU-GM per 7.5×10^4 mouse bone marrow cells
	29 ± 1
10^{-8} M PGE_1	18 ± 2
10^{-8} M PGE_1, dialyzed	33 ± 2

Note: Colony-stimulating activity in 10% (v/v) supernate from 24-hr cultures of adherent cells derived from 1×10^5 BDF_1 peritoneal cells. Prostaglandin E_1 was added at culture initiation and was present throughout the duration of the culture. The indicated sample was dialyzed against 3 changes of quarter-strength phosphate-buffered saline for 48 hr at 4°C, using membrane tubing having a 3500 mol wt cutoff.

supernates from cultures of mouse macrophages and human monocytes confirm the coincident production of both activities (Fig. 2).

Inhibition of prostaglandin synthesis by use of the cyclooxygenase inhibitor indomethacin in culture results in the detection of higher levels of GM-CSF activity in culture supernates. Similar results are obtained if monocyte-macrophage culture supernates are dialyzed to remove prostaglandin (Fig. 2). These results indicate an effect of prostaglandin at the level of the proliferating stem cell and not at the level of GM-CSF production. The inability of PGE to affect macrophage GM-CSF production was confirmed by adding exogenous PGE to cultures of mouse macrophages during incubation and subsequently dialyzing to remove the prostaglandin (Table 1). The level of GM-CSF activity following dialysis was equal to or slightly greater than the control. The enhancement of GM-CSF levels following dialysis results from the elimination of contaminating prostaglandin produced during the culture incubation.

The ability of PGE to inhibit the proliferation of myeloid progenitor cells was assayed directly by the addition of authentic PGE_1 to cultures of mouse bone marrow cells stimulated by WEHI-3 GM-CSF (Fig. 3). The addition of PGE_1 at concentrations of 10^{-5} to 10^{-8} M results in a dose-dependent inhibition of total colony formation. However, morphological analysis of single colonies indicates that macrophage colonies are significantly more sensitive to inhibition than either neutrophil or mixed colonies. The preferential inhibition of macrophage

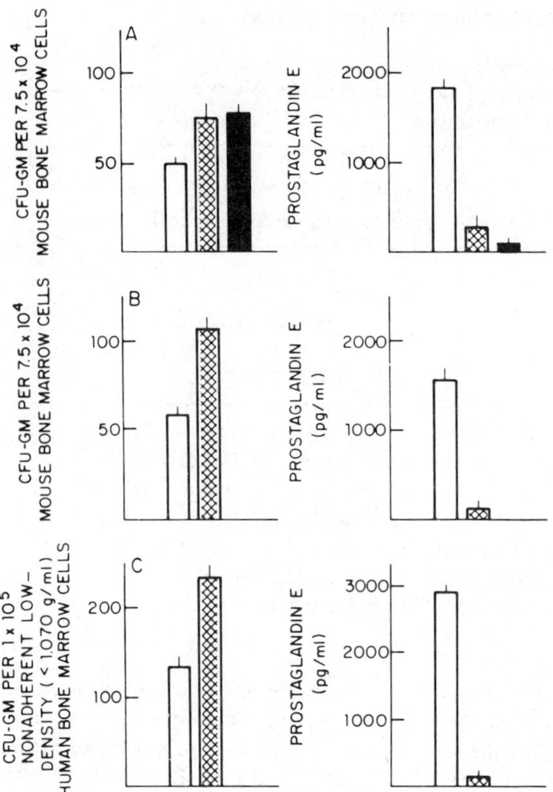

FIG. 2 Measurement of GM-CSF and prostaglandin E activity produced by adherent murine peritoneal macrophages and human peripheral blood monocytes. Culture supernates and macrophage feeder layers were prepared in the absence (□) and presence (▨) of 10^{-6} M indomethacin. Some culture supernates were prepared in the absence of indomethacin and were dialyzed to remove prostaglandin (■). A: Simultaneous determination of GM-CSF and prostaglandin E in 24-hr-culture supernates from adherent macrophages derived from 1×10^5 resident BDF_1 mouse peritoneal cells. Prostaglandin E was assayed in 1.0-ml-culture supernates. Granulocyte-macrophage CSF activity was determined in 10% (v/v) supernate. B: Colony formation in response to GM-CSF produced by feeder layers of adherent cells from 1×10^5 resident BDF_1 mouse peritoneal cells. Prostaglandin E measurements were performed on parallel 24-hr liquid cultures. C: Granulocyte-macrophage CSF and prostaglandin E levels in cell-free 48-hr supernates from cultures of adherent human blood monocytes. Peripheral blood mononuclear cells were isolated by neutral density centrifugation in bovine serum albumin (density 1.070 g/ml). There were 1×10^6 mononuclear cells seeded per culture and washed after 90 min at 37°C, after which fresh media was added. Colony-stimulating activity was assayed in 10% (v/v) supernate, prostaglandin E in 1.0 ml culture supernate.

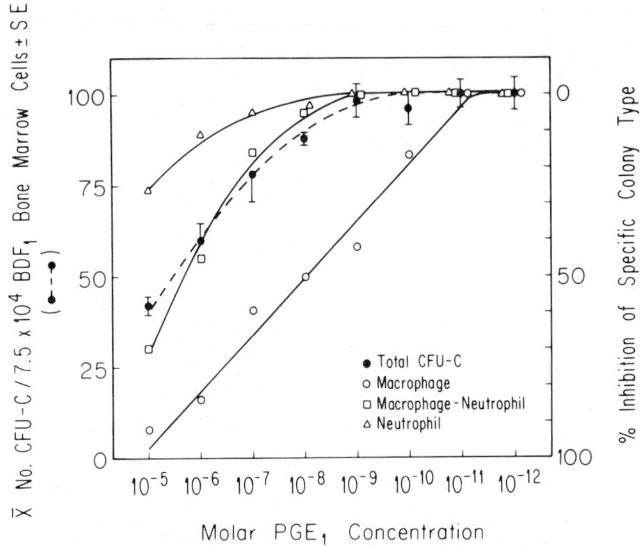

FIG. 3   The effect of prostaglandin E on total (•) and morphologically
defined mouse bone marrow colony formation stimulated by WEHI-3
GM-CSF. There were 100 sequential colonies for each point transferred to glass slides and morphologically identified as being macrophage (○), mixed macrophage-neutrophil (□), or pure neutrophil (△)
in composition. Total colony formation is expressed as the absolute
number of colonies. Morphologically defined colony formation is expressed in terms of percentage inhibition at each molar prostaglandin
concentration.

colony formation was further confirmed using CSF preparations differing in their ability to stimulate distinct colony types. Thus, macrophage colonies stimulated by the monocytoid specific L cell CSF are
extremely sensitive to inhibition by exogenously added PGE ($ID_{50} = 5 \times 10^{-9}$ M) (12), whereas granulocyte colonies stimulated by the WEHI-3
granulocytic CSF subtype are essentially resistant to inhibition ($ID_{50} > 10^{-5}$ M) (12). Mixed neutrophil-macrophage colony formation was
found to be intermediate between pure neutrophil and pure macrophage
colonies as a result of the effect of prostaglandin on the monocytic
component of these colonies. The sensitivity of colony formation to inhibition by PGE was not dependent on CSF concentration, being consistent throughout the dose response curves for both CSF subtypes.
The clonal proliferation of the peritoneal M-CFC population was likewise found to be sensitive to the inhibitory effects of exogenously

TABLE 2 The Effects of Resident Peritoneal Macrophages on GM-CFC Proliferation

Peritoneal cell concentration[a]	INDO (10^{-6} M)	Mean GM-CFC per 7.5×10^4 Mouse bone marrow cells	Colony morphology[a]		
			Macrophage	Mixed macrophage neutrophil	Neutrophil
5×10^4	−	43 ± 2	4	36	3
	+	62 ± 1	31	28	3
1×10^5	−	56 ± 3	6	39	11
	+	94 ± 3	49	36	9
2.5×10^5	−	31 ± 2	2	20	9
	+	74 ± 2	33	33	9
5×10^5	−	28 ± 2	3	16	9
	+	63 ± 4	22	38	5

[a]The number of resident B6D2F1 murine peritoneal cells seeded per culture. Cells were allowed to adhere for 90 min, were washed 3 times with phosphate-buffered saline, and were overlayed with 1.0 ml of 0.5% agar medium and subsequently with 7.5×10^5 mouse bone marrow cells in 1.0 ml of 0.3% agar medium.

[b]Differential colony morphology was determined by analysis of 100 sequential colonies transferred to microscope slides and stained with 0.6% orcein in 60% acetic acid. Data are expressed as the number of colonies identified as having the indicated morphology.

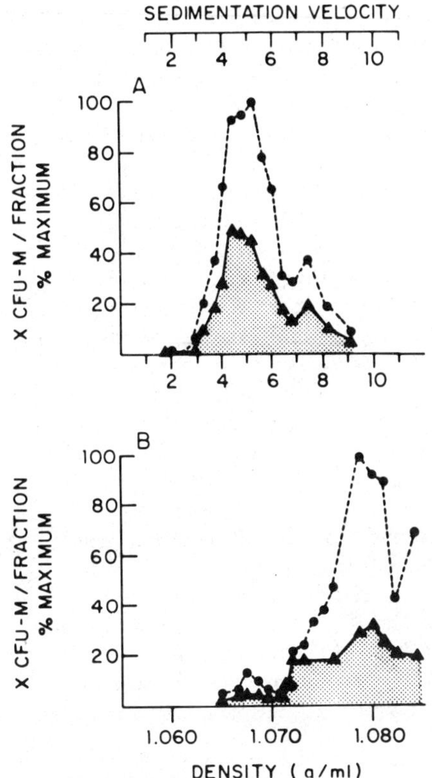

FIG. 4   A: Velocity sedimentation distribution of GM-CFC stimulated by L cell M-CSF in the absence (●) and presence (▲) of 10^{-8} M prostaglandin E_1. B: Buoyant density distribution of proliferating macrophage colonies stimulated by WEHI-3 GM-CSF in the absence (●) and presence (▲) of 10^{-8} M prostaglandin E_1. Macrophage colonies were determined by morphological analysis of intact dehydrated cultures after glutaraldehyde fixation and staining with Harris' Hematoxylin. The total number of morphologically identifiable pure macrophage colonies in each of three replicate cultures was determined for each point. Data are expressed as the number of GM-CFC per fraction as a percentage of maximum. Colony-forming capacity was determined using 2.0×10^4 separated bone-marrow cells per culture and colony incidence was adjusted to the total number of cells in each fraction.

added PGE_1, with 50% inhibition of colony formation evident with prostaglandin E_1 concentrations between 10^{-9} and 10^{-10} M.

The studies described clearly indicate that macrophage-derived CSF and PGE play a role in the proliferation of GM-CFC. Furthermore, using exogenously added factors, the inhibitory effects of PGE were confirmed and extended to demonstrate a selective effect on monocyte-macrophage proliferation. These and similar studies suggest a central role for monocytes in regulating monocytopoiesis. The capacity of macrophages to directly modulate GM-CFC proliferation in vitro was assayed in bilayer agar culture (Table 2). In the absence of exogenously added GM-CSF, feeder layers of resident peritoneal macrophages stimulate the proliferation of bone marrow GM-CFC in agar overlays, with maximal colony formation observed with adherent macrophages derived from 1×10^5 peritoneal cells. Increasing the number of feeder cells beyond this point results in a decline in total colony formation. However, the addition of indomethacin to the agar feeder layers at the start of the culture augments colony formation at all points tested and greatly reduces the decline in colony numbers at high peritoneal cell concentrations. More dramatic than the effect of indomethacin on total colony formation is the effect on monocyte-macrophage colony formation. Inhibition of macrophage prostaglandin synthesis results in 7-16-fold increases in monocytoid cloning efficiency.

The preferential sensitivity of murine monocytoid colonies was likewise found for human monocyte-macrophage colonies (35). Proliferating day 7 and day 14 monocytic clones are sensitive to prostaglandin inhibition, with 3×10^{-9} and 9×10^{-8} M PGE_1 concentrations required for 50% inhibition, respectively. The greater molar prostaglandin requirement for inhibition of day 14 monocyte-macrophage proliferation reflects the immaturity of this progenitor cell in relation to day 7 GM-CFC (17).

IV. Heterogeneity of Colony-Forming Cells

Separation of murine bone marrow cells by velocity sedimentation at unit gravity indicates that GM-CFC giving rise solely to monocyte-macrophage colonies in the presence of M-CSF display a considerable size heterogeneity (Fig. 4a). Monocyte-macrophage colony formation could be detected throughout the sedimentation range of 3 to 9 mm/hr. In the presence of 10^{-8} M PGE_1, inhibition of colony formation was observed throughout the sedimentation range; however, those colony-forming cells sedimenting in the range of 4 to 6 mm/hr, and coincident with maximal colony formation, were most sensitive to inhibition. The heterogeneity of monocytoid-committed GM-CFC with respect to inhibition by PGE was most apparent following equilibrium density centrifugation through a continuous bovine serum albumin gradient (Fig. 4b). Morphologically identified macrophage colonies could be detected over a density range of 1.066 to 1.084 g/ml, with peak activity corresponding to a density of 1.079 g/ml. However, sensitivity to inhibition by 10^{-8} M PGE_1 is found only in those monocytoid clones in the

TABLE 3 Sensitivity of Various Granulocyte-macrophage Progenitor Cells to Inhibition by PGE

Source of monocyte-macrophage colony-forming cells	Molar prostaglandin E_1 concentration required for 50% inhibition of cloning
Bone marrow GM-CFC	6×10^{-9}
Peritoneal M-CFC	5×10^{-10}
Continuous marrow culture GM-CFC	5×10^{-8}
Mixed neutrophil-macrophage colonies	7×10^{-5}

density range of 1.074 to 1.084 g/ml. In addition, the differential sensitivity of a subclass of macrophage colonies cloned in the absence of red blood cell hemolysate has also been reported (33). These studies suggest that the sensitivity of monocyte-macrophage colony-forming cells to inhibition by PGE is an intrinsic property of the specific colony-forming cells.

A second level of heterogeneity is observed between monocyte-macrophage colony-forming cells grown under different conditions (Table 3). Comparison of the molar PGE concentration required for 50% inhibition of in vitro cloning indicates that monocyte-macrophage colony formation from the peritoneal M-CFC and bone marrow GM-CFC populations are most sensitive to PGE inhibition, although the M-CFC population appears more sensitive. The sensitivity of the peritoneal M-CFC population to inhibition, and their derivation from an anatomical site rich in prostaglandin-producing macrophages, may explain their extremely low incidence under resident conditions. Enrichment for M-CFC following thioglycollate injection may reflect the fact that the induced exudate macrophages are poor prostaglandin producers (34, 35).

Equivalent inhibition of macrophage colony formation from GM-CFC harvested from continuous bone marrow suspension cultures requires approximately a one log greater concentration of prostaglandin. Continuous suspension culture of murine bone marrow permits the continued maintenance of pluripotent stem cells and the differentiation of GM-CFC and mature cell forms for up to 20 weeks from a single bone marrow inoculum. The diminished responsiveness of this population of colony-forming cells may reflect prior exposure to stimulatory and inhibitory influences in the suspension culture.

Inhibition of mixed macrophage-neutrophil colony formation requires approximately three log greater concentrations of PGE. In the presence of prostaglandin, mixed colonies are predominantly neutrophil

in composition; however, some mixed colony macrophages persist even
at concentrations of PGE that totally inhibit pure macrophage colony
formation. The resistance of this macrophage population may be intrinsic or may be a consequence of intracolony microenvironmental
influences.

V. Specificity of Colony Formation to Inhibition by Prostaglandin E

In contrast to the heterogeneity of GM-CFC to inhibition, they are
relatively homogeneous with respect to prostaglandin specificity. By
far, GM-CFC proliferation is most sensitive to inhibition by prostaglandins of the E series (Table 4). In comparison, two log greater
concentrations of the A series prostaglandins are required for equivalent inhibition. However, recent mass spectral gas-liquid chromatographic studies have failed to detect circulating levels of prostaglandin
A in human plasma (36,37), suggesting that prostaglandin A is not
formed enzymatically in the body but, rather, results from the chemical dehydration of prostaglandin E. It may be, therefore, that as
prostaglandin E degrades to the more stable A series prostaglandin,
its inhibitory effect can still be exerted. Of interest is the fact that
prostaglandin D_2 is active in inhibiting monocytopoiesis, albeit to a
lesser degree than prostaglandin E. The role of this prostaglandin is
relatively unknown, since it occurs prominently only in the brain and
during cardiac anaphylaxis. Overall, the E series prostaglandins are
produced in the largest quantities within the hematopoietic system,
and their role as regulators of monocytopoiesis is supported by the
sensitivity of monocytoid-committed colony-forming cells to their
effects.

VI. The Macrophage Connection: Dualistic Regulation of Monocytopoiesis

The regulatory interactions involving diffusible stimulatory and inhibitory activities elaborated by monocytes and macrophages which
affect the proliferation of myeloid progenitor cells, namely GM-CSF
and PGE, indicate that these cells may be of central importance in the
modulation of myelopoiesis. These observations suggest a unique
ability of these cells to control the proliferation of their own progenitor
cells. However, control of monocytopoiesis by coincident production of
two opposing biological activities lacks physiological significance, unless it can be shown that mechanisms exist so that the levels of these
compounds can be modulated under both steady-state conditions and
in response to perturbation. The simultaneous production of GM-CSF

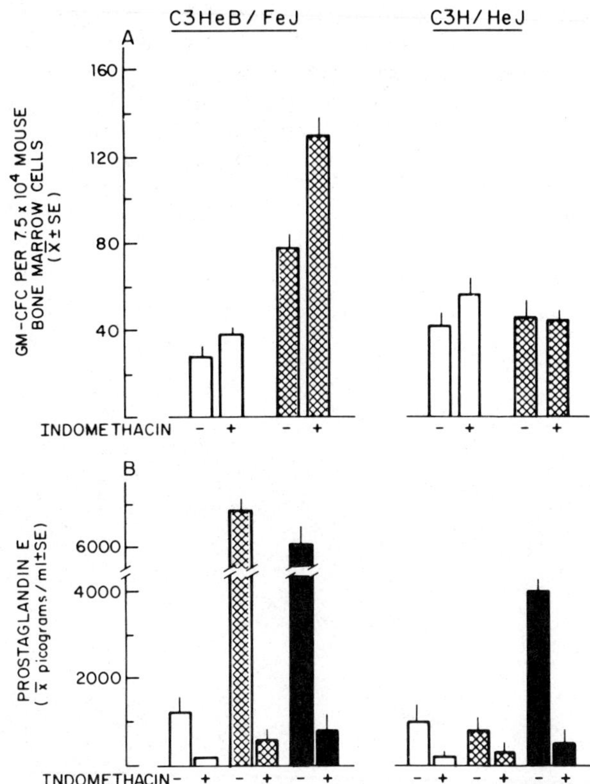

FIG. 5   Comparison of constitutive and inducible GM-CSF and prostaglandin E synthesis by peritoneal macrophages from C3Heb/FeJ and
C3H/HeJ mice. A: Adherent macrophages from 1×10^6 resident peritoneal cells from each strain of mice were incubated in the absence and
presence of 10^{-6} M indomethacin for 24 hr. Supernatant media at 10%
(v/v) were tested for constitutive GM-CSF activity (□) and after induction by 1.0 μg/ml bacterial LPS (▨). B: Prostaglandin E concentration
in 1.0 ml culture supernates as described above. Control (□), 1.0
μg/ml bacterial LPS (▨), and 1:20 dilution WEHI-3 GM-CSF (■).

and PGE by monocytoid cells does not fit this criteria unless they are
mutually interrelated.

Previous studies (Fig. 2 and Table 1) indicate that PGE is without
effect on monocyte-macrophage GM-CSF production. However, the
addition of media containing GM-CSF to cultures of mouse macrophages
results in elevated PGE levels (38). Moreover, endotoxin, which ele-
vates serum CSF levels (39) and stimulates murine macrophage (27)

TABLE 4   Effects of Various Prostaglandins on Human GM-CFC Proliferation

Prostaglandin	Molar concentration producing 50% inhibition of in vitro cloning
Prostaglandin H_2 [U-44069]	5.8×10^{-6}
Prostaglandin H_2 [U-44619]	4.8×10^{-6}
Thromboxane B_2	$> 10^{-5}$
Prostaglandin I_2 [a]	$> 10^{-5}$
6-keto-prostaglandin $F_1\alpha$	$> 10^{-5}$
Prostaglandin D_1	8.5×10^{-7}
Prostaglandin D_2	3×10^{-8}
Prostaglandin E_1	4×10^{-9}
Prostaglandin E_2	7×10^{-9}
Prostaglandin A_1	5.6×10^{-7}
Prostaglandin A_2	3.5×10^{-7}
Prostaglandin $F_1\alpha$	$> 10^{-5}$
Prostaglandin $F_2\alpha$	$> 10^{-5}$

[a]PGI_2 was stabilized in pH 9.2 tris buffer before addition to agar cultures. The buffer was without significant effect on GM-CFC proliferation.

and human monocyte (28) GM-CSF production, was found to likewise augment PGE production (30). These preliminary observations suggested a link between the production or release of GM-CSF and PGE synthesis.

A putative link between CSF and PGE production was analyzed by determining the absolute levels of GM-CSF and PGE produced by mouse peritoneal macrophages both constitutively and after induction by bacterial lipopolysaccharide (LPS). The congenic LPS responder

TABLE 5   The Effects of Lactoferrin on Mouse Macrophage GM-CSF and Prostaglandin E Production

Macrophage concentration[a]	Colony-stimulating factor[b] (mean CFU-GM per 7.5×10^{-4} mouse bone marrow cells)		Prostaglandin E (pg/ml)	
	$-LF^c$	$+LF$	$-LF$	$+LF$
5×10^4	7 ± 1	5 ± 1	252	172
1×10^5	17 ± 1	11 ± 1	306	79
2.5×10^5	23 ± 3	13 ± 2	1564	374
5×10^5	33 ± 1	17 ± 1	2154	1751
1×10^6	24 ± 2	13 ± 2	4775	3515

[a]Adherent cells derived from the number of resident peritoneal cells indicated.

[b]GM-CSF activity in 10% (v/v) supernatant.

[c]LF = 10^{-8} M 100% Fe-saturated lactoferrin.

and nonresponder mice, C3Heb/FeJ and C3H/HeJ, respectively, were used as a source of resident peritoneal macrophages. In the absence of bacterial LPS, constitutive levels of both GM-CSF and PGE could be detected in peritoneal cell culture supernates from the C3Heb/FeJ and C3H/HeJ mice (Fig. 5). In contrast, the addition of 1.0 µg/ml of bacterial LPS markedly stimulates the production/release of GM-CSF and synthesis of PGE by C3Heb/FeJ mice, but is without effect on C3H/HeJ macrophages. Thus, the LPS hyporesponsiveness of C3H/HeJ mice extends equally to macrophage production of GM-CSF and PGE. In the presence of indomethacin, the absolute detectable titer of GM-CSF in supernates from C3Heb/FeJ mice was found to be significantly greater, confirming the effects of PGE at the proliferating stem cell level (Fig. 5). Indomethacin was without effect on GM-CSF titer in bacterial LPS-stimulated C3H/HeJ macrophage culture supernates, reflecting the lack of inducible PGE synthesis in these cultures.

The addition of GM-CSF provided by conditioned media from the WEHI-3 myelomonocytic cell line stimulates PGE synthesis by macrophages from both strains of mice. The inability of bacterial LPS to induce PGE synthesis by C3H/HeJ macrophages can be bypassed by the

TABLE 6   PGE Production by Resident Murine Peritoneal
Macrophages after Stimulation by WEHI-3 Colony-Stimulating
Activities

CSF dilution	PGE[a]		
	WEHI-3CM	DEAE breakthrough (G-CSF)	DEAE elute (M-CSF)
Control	65 ± 11	65 ± 11	65 ± 11
1:2 (1.0)[b]	2030 ± 12	186 ± 112	4093 ± 711
1:4	1504 ± 180	19 ± 16	1485 ± 78
1:8	1199 ± 76	23 ± 12	1793 ± 93
1:16	1131 ± 64	24 ± 24	1445 ± 174
1:32	897 ± 13	24 ± 24	1801 ± 1

[a]Radioimmunoassay measurements of PGE in cell-free 24-hr supernates.
The results are expressed as mean concentration of PGE (picograms
per milliliter) ± SE elaborated by adherent macrophages derived from
cultures of 2.5×10^5 BDF_1 PC.

[b]Concentration of CSF which maximally stimulates CFU-GM proliferation.

Source: Ref. 12.

addition of GM-CSF. These studies indicate that macrophage synthesis
of PGE, at least with respect to stimulation by bacterial LPS, is
dependent upon a mechanism associated with GM-CSF production.
Likewise, the addition of other agents known to stimulate GM-CSF
production, concanavalin A, zymosan, and poly I-poly C, lead to PGE
synthesis by macrophages from both strains of mice (data not shown).

Any mechanism for macrophage PGE synthesis as a consequence of
GM-CSF production/release requires that the stimulatory activity, GM-
CSF, appear earlier in a temporal sequence. Kinetic analysis of GM-
CSF and PGE synthesis by mouse macrophages following bacterial LPS
induction indicate that GM-CSF levels were greatly augmented within
3 hr, reaching a plateau within 6 hr of exposure. Stimulation of GM-
CSF production is soon followed by accumulation of PGE, reaching
maximum at 24 hr (40).

A third level of evidence for a role of GM-CSF in the induction of
PGE synthesis by macrophages is provided by studies using lactoferrin, an iron-binding glycoprotein found in the secondary granules

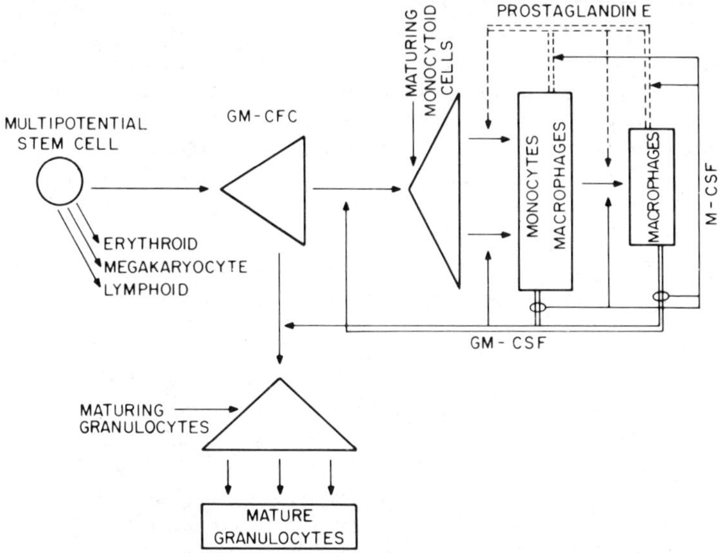

FIG. 6 Schematic representation of the control of monocytopoiesis. Solid lines indicate stimulation, dotted lines indicate inhibition. Double lines signify source of factor.

of polymorphonuclear neutrophils. In its iron-saturated form, lactoferrin inhibits monocyte-macrophage GM-CSF production (41). The inclusion of 10^{-8} M iron saturated lactoferrin in 48-hr cultures of murine macrophages effectively reduces PGE synthesis (Table 5). Likewise, GM-CSF production was simultaneously reduced. It would appear that lactoferrin-mediated reduction of PGE synthesis could result from the reduction of GM-CSF levels. The addition of bacterial LPS which overcomes the effects of lactoferrin on GM-CSF production results in elevated levels of both GM-CSF and PGE (not shown).

The evidence that different CSF preparations stimulate colony formation differing in prostaglandin specificity suggests that different CSF may have the differential capacity to stimulate macrophage prostaglandin production. To test this hypothesis, the unseparated and partially purified CSF from WEHI-3-conditioned media were tested for their ability to stimulate PGE synthesis by resident mouse peritoneal macrophages. Serum-free WEHI-3 CM was further purified by ion-exchange chromatography on DEAE Sephadex A25 to obtain two fractions, G-CSF and M-CSF, enriched in their ability to stimulate predominantly granulocytic and monocytic colony formation, respectively. Radioimmunoassay measurements on cell-free 24-hr supernates demonstrates that increasing concentrations of unseparated WEHI-3 GM-CSF

and partially purified M-CSF stimulate macrophage PGE synthesis
(Table 6). The WEHI-3 G-CSF which stimulates predominantly granulocytic colony formation does not have the capacity to stimulate macrophage PGE production. In similar experiments, mouse L cell CSF also
stimulates PGE synthesis (not shown). It therefore appears that the
preferential sensitivity of macrophage colonies to inhibition by PGE is
complemented by the selective ability of CSF preparations containing
monocytoid-specific colony-stimulating activity to stimulate PGE production. These results indicate that a specific compartmental regulatory
mechanism may exist whereby monocytes and mature tissue macrophages regulate the proliferation of their specific progenitor cells
(Fig. 6).

The in vitro regulatory influences of GM-CSF and PGE suggest
one model which may explain both steady-state control of macrophage
differentiation in vivo and the response of the host to perturbations
such as antigenic challenge, bacterial infection, or transient endo-
toxemia. The modulation of monocytopoiesis by macrophage-derived
factors applies both locally, as well as peripherally, within the marrow
microenvironment as a consequence of marrow monocytoid cells upon
GM-CFC mediated by monocyte-macrophage modulation of M-CFC. In
the equilibrium state, monocytoid differentiation is governed by the
balance between the positive stimulus provided by GM-CSF and the
negative influences of PGE produced as a consequence of macrophage
surveillance of GM-CSF levels. Antigenic stimulation or bacterial infection leads to increased myeloid progenitor cell proliferation in response to increasing GM-CSF levels. Elevated GM-CSF levels result
from direct induction of GM-CSF synthesis by macrophages, as well as
in response to lymphokine. In addition, GM-CSF synthesis/release by
activated lymphocytes has been reported and may provide for increased
numbers of macrophages required for immunological reactions.

In the presence of high GM-CSF levels, macrophage prostaglandin
E production increases, thereby limiting monocytopoiesis and slowing
the accumulation of new GM-CSF producing monocytic cells. Upon
elimination of the source of stimulation, GM-CSF and PGE levels decline. Diminution of GM-CSF production occurs primarily in response
to lactoferrin released from polymorphonuclear neutrophils as a consequence of antigenic and bacterial stimulation primarily via phagocytosis. Lactoferrin serves to reduce GM-CSF production and, coin-
cidentally, PGE synthesis, thereby facilitating a return to basal
steady-state conditions.

Acknowledgments

Supported by grants CA-28512 and CA-19052 from the National Cancer
Institute, DHEW, and the Gar Reichman Foundation.

References

1. E. R. Unanue, *Immunol. Rev. 40:*227 (1978).
2. A. S. Rosenthal, *Immunol. Rev. 40:135* (1978).
3. J. B. Hibbs, Jr., H. A. Chapman, Jr., and J. B. Weinberg, *J. Reticuloendothel. Soc. 24:549* (1978).
4. M. N. I. Walters and J. M. Papadimitriou, *CRC Crit. Rev. Toxicol. 377* (1978).
5. C. F. Nathan, H. W. Murray, and Z. A. Cohn, *N. Engl. J. Med. 303:*622 (1980).
6. D. S. Nelson, ed., *Immunobiology of the Macrophage,* Academic, New York, 1976.
7. M. A. S. Moore, and N. Williams, *J. Cell Physiol. 80:*195 (1972).
8. P. A. Chervenick and A. F. LoBuglio, *Science 178:*164 (1972).
9. D. W. Golde, T. N. Finley, and M. J. Cline, *Lancet ii:*1397 (1972).
10. L. M. Pelus and R. S. Bockman, *J. Immunol. 123:*2118 (1979).
11. J. L. Humes, R. J. Bonney, L. M. Pelus, M. E. Dahlgren, S. J. Sadowski, F. A. Kuehl, Jr., and P. Davies, *Nature (Lond.) 269:*149 (1977).
12. L. M. Pelus, H. E. Broxmeyer, J. I. Kurland, and M. A. S. Moore, *J. Exp. Med. 50:*277-292 (1979).
13. D. Metcalf, *Hematopoietic Colonies,* Springer-Verlag, Heidelberg, 1978.
14. C. C. Stewart, In *Macrophage Regulation of Immunity* (E. Unanue and A. S. Rosenthal, eds.), Academic, New York, 1980.
15. N. Jacobsen, H. E. Broxmeyer, E. Grossbard, and M. A. S. Moore, *Cell Tissue Kinet. 12:*213 (1979).
16. G. R. Johnson, C. Dresch, and D. Metcalf, *Blood 50:*823 (1977).
17. L. M. Pelus, H. E. Broxmeyer, and M. A. S. Moore, *Cell Tissue Kinet. 14:*515 (1981).
18. D. Metcalf, *Proc. Natl. Acad. Sci., U.S.A. 77:*5327 (1980).
19. S. H. Chan, D. Metcalf, and E. R. Stanely, *Br. J. Haematol. 20:*329 (1971).
20. W. Robinson, D. Metcalf, and T. R. Bradley, *J. Cell Physiol. 69:*83 (1967).
21. N. A. Nicola, A. W. Burgess, and D. Metcalf, *J. Biol. Chem. 254:*5290 (1979).
22. N. A. Nicola, D. Metcalf, G. R. Johnson, and A. W. Burgess, *Blood 54:* 614 (1979).
23. E. R. Stanely, D. M. Chen, and H. S. Lin, *Nature (Lond.) 274:*168 (1978).
24. G. R. Johnson and A. W. Burgess, *J. Cell Biol. 77:*35 (1978).

25. N. Williams, R. R. Eger, M. A. S. Moore and N. Mendelsohn, *Differentiation* *11*:59 (1978).
26. A. W. Burgess and D. Metcalf, *Blood* *56*:947 (1980).
27. A. C. Eaves and W. R. Bruce, *Cell Tissue Kinet.* *7*:19 (1970).
28. M. J. Cline, B. Rothman, and D. W. Golde, *J. Cell Physiol.* *84*:193 (1974).
29. M. A. S. Moore and J. I. Kurland, In *Progress in Differentiation Research* (N. Muller-Berat, ed.), North-Holland, Amsterdam, 1976.
30. J. I. Kurland and R. S. Bockman, *J. Exp. Med.* *147*:952 (1978).
31. L. M. Pelus and H. R. Strausser, *Life Sci.* *20*:903 (1977).
32. J. S. Goodwin and D. R. Webb, *Clin. Immunol. Immunopathol.* *15*:106 (1980).
33. N. Williams, *Blood* *53*:1089 (1979).
34. L. M. Pelus and M. A. S. Moore, in *Methods for Studying Mononuclear Phagocytes* (D. O. Adams, ed.), Academic, New York, 1981.
35. J. L. Humes, S. Burger, M. Calvage, F. A. Kuchl, Jr., P. D. Wightman, M. E. Dahlgren, P. Davies, and R. J. Bonney, *J. Immunol.* *124*:2110 (1980).
36. J. C. Frolich, B. J. Sweetman, K. Carr, J. W. Hollifield, and J. A. Oales, *Prostaglandins* *10*:185 (1975).
37. K. Green and S. Steffenrud, *Anal. Biochem.* *76*:606 (1976).
38. J. I. Kurland, H. E. Broxmeyer, L. M. Pelus, R. S. Bockman and M. A. S. Moore, *Blood* *52*:388 (1978).
39. P. J. Quesenberry, A. A. Morley, F. Stohlman, R. Richard, D. Howard, and M. Smith, *N. Engl. J. Med.* *286*:277 (1972).
40. J. I. Kurland, L. M. Pelus, P. Ralph, R. S. Bockman, and M. A. S. Moore, *Proc. Natl. Acad. Sci. U.S.A.* *76*:2326 (1979).
41. H. E. Broxmeyer, A. Smithyman, R. R. Eger, P. A. Meyers, M. DeSousa, *J. Exp. Med.* *148*:1052 (1978).

6

Interactions of Lectins and Mononuclear Phagocytes

PAUL J. EDELSON*   Harvard Medical School, Boston, Massachusetts

MARC ALFANT[†]   Harvard School of Dental Medicine, Boston, Massachusetts

I. Background

The macrophage is the central component of the mononuclear phago-
cyte system, as the current incarnation of the old reticuloendothelial system is called (1). The biology of the macrophage has recently been reviewed (23), but this section will briefly cover the
key aspects of the topic.

Macrophages are descended from bone marrow precursors.
These generate cells which, after spending a brief adolescence in
the circulation as monocytes, migrate into the tissues and serous
cavities and assume their mature identity as macrophages. Macrophages, along with the polymorphonuclear leukocyte, or neutrophil,
have been referred to by Professor Rabinovitch as "professional phagocytes" because they are extremely efficient at ingesting particulate
material. The basis for this enhanced endocytic activity is in part
due to the presence of specialized receptors on the plasma membrane
which recognize either the F_C portion of the IgG molecules or the
large fragment of the third complement component, C3b. Either of
these molecules can act as a ligand to promote the binding of
various particles to the plasma membrane, but, except in the activated macrophage, only IgG promotes ingestion—that is, only IgG is
normally opsonic.

Although these receptors may increase endocytic activity
several orders of magnitude, the basal endocytic rate of these cells,
as measured by their unstimulated rate of fluid uptake, is also much
higher than it is for other cell types. This enhanced endocytic
activity makes a qualitative difference in the physiology of macro-

---

*Present affiliation: Cornell Medical College, Ithaca, New York
†Present affiliation: University of Florida College of Dentistry, Gainesville,
Florida

phage plasma membrane which needs to be considered in understanding how lectins interact with mononuclear phagocytes.

A second characteristic of the macrophage is its well-developed
lysosomal systems which give it a substantial capacity to degrade ingested materials. For a long while this capacity was so impressive that
it was considered the sole function of these cells. Lysosomal hydro-
lases are delivered to incoming endocytic vacuoles containing ingested
material, and hydrolytic degradation takes place in these hybrid
phagolysosomal vacuoles. Undegraded material appears to persist in
the cells for the rest of their lives. Because no evidence for the exo-
cytosis of this debris was ever obtained, it was generally assumed
that the interaction of the macrophage with its environment was essentially one-way, inwards toward the cell cytoplasm.

However, over the past several years, a broad range of secretory
activities have been described for resident and activated macrophages.
These cells secrete enzymes, including lysozyme and neutral proteases,
inflammatory mediators, such as prostaglandins, SRS-A (leukotriene
C), and activated oxygen products, and components of the complement
and clotting systems. Secretion appears to be a major macrophage
function, and its regulation by materials, like lectins, which interact
with the plasma membrane, may tell us a great deal about the patho-
physiology of the inflammatory response.

The biology of the macrophage, as a *cell*, is a key perspective for
understanding the basis for its role in inflammation and immunity.
This cell biologic approach has already been extremely fruitful and
seems likely to continue to offer us a coherent framework for analyzing
macrophage physiology.

II. Early Observations: In Vivo and In Vitro

Lectins initially entered the immunology laboratory as in vitro tools
for stimulating lymphocyte responses. However, in vivo experiments
with lectins were carried out in order to assess the pathophysiologic
significance of their stimulatory effects. Some of the earliest work in
this area was carried out by Jennings and Hughes (4), who injected
phytohemagglutinin (PHA) into the mouse peritoneal cavity and examined the cellular response. They found that the macrophages recovered after 4 days of intraperitoneal injections qualitatively appeared
larger, more vacuolated, and more strongly adherent to glass surfaces
than the usual resident population. These observations are suggestive
of a population of cells which have been exposed to an inflammatory
stimulus, although the changes are neither quantitatively characterized nor sufficiently specific to establish this point. The authors
make the very intriguing observation that, unlike unstimulated cells,
the PHA-stimulated macrophages bind and ingest rabbit or human

erythrocytes in the absence of serum. Mouse erythrocytes are also bound, but are not ingested. Unfortunately it is not clear from this report whether PHA still present on the macrophage surface might be mediating these phenomena, or whether they represent a basic change in the physiology of the plasma membrane of these cells. Interestingly, concanavalin A (ConA) is also able to generate macrophages which ingest rabbit erythrocytes in serum-free medium (5). Here again, mouse or sheep cells are not ingested.

Not surprisingly, other work supports the concept that lectins can act as inflammatory stimuli. For example, Raz et al. (6) reported that ConA injected intraperitoneally provokes a macrophage exudate, with about a 10-fold increase in cell yield, and the generation of a population of cells with 2- to 4-fold elevated levels of acid phosphate and at least a 90% reduction in 5'nucleotidase activity. The latter marker appears to be particularly well correlated with the generation of an inflammatory population (2,7).

There are several mechanisms by which lectins may provoke an inflammatory response, and at present none have been either clearly implicated or entirely ruled out. They may act simply as foreign proteins, the way serum albumin does, they may directly interact with peritoneal macrophages or precursor mononuclear phagocytes, or they may stimulate macrophages indirectly as a result of their effects on peritoneal or circulating lymphocytes.

In addition to their inflammatory effects, the other interesting early observation made was that lectins may promote giant cell formation as a result of macrophage fusions. Berman and Stulberg (8) noted that cultivated human peritoneal blood monocytes will fuse in the presence of PHA or ConA, and Smith and Goldman (9) reported that both PHA and ConA can promote the fusion of human colostral macrophages but not of mouse peritoneal macrophages. In the case of ConA, the fusion effect depended on the sugar-binding specificity of the lectin, being inhibited by either α-methylmannose or α-methylglucose. The process was slow, taking 6-18 hr for multinucleated cells to appear in cultures of cells containing lectin. However, the formation of these giant cells progressed over several days until aggregates of 50 or more cells were formed. Pokeweed mitogen, in contrast, did not cause the formation of the multinucleated giant cells.

Chambers (10) has reported that hamster peritoneal macrophages are also stimulated to fuse by ConA or PHA and suggested that the mechanism for this phenomenon may be related to the cross-binding of two cells by multivalent lectin, which each cell simultaneously attempts to ingest. It is, however, quite possible that the lectin has a more generalized physiologic effect on the macrophage membrane, causing it to be fusion prone upon encountering any other biologic membrane. There is, in fact, much information on membrane effects of the lectins, which is detailed below.

III. Lectin Binding: Qualitative and Quantitative Aspects

Although the earlier work suggested that lectins can interact with
macrophages, it was a very important advance to know that lectins
can bind specifically to macrophage plasma membranes. Allen et al.
(10) reported that ConA could mediate the attachment of *Bacillus
subtilis* to the surface membranes of mouse peritoneal macrophages.
The experiments were carried out by exposing the cells first to the
lectin, and then adding the bacteria. Large numbers of organisms
attached themselves to the macrophages, indicating that the lectin
was bound to the cell surface. At about the same time, Mallucci (11),
using fluorescein-labeled lectins, also concluded that lectins can bind
to macrophage surfaces.

These qualitative results were strengthened by subsequent quantitative studies of ConA binding carried out by Lutton (12). He prepared ^{125}I-labeled ConA and examined its ability to bind to mouse
peritoneal macrophages which had been allowed to adhere to glass
cover slips. Although the binding studies were carried out at 18°C,
the temperature at which pinocytosis may still proceed (13), Lutton
appeared to have reasonable saturation kinetics for his binding assay.
In addition, either unlabeled ConA or α-methylmannose were effective
competitors of cell binding, suggesting that his assay represented a
valid measure of specific ConA binding to sugar residues on the surfaces of the macrophages. Based on the specific activity of the lectin
preparation, and the number of counts bound per cover slip, it appears that at saturation, approximately 10^7 molecules of ConA were
bound per cell. Stimulating the cells to spread with trypsin or dithio-
threitol did not affect the amount of lectin bound, but after extensive
ingestion of polyvinyltoluene or titanium dioxide particles, the cell's
binding capacity was reduced about 25-35%. Recovery of this loss of
binding took about 8 hr in medium supplemented with serum or beef
heart infusion but did not occur when cells were maintained in unsup-
plemented medium for up to 24 hr. Cyclohexamide could also block recovery. In a subsequent paper, Lutton (14) briefly reported that
peritoneal cells obtained after endotoxin stimulation appear to bind
about the same amount of lectin as do unstimulated macrophages. However, endotoxin-stimulated populations appear to be quite heterogeneous in several respects (15), and it is therefore possible that a population of cells with very different binding characteristics might have
been overlooked in this assay.

There is some interesting information that the distribution of
ConA binding sites in the macrophage-like cell line J774.1, and in
CHO cells, may be cell-cycle associated (16), but there are no quantitative data on possible changes in the numbers of binding sites as a
function of cell cycling.

IV. Cell Biology of Lectin-Macrophage Interactions

Loor and Roelants (17) conducted a survey of the fate of various
ligands allowed to interact with the macrophage plasma membrane. In
that study they noted that fluorescein or rhodamine conjugates of
ConA, pokeweed mitogen, or phytohemagglutinin will bind to mouse
peritoneal macrophages in culture. They also observed a redistribution and accumulation of fluorescent material under conditions where
endocytosis was allowed to proceed, which they described as capping
followed by endocytic internalization of the ligand. Lutton (12), too,
had previously noted that fluoresceinated ConA would apparently bind
to mouse peritoneal macrophages, and Mallucci (11) and Allen et al.
(18) had reported similar observations. However, in general these
studies did not look at the effects which lectin binding had on the
cell, and most especially on the fate of the plasma membrane to which
it bound.

We (19,20) therefore looked at these two questions in some detail. Our initial observation was that, when macrophages are exposed
to ConA at concentrations of 5-50 μg/ml for 30 min at 37°C, they develop large numbers of phase-lucent cytoplasmic vacuoles. By electron
microscopy it was clear the vacuoles were bounded by membrane, and
that they contained various marker molecules which had been included
in the extracellular incubation medium, including horseradish peroxidase, colloidal gold, and thorotrast. In addition, the membrane itself
carried the plasma membrane ATPase, conclusively demonstrating that
these vacuoles were pinosomes derived by endocytosis from the plasma
membrane. We also showed that these pinosomes were derived precisely from those areas of membrane to which ConA bound and that the
lectin could be identified by electron microscopy as being in continuous
association with the inner leaflet of the vesicle membrane.

Next, we measured the pinocytic rate of mouse peritoneal macrophages exposed to ConA, using the quantitative uptake of horseradish
peroxidase (21) as well as the uptake of ^{125}I-labeled bovine serum
albumin. Macrophages exposed to ConA pinocytose at a rate of 92.2
nl/hr per 10^6 cells, compared with a control rate of 27.3 nl/hr, an increase of about 3.4 times. This increase was completely prevented
when α-methylmannose (50 mM) was included in the incubation medium.
This pinocytotic stimulation depended upon the continuous presence
of ConA in the medium and stopped promptly when the cells were
rinsed and placed in a lectin-free environment.

The second issue examined was the fate of these vacuoles once
they formed. Cells exposed for 60 min to ConA, to permit vacuole formation, and then placed in a lectin-free medium continued to show many
vacuoles for up to 48 hr of incubation. Since most pinosomes fuse with
lysosomes within minutes of their formation (13), this behavior suggested to us that these vesicles might be failing to fuse with lysosomes

and might persist as primary endocytic vesicles. This is in fact so.
Neither primary lysosomes, as assessed by staining for acid phos-
phatase, or secondary lysosomes containing such preloaded markers
as horseradish peroxidase, colloidal gold, or thorotrast, fuse with
ConA-stimulated vesicles. In addition, we documented this fusion
failure biochemically by showing a prolonged survival of horseradish
peroxidase or ^{125}I-labeled albumin which had been engulfed in these
pinosomes. The continuing association of the lectin with the inner
face of the vacuole membrane was essential for the inhibition of fusion.
When the lectin was competitively displaced by allowing mannose to in-
fuse into the cells, fusion was allowed to proceed normally.

Goldman (22) also noted the development of cytoplasmic vesicles
in ConA-treated macrophages and their persistence for up to 48 hr in
culture. She also identified these vesicles as pinosomes because their
formation was inhibited by azide or low temperature. However, she
has claimed that there is no inhibition of pinolysosome formation and
that these vesicles fuse normally with lysosomes (23).

Several other lectins may also promote vesicle formation (Edelson,
unpublished observations, Goldman et al., Ref. 24), but not all
lectins are equally effective. Phytohemagglutinin and waxbean lectin
are quite active, but soybean agglutinin and peanut and lotus lectins
appear to be inactive. Such differences may not have any deep significance and may only reflect the relative availability of various types
of sugar residues on the mouse cell surface.

The mechanisms of these two effects, stimulation of pinocytosis
and inhibition of lysosomal fusion, are still unknown. In fact, it might
even seem a paradox that an agent may promote fusion processes at
the plasma membrane, in order for pinosomes to form, and then inhibit fusions in the cytoplasm between these vesicles and lysosomal
granules. The paradox though may be more apparent than real, since
the fusions involve opposite faces of the plasma membrane and may
proceed by quite different mechanisms. Even if they involve very
similar, or identical, molecular processes, it is quite possible that a
key molecular species has been so completely tied-up in the first fusion process that it is unavailable to participate in a second event.

In fact, it appears that the ability to cross-link membrane components may be essential for the ConA effect. Petty (25) has reported that ConA labeled for electron microscopy with cationized
ferritin collects in microclusters on the surface of guinea pig macrophages before it is pinocytosed. These aggregates do not seem to
represent preexisting clusters of ConA binding sites, since ConA was
distributed more uniformly on cells which had been pretreated briefly
with 1% glutaraldehyde to inhibit redistributions in the plane of the
membrane. Surface aggregates were not seen when succinylated ConA
was used, but reappeared when cells coated with succinyl ConA were
then exposed to an anti-ConA antiserum. We have recently observed

that, unlike ConA, succinyl ConA does not enhance endocytic activity
(26). Petty and Ware (27) have also noted a change in surface charge
of cells to which ConA is bound. This change, too, is not seen with
succinyl ConA. It is possible that charged species to which ConA
binds are important in controlling membrane fusion at either the plasma membrane or lysosomal level (7).

V. Biochemical Effects of Lectins

ConA can stimulate the production of activated oxygen species,
superoxide anion, hydroxyl radical, and peroxide by a variety of
phagocytic cells. Rossi and his colleagues (28) drew attention to its
ability to do this in the peritoneal and alveolar macrophages of both
the guinea pig and the rabbit. They have argued that this effect is
due to the activation of an NADPH-dependent oxidase associated with
an increase in the V_{max} of the enzyme.

Because ConA bound to large sepharose beads is also effective in
stimulating this system, these workers have argued that the phenomenon is related strictly to the interaction of the lectin with the cell
surface (29). Cuatrecasas has pointed out, though, that material
bound to sepharose by cyanogen bromide may slowly dissociate into
the fluid phase, and that these small amounts of soluble material may
actually be responsible in some cases for the effects attributed to
bound agents. Soluble ConA is a potent endocytic stimulator (7), and
it is possible that the endocytic activity triggered by the lectin leads
indirectly to the stimulation of oxygen metabolism.

The phenomenon of metabolic stimulation by ConA is, however, a
complex one, and the precise biochemical pathway responsible for it
is still unknown. It seems that the sugar-binding site on the ConA
molecule is essential to the process, since α-methylmannose, α-methylglucose, or mannan will each inhibit the effect. The stimulation probably depends upon repeated triggering at the cell surface, since
even after the burst has been promoted, the addition of competitive
sugars can reverse some of the stimulation. Interestingly, the activation of macrophages seems to depress their responsiveness to ConA.
BCG-stimulated rabbit alveolar macrophages show less of a respiratory
response to ConA than do unstimulated alveolar cells (29). Since it is
clear now that activated cells are fully capable of producing hydrogen
peroxide (see, for example, Ref. 30), this may be related either to
the number of ConA binding sites which these cells bear, or to a difference in physiology of their plasma membranes. One complicating
factor in analyzing these experiments is that many of these observations were made on cell suspensions where, upon addition of the lectin, the cells agglutinated. Although qualitatively this did not appear
to be substantially different from the behavior of resident cells, it

might be interesting to know whether the apparent hyporesponsiveness
of the activated cells to ConA persists when the cells are allowed to
attach to a surface before exposure to the lectin.

Yasaka and Kambara (31) report similar conclusions in experiments with guinea pig peritoneal cells elicited with either paraffin oil
or glycogen. They note, in addition, that succinyl ConA was as effective as ConA in promoting the consumption of oxygen, although both
were much more effective in neutrophils than in macrophages. Since
succinyl ConA is not an endocytic stimulus (26), this work suggests
that the binding or rearrangement of various membrane components
may be sufficient to explain the metabolic effect of the lectins, although one might want additional information characterizing the
succinyl ConA preparation used in these studies before accepting
these conclusions firmly.

Lectins, particularly ConA, have also been reported to have an
effect on cellular cyclic AMP metabolism. It seems that, although exposure to ConA will not directly affect intracellular cAMP levels, it
will sensitize the cells to give an enhanced response to cAMP stimula-
tors. Gemsa et al. (32) observed that ConA will sensitize casein-
stimulated rat peritoneal cells to the effects of prostaglandins (E_1,
E_2, A_1, and A_2) as well as to isoproterenol and cholera toxin. The
effect appeared to depend upon a ConA-sugar interaction, since α-
methylmannose inhibited the ConA sensitization and lentil lectin, a
protein with the same sugar specificity as ConA, was also effective.
The mechanism involved was not established, although it did not appear that either a lectin-induced reduction of cAMP excretion or an
inhibition of the cAMP phosphodiesterase was involved.

Grunspan-Swirsky and Pick (33) reached similar conclusions
using guinea pig macrophages which had been elicited with light
paraffin oil. These workers also examined responses to prostaglandin
E (PGE), as well as to isoproterenol, and reported that ConA appears
to sensitize the cells to these agents without having any effect on
basal cAMP levels. However, in contrast to Gemsa's work, these
authors reported only a very modest effect on the sensitivity of cells
to cholera toxin. In addition, they found that neither succinyl ConA
nor ConA bound to sepharose beads was effective, paralleling previous
results with lymphocyte cAMP, as the authors point out. Like the previous workers, these authors also suggested that the lectin effect was
on cAMP synthesis, although direct measurements of synthetic rates
needed to be made.

It is interesting that Gemsa and his colleagues (34) have found
that a similar sensitization to the effects of PGE occurs with phagocytosis. ConA is of course a potent endocytic stimulus, whereas
succinyl ConA is not. It is, therefore, possible that all the sensitizing
agents work through a common mechanism associated with their promotion of endocytic activity. One candidate mechanism might be the

generation of prostaglandins, but this seems unlikely, since latex, which does not promote prostaglandin production, is also effective in sensitizing cells to PGE-induced elevations in cAMP cells. In addition, zymosan appears able to sensitize cells even in the presence of indomethacin, which inhibits prostaglandin synthesis.

The effects of ConA on the secretion of the neutral protease plasminogen activator have been reported by Vassalli and his colleagues (35). Plasminogen activator is secreted by activated, or thioglycollate-stimulated, macrophages, but not by either resident or endotoxin-induced cells. The regulation of synthesis and secretion, however, is complex, since a phagocytic stimulus will promote the secretion of the enzyme by endotoxin-induced cells but not by resident cells (for a review, see Ref. 36).

Vassalli and his coworkers report that ConA can stimulate the secretion of plasminogen activator from either endotoxin-induced or resident cells, although the lag time for secretion is somewhat longer for resident cells. The ConA effect is inhibited by steroids, prostaglandins, colchicine, imblastine, or choleratoxin. Waxbean agglutinin is also an effective stimulator of the enzyme, but wheat germ agglutinin is not. Actinomycin D (3 µg/ml) can inhibit the induction in resident cells, suggesting that the effect depends upon new RNA synthesis. This is supported by the result that tritiated uridine incorporation is also enhanced by the lectin, although changes in transport rates or uridine pool size were not ruled out in this work. The material secreted appears identical to that secreted by thioglycollate-stimulated cells. It appears as at least two species, one of 28 kilodaltons and another producing a doublet band at 48 kilodaltons on SDS polyacrylamide gels. In these studies ConA appeared to have little effect on lysosomal enzymes, and what effect occurred was not consistent when resident cells were compared with thioglycollate-stimulated cells. There was also only a very modest effect on lysozyme secretion. This work suggests that either interactions at the plasma membrane or endocytic activity, particularly with an inhibition of lysosomal fusion, may regulate the transcription of the macrophage genome, a very intriguing idea and one very much deserving of further work.

VI. Effects of Lectins on Phagocytosis

Although, as discussed above, some lectins are able to strikingly enhance pinocytosis, their effects on phagocytosis are far less straightforward. Two sorts of experiments have been carried out to examine this question. In one type, macrophages which have been treated with ConA are then challenged with red blood cells, latex spheres, or other particles, and their phagocytic capacity is measured. In the

second type, particles are coated with a lectin and their ingestibility
is examined in what is a test of the lectin's opsonic activity.

We (19) found that mouse macrophages which had been exposed to
50 µg/ml Con A for 1 hr showed no change in the average number of
IgG-coated sheep red blood cells which they would subsequently ingest, nor was there any qualitative change in their ingestion of latex
or zymosan particles. Cam (37) obtained the same results using a
quantitative assay of latex uptake. Friend and her colleagues (38)
reported the opposite results, using an apparently identical system.
They reported that ConA in concentrations as low as 10 ng/ml markedly inhibited both the adherence and uptake of polystyrene particles
by cultures of mouse peritoneal macrophages. We have found that when
cells are exposed to very substantial concentrations of ConA they may
round up and reduce their phagocytic activity, at least temporarily.
We suspect that this is due to the reduced surface area which these
rounded cells seem to display, and perhaps also to a reduction in
endocytic activity when a large fraction of plasma membrane in inter-
nally sequestered in large ConA pinosomes. However, even under
these fairly extreme conditions we have never seen a decrease in the
amount of latex adherent to the cells. Friend et al. suggested that
the diminished uptake which they reported is due to a postulated increase in the rigidity of the membrane caused by extensive cross-
linking of membrane components by ConA. One might expect that a
decrease in membrane deformation would not be compatible with the
rise in pinocytic activity which ConA promotes.

ConA is able to act as an opsonin for such otherwise unphago-
cytosed particles as sheep erythrocytes. Goldman and Cooper (39) reported that ConA can promote both the attachment and ingestion of
mouse red blood cells to mouse macrophages. They found that simply
coating the red cells with lectin was enough to cause them to bind to
the macrophages; however, it was necessary to add ConA to the medium as well for the cells to be ingested. We (Edelson, unpublished
observations) have made similar observations with sheep erythrocytes.
In our case we found that the cells would be ingested if both the red
cells and the macrophages were exposed to ConA before mixing the two
cell types.

It was never clear to us whether the failure of ConA-coated particles to be routinely ingested was simply due to a limited number of
ConA binding sites on the phagocytic cells, or whether there was
some necessary spatial arrangement or rearrangement which ConA,
once it was bound to a red cell surface, was less able to promote. It
would be interesting to examine the fate of ConA-coated particles on
which the ConA could not aggregate—zymosan or glutaraldehyde-
treated erythrocytes are examples—to see whether under these conditions ConA might not be a more efficient opsonin.

Goldman and Cooper (40), in a more extensive paper, reported on the details of the red blood cell system. In this paper they argued that the density of ConA molecules on the red cell surface is the key determinant of uptake, but they did not try to directly assess this proposal experimentally. Goldman and Bursuker (41), in a follow-up paper, do, however, provide some additional information which would support this idea. In this paper they compare the effects of wheat germ agglutinin (WGA), a more efficient red cell opsonin than is ConA. These workers argue that this is because WGA sites are more abundant and more widely distributed on macrophage membranes than are ConA sites. Again, this seems a plausible suggestion, but one not yet firmly established by experimental studies.

Perhaps one of the most important conclusions to be drawn from this work concerns the nature of immune opsonization. By showing that such nonspecific molecules as ConA or WGA are effective opsonins, these experiments teach that we do not need to invoke any more elaborate mechanisms to understand IgG-mediated ingestion than simply the ability of the molecule to bind simultaneously the particle and mobile binding sites on the cell membrane. Membrane flexibility and the physicochemical determinants of membrane fusion will apparently do the rest.

VII. Effects on the Physiology of Macrophage Defenses

The effects of lectins on lymphocyte-mediated cytotoxicity has been widely studied, but far less has been reported on their effects on macrophage antitumor activity. Inoue et al. (42) noted that ConA could promote the attachment of Ehrlich ascites tumor cells to mouse peritoneal macrophages, and that this interaction could be blocked by the appropriate sugars. However, these workers did not report any further details about the effects of such binding on the survival of the tumor cells or their ultimate fate.

Toh and his colleagues (43) looked particularly at the cytotoxicity of rat peritoneal macrophages for a methylcholanthrene-induced sarcoma (KMT-114) when these cells were exposed to ConA. They found that ConA appeared to enhance the antitumor activity of peritoneal macrophages. However, the assessment was made by measuring the ability of the tumor cells to incorporate tritiated thymidine, which may not distinguish cytostatic from genuinely cytotoxic activities. The authors do, though, include phase contrast photographs of their cultures which suggest that there is a loss of tumor cells when they are exposed to macrophages.

ConA may also affect the interaction of macrophages with viruses. For some time now, Bang and his colleagues have studied a very interesting infection caused by the mouse hepatitis virus (MHV).

Resistance to this agent may be genetically conferred, and this characteristic of a given strain is reproduced in explanted macrophages of that strain. In this system, Weiser and Bang (44) reported that ConA-elicited peritoneal macrophages from genetically susceptible mouse strains are resistant to MHV, and that the administration of ConA to susceptible mice reduces their mortality after infection with MHV.

The mechanisms by which ConA may accomplish this protection are not clear. When ConA is injected into the peritoneal cavity along with the mouse hepatitis virus, there is no protective effect, but when the virus is injected 3 days after the lectin, there is about a 60% survival rather than a 100% mortality.

When ConA-elicited cells are removed from the peritoneal cavity and examined in culture, it appeared that, unlike the thioglycollate-induced cells which were uniformly susceptible to virus, the ConA-stimulated cells are heterogeneous. Obviously, the basis for the restriction or permissiveness of viral infection in the two ConA subpopulations is a key question. One might imagine that this heterogeneity reflects the heterogeneous histories of the inflammatory cells: some representing newly emigrated monocytes which perhaps develop into activated macrophages as a result of the inflammatory stimulus, whereas others were resident cells present in the peritoneal cavity before the lectin was injected. These two populations are physiologically quite different (for a recent review, see Ref. 3). Their interactions with viruses may be different at many levels of cell organization, from the plasma membrane binding sites to the presence or absence of a required thymidine kinase.

Perhaps one of the most intriguing observations in this paper is that the supernate of a ConA-stimulated spleen cell suspension will also confer resistance on susceptible macrophages. However, the supernate of a mixed lymphocyte reaction involving allogeneic cells has exactly the opposite effect—it will make resistant cells susceptible to virus. As the authors very appropriately point out, we should not assume that in this case the effects of the lectin on resistance are related to a direct action on the macrophages. An indirect effect via lymphocytes, or perhaps even other cell types, is also a real possibility.

References

1. R. van Furth, *Mononuclear Phagocytes*, F. A. Davis, Philadelphia, 1970.
2. P. J. Edelson, Monocytes and macrophages: Aspects of their cell biology. in *The Cell Biology of Inflammation* (G. Weissmann, ed.), Elsevier North-Holland, Amsterdam, 1980, pp. 469-495.

3. P. J. Edelson, Macrophage plasma membrane enzymes as differentiation markers of macrophage activation. *Lymph. Rep.* (in press).

4. J. F. Jennings and L. A. Hughes, The effect of phytohemagglutinin on phagocytosis in the mouse peritoneal cavity. *J. Reticuloendothel. Soc.* 7:617-626 (1970).

5. C. W. Smith and A. S. Goldman, Effects of concanavalin A and pokeweed mitogen in vivo on mouse peritoneal macrophages. *Exp. Cell Res.* 73:394-398 (1972).

6. A. Raz, A. Sharon, and R. Goldman, Characterization of an in vivo induced peritoneal macrophage population following intraperitoneal injection of concanavalin A. *J. Reticuloendothel. Soc.* 22:445-460 (1977).

7. P. J. Edelson and Z. A. Cohn, Endocytosis: Regulation of membrane interactions. *Cell Surf. Revs.* 5:387-405 (1978).

8. L. Berman and C. S. Stulberg, Primary cultures of macrophages from normal human peripheral blood. *Lab. Invest.* 11:1322-1331 (1962).

9. C. W. Smith and A. S. Goldman, Macrophages from human colostrum. Multinucleated giant cell formation by phytohemmagglutinin and concanavalin A. *Exp. Cell Res.* 66:317-320.

10. T. J. Chambers, Fusion of hamster macrophages produced by lectins. *J. Pathol.* 123:53-61 (1977).

11. L. Mallucci, Binding of concanavalin A to normal and transformed cells as detected by immunofluorescence. *Nature (New Biol.)* 233:241-242 (1971).

12. J. D. Lutton, The effect of phagocytosis and spreading on macrophage surface receptors for concanavalin A. *J. Cell Biol.* 56:611-617 (1973).

13. R. M. Steinman, S. E. Brodie, and Z. A. Cohn, Membrane flow during pinocytosis. A stereologic analysis. *J. Cell Biol.* 68:665-687 (1976).

14. J. D. Lutton, The binding of ^{125}I-concanavalin A to normal and endotoxin stimulated peritoneal macrophages. *Experientia 31*: 370-371 (1975).

15. C. Bianco and P. J. Edelson, Characteristics of the activated macrophage, in *Immune Effector Mechanisms in Disease* (M. E. Weksler, ed.), Grune and Stratton, New York, 1978, pp. 1-8.

16. R. D. Berlin, J. M. Oliver, and R. J. Walter, Surface functions during mitosis. I. Phagocytosis, pinocytosis and mobility of surface-bound ConA. *Cell 15*:327-341 (1978).

17. F. Loor and G. E. Roelants, The dynamic state of the macrophage plasma membrane. Attachment and fate of immunoglobulin, antigen and lectins. *Eur. J. Immunol.* 4:649-660 (1974).

18. J. M. Allen, G. M. W. Cook, and A. R. Poole, Action of concanavalin A on the attachment stage of phagocytosis by macrophages, *Exp. Cell Res.* 68:466-471 (1971).

19. P. J. Edelson and Z. A. Cohn, Effects of concanavalin A on mouse peritoneal macrophages. I. Enhancement of endocytosis and inhibition of phago-lysosome formation. *J. Exp. Med. 140:* 1364-1386 (1974).

20. P. J. Edelson and Z. A. Cohn, Effects of concanavalin A on mouse peritoneal macrophages. II. Metabolism of endocytized protein and reversibility of the effects by mannose. *J. Exp. Med. 140:* 1387-1403 (1974).

21. R. M. Steinman and Z. A. Cohn, The interaction of soluble horseradish peroxidase with mouse peritoneal macrophages in vitro. *J. Cell Biol. 55:* 186-204 (1972).

22. R. Goldman, Induction of vacuolation in the mouse peritoneal macrophage by concanavalin A. *FEBS Letters 46:* 203-208 (1974).

23. R. Goldman and A. Raz, Concanavalin A and the in vitro induction in macrophages of vacuolation and lysosomal enzyme synthesis. *Exp. Cell. Res. 96:* 393-405 (1975).

24. R. Goldman, N. Sharon and R. Lotan, A differential response elicited in macrophages on interaction with lectins. *Exp. Cell. Res. 99:* 408-422 (1976).

25. H. R. Petty, Response of the resident macrophage to concanavalin A. Alterations of surface morphology and anionic site distribution. *Exp. Cell Res. 128:* 439-454 (1980).

26. M. Alfant, P. J. Edelson, and J. Aronson, Mechanism of concanavalin A stimulation of pinocytosis in mouse macrophages, International Association for Dental Research, Annual Meeting, Chicago, Illinois, abstract, 1981.

27. H. R. Petty and B. R. Ware, Macrophage response to concanavalin A: Effect of surface crosslinking on the electrophoretic mobility distribution. *Proc. Natl. Acad. Sci. U.S.A. 76:* 2278-2282 (1979).

28. F. Rossi, G. Zabucchi, and D. Romeo, Metabolism of phagocytosing mononuclear phagocytes. in *Mononuclear Phagocytes in Immunity, Infection and Pathology* (R. van Furth, ed.), Blackwell, Oxford, 1975, pp. 441-460.

29. D. Romeo, M. Jug, G. Zabucchi, and F. Rossi, Perturbation of leukocyte metabolism by nonphagocytosable concanavalin A coupled beads. *FEBS Letters 42:* 90-93 (1974).

30. C. F. Nathan, The release of hydrogen peroxide from mononuclear phagocytes and its role in extracellular cytosis. in *Mononuclear Phagocytes: Functional Aspects* (R. van Furth, ed.), Martinus Nijhoff, The Hague, 1980, pp. 1165-1182.

31. T. Yasaka and T. Kambara, Effects of concanavalin A and its succinylated derivative on the oxidative metabolism of guinea pig peritoneal macrophages. *Biochim. Biophys. Acta. 508:* 306-312 (1978).

32. D. Gemsa, L. Steggeman, G. Till, and K. Resch, Enhancement of the PGE, response of macrophages by concanavalin A and colchicine. *J. Immunol. 119*:524–529 (1977).

33. A. Grunspan-Swirsky and E. Pick, Facilitation of adenylate cyclase stimulation in macrophages by lectins. *Cell. Immunol. 45*: 415–427 (1979).

34. D. Gemsa, M. Seitz, W. Kramer, G. Tiu, and K. Resch, The effects of phagocytosis, dextran sulfate, and cell damage on PGE, sensitivity and PGE, production of macrophages. *J. Immunol. 120*:1187–1194 (1978).

35. J. D. Vassalli, J. Hamilton and E. Reich, Macrophage plasminogen activator: Induction by concanavalin A and phorbal myristate acetate. *Cell 11*:695–705.

36. S. Gordon, The secretion of lysozyme and a plasminogen activator by mononuclear phagocytes, in *Mononuclear Phagocytes in Immunity, Infection and Pathology*, (R. van Furth, ed.), Blackwell, Oxford, 1975, pp. 463–473.

37. V. Cam, Quantitative studies of phagocytosis by mouse peritoneal macrophages: Energy requirements and additional characteristics, Ph.D. thesis, New York University, 1977.

38. K. Friend, R. D. Ekstedt, and J. L. Duncan, Effect of concanavalin A on phagocytosis by mouse peritoneal macrophages. *J. Reticuloendothel. Soc. 17*:10–19 (1975).

39. R. Goldman and R. A. Cooper, Concanavalin A mediated attachment and ingestion of red blood cells by macrophages, *Isr. J. Med. Sci. 11*:1183–1184, abstract (1975).

40. R. Goldman and R. A. Cooper, Concanavalin A mediated attachment and ingestion of red blood cells by macrophages. *Exp. Cell Res. 95*:223–231 (1975).

41. R. Goldman and I. Bursuker, Differential effects of lectins mediating erythrocyte attachment and ingestion by macrophages. *Exp. Cell Res. 103*:279–294 (1976).

42. M. Inoue, M. Mori, K. Utsumi and S. Seno, Role of concanavalin A in tumor cell agglutination and adhesion to macrophages. *GANN 63*:795–799 (1972).

43. K. Toh, N. Sato and K. Kikuchi, Effect of concanavalin A on the cytotoxicity of rat peritoneal macrophages. *J. Reticuloendothel. Soc. 25*:17–28 (1979).

44. W. Y. Weiser and F. B. Bang, Blocking of in vitro and in vivo susceptibility to mouse hepatitis virus. *J. Exp. Med. 146*:1467–1472 (1977).

45. P. J. Edelson and Z. A. Cohn, 5'nucleotidase activity of mouse peritoneal macrophages. I. Synthesis and degradation in resident and inflammatory populations. *J. Exp. Med. 144*:1581–1595 (1976).

46. Literature review completed December, 1981.

7

Studies on the Nonspecific Regulation of Immunocompetent Cell Function by Prostaglandins

DAVID R. WEBB, KENNETH J. WIEDER,* and IRENE NOWOWIEJSKI
Roche Institute of Molecular Biology, Nutley, New Jersey

I. Introduction

As can be ascertained from a glance at current literature, the role
that prostaglandins (PG) play in regulating the immune response is
receiving increasing attention (1). The purpose of this chapter will
be to review the evidence gathered in this laboratory and by others
concerning the involvement of products of the PG pathway in normal
immune responses involving both humoral and cell-mediated immunity.
We will not discuss the possible role of PG in tumor immunity or
other disease states which has recently been reviewed elsewhere.
Finally, we will present a summary model whose purpose will be to
provide an idea of how PG-mediated control may relate to other
control mechanisms which regulate immunocompetent cell function.

The central dogma of cellular immunology—that the immune
response is the result of positive and negative cell interactions—is
well established. What has proved to be more difficult is the sorting
out of the various subpopulations of cells and the kinds of signals
these cells give and receive. Among the T lymphocyte population,
various cell functions, e.g., helper, suppressor, and cytotoxic
killer cell, have been associated with certain antigens expressed on
the cell surface. One of the most useful family of cellular antigens
has been the Lyt antigens in which $Ly\text{-}1^+2^-,3^-$, $Ly\text{-}1^-2^+,3^+$, or
$Ly\text{-}1^+2^+,3^+$ cells can be roughly associated with helper, suppressor
or killer, and regulatory cell function, respectively (2). Additional
Lyt phenotypes, as well as other surface markers (Qa, for example),
have allowed for further divisions. In addition to these classifica-

---

Present affiliation: Du Pont-Ne Mours, Glenolden, Pennsylvania

tions, it is also possible to separate T cell populations on the basis
of physical characteristics, e.g., adherence to various substrates
(3-5) and buoyant density (6), or by use of the fluorescence-
activated cell sorter (7).

In our laboratory we have found the property of adherence to
glass wool useful in the isolation of splenic lymphocyte subpopulations
with discrete functions (8,9). For example, almost all T helper cells
are nonglass adherent and pass through glass fiber filter columns
(although this population contains both $Ly-1^+2^-,3^-$ and $Ly-1^-2^+,3^+$
cells, the function of these $Ly-1^-2^+,3^+$ cells is unknown). The glass-
adherent T cells seem to be exclusively involved in suppressor cell
activity, although it is not clear whether some cells are suppressor inducers or actually functional suppressor cells. At the time these investigations were being initiated, it was not known whether lymphocytes had the capacity to make prostaglandins. Indirect evidence using
highly purified lymphocyte populations and inhibitors of prostaglandin
synthesis suggested that they could do so, and therefore experiments
were carried out by us to study this issue (9). As may be seen by the
data in Table 1, both adherent and nonadherent lymphocytes make PG
in response to a mitogenic stimulus. On the other hand, purified
macrophages in this strain of mice (C57B1/6) showed no increased PG
production following exposure to phytohemagglutinin (PHA). Recently,
Bauminger (10) has looked at the capacity of thymic lymphocytes to
generate PG and has provided evidence that these cells as well make
PG. Further investigations using mitogen-stimulated or control splenic
lymphocytes (D. R. Webb and M. Bailey, unpublished observations)
exposed to radiolabeled arachidonic acid have shown that the major
products of arachidonic acid metabolism are metabolites of the lipoxygenase pathway, e.g., the hydroxy fatty acids.

In a series of papers from Parker's laboratory, it has become
clear that lymphocytes may also generate thromboxanes (11,12). The
presence of these compounds implies an active cyclooxygenase which
is required to provide the endoperoxide intermediate necessary for
either prostaglandin or thromboxane synthesis (see Fig. 1). Thus it
would appear undeniable that lymphocytes possess the metabolic machinery necessary to generate the products of the prostaglandin and
hydroxy fatty acid pathways.

It has been known for some time that macrophages make and release PG in response to a variety of stimuli (13,14). It has recently
been reported that they also make leukotriene C, which has been
identified as being SRS-A in mast cells activated by IgE-antigen complexes (15,16). Thus it is clear that the major classes of immunocompetent cells, lymphocytes and macrophages, may make and release products of the PG pathway. In the remaining sections we shall consider
the role of these products in regulating cell function.

TABLE 1 Stimulation of Prostaglandin Levels by PHA in Spleen Cell Subpopulations

Cell Population	Culture Time		Average net iPG (ng/culture)[a]		
NAL	24		2.74 ± 0.9	P	0.005
	48	(5)	6.82 ± 2.0	P	0.005
	72		5.0 ± 3.1	P	0.005
GAT	24		1.27 ± 0.1	P	0.05
	48	(3)	1.27 ± 2.1	P	0.005
	72		5.4 ± 2.1	P	0.005
NAL/GAT (1:1)	24		1.4 ± 0.01	P	0.05
	48	(2)	10.0 ± 4.2	P	0.005
	72		11.1 ± 0.1	P	0.005

Cell Population	Culture Time		Average net $PGF_{2\alpha}$ (ng/culture)[a]		
NAL	24		0.45 ± 0.1	NS	
	48	(4)	0.55 ± 0.1	NS	
	72		0.15 ± .01	NS	
GAT	24		No net change		
	48	(2)	No net change		
	72		No net change		
NAL/GAT (1:1)	24		3.9 ± 0.2	P	0.05
	48	(2)	2.6 ± 0.1	P	0.05
	72		4.9 ± 0.5	P	0.05

[a]These values represent the mean PG levels from several experiments. In each experiment, cultures were prepared in duplicate or triplicate and were incubated with or without mitogen for varying times. At the end of the incubation period, the cultures were assayed for PG as described previously. The net PG value was obtained by subtracting the mean PG level in control (non-mitogen-treated) cultures from the mean PG level in mitogen-treated cultures for each individual experiment. The PG levels depicted here represent the average net PG levels of the several experiments ± standard error. The numbers in parentheses indicates the number of separate experiments performed from which the average values were obtained. The average basal levels of iPG in NAL (24-72 hr) was 0.62 ± 0.18 ng; GAT basal levels were 5.56 ± 1.07 ngs; and NAL/GAT basal level averaged at 4.23 ± 1.61 ng; basal level of N/GAT: PG was 1.06 ± 0.07 ng/culture. Calculation of levels of significance was performed using analysis of variance (ANOVA). NS = not significant.

Source: Ref. 9.

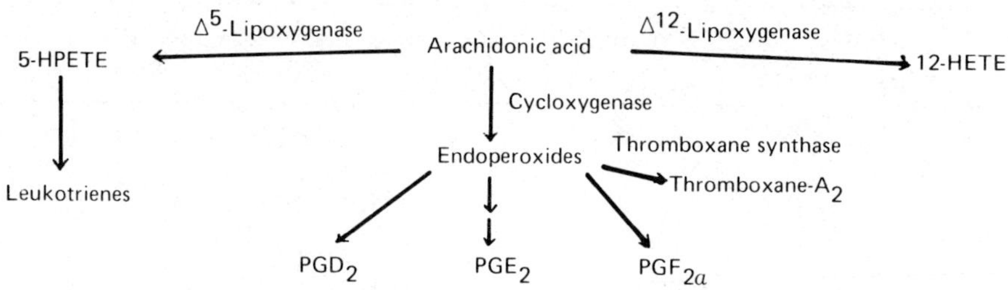

FIG. 1   Pathway of arachidonic acid metabolism.

II. Role of PG in Controlling Lymphocyte Activation by Mitogens

Over the past 10 years numerous investigators have explored questions related to biochemical requirements for lymphocyte activation
(17). Although a great amount of information has been obtained, it is
still not clear what the nature of the signals are which activate and
control the conversion of a resting lymphocyte into a cell which will
either undergo mitogenesis and differentiation or follow some other
pathway leading to quiescence. Recent reports from Kelly et al. (11)
and Parker et al. (12) suggest that the generation of thromboxanes or
possibly hydroxy fatty acids during the early stages of lymphocyte
activation may be obligatory in order for T lymphocytes to complete
one round of replication. That such products may also have a role in
cell signaling will be addressed below. In terms of negative regulation, Goodman and Weigle (18) have shown that arachidonic acid oxidized by lipoxidase becomes a potent inhibitor of both T cell and B
cell mitogenesis. Thus at the level of the single cell, in the absence
of other cell types there are possible negative and positive control
elements.

Of course, under normal circumstances a given set of cells are
activated in the presence of a variety of other cell subpopulations.
This makes the process of activation enormously complicated. As may
be seen from other chapters, there are several proteins which appear
to play a central role in lymphocyte activation. Chief among these are
interleukin 1 (or LAF) and interleukin 2 (TAF or TCGF). As will be
detailed in another chapter, it now appears that following stimulation
by antigen or mitogen, macrophages produce IL-1 which activates a
population of T lymphocytes ($Ly-1^+2^-,3^-$) to produce IL-2 which
stimulates blastogenesis and continued growth in T lymphocytes bear-
ing IL-2 receptors. There is another factor very closely related or
identical to IL-1 which may activate B cells (19,20). Coupled with
these positive signal elements are negative signals generated by activated macrophages and lymphocytes. Among these are products of the
PG pathway. In studies on mitogen-stimulated spleen cell subpopula-

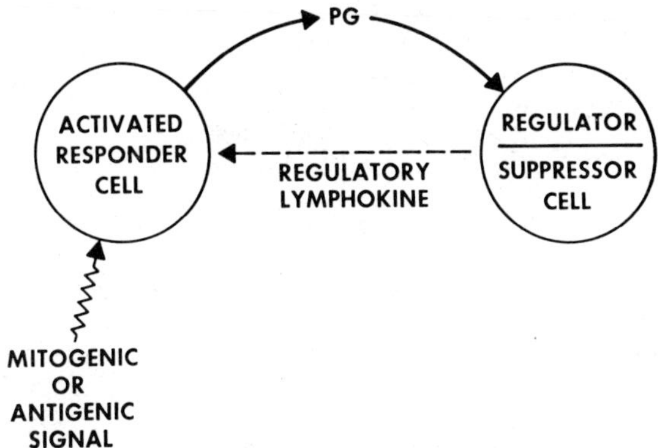

FIG. 2   Hypothetical role of prostaglandin in the control of immuno-competent cell function. (From Ref. 22.)

tions, we have been able to identify a glass-adherent, splenic T cell which can be stimulated directly by PGE_1 or PGE_2 to become a non-specific (i.e., nonantigen-specific) suppressor cell (8,9). This suppressor cell produces a low molecular weight suppressor molecule which can inhibit blastogenesis in antigen- or mitogen-stimulated T cells and B cells (21). Experiments have also shown that this suppressor cell can be induced by mitogen-stimulated nonglass-adherent T cells. This mode of induction is dependent on the inducer cells being able to synthesize products of the prostaglandin pathway (8,9). These results led us to formulate a minimal model of feedback loop regulation in which the inducer cell signals its activation via a PG product to the suppressor cell (see Fig. 2) that in turn releases its suppressor which can feedback and block the activation of the inducer cell. Our original experiments showed that this loop could be blocked by inhibitors of PG synthesis which inhibited cyclooxygenase-catalyzed conversion of arachidonic acid to endoperoxide (22). Subsequently, we have carried out a series of experiments using 1-substituted imidazole derivatives which block conversion of endoperoxides to thromboxanes but which allow synthesis of PG to go on. These data (Webb and Nowowiejski, in preparation) confirm the observations of Kelly et al. (11) and Parker et al. (12) that inhibition of thromboxane synthesis can inhibit blasto-genesis. However this is true only for nonglass-adherent T cells; the glass-adherent T cells remain unaffected or show slightly enhanced blastogenesis when thromboxane synthesis is inhibited. The effects of the thromboxane synthetase inhibitors on the feedback suppression loop is variable. This suggests that possibly PG and/or thromboxane may activate the suppressor cell.

The possible contribution of the macrophage to the control of the PG-mediated suppressor loop has also been studied (Webb and

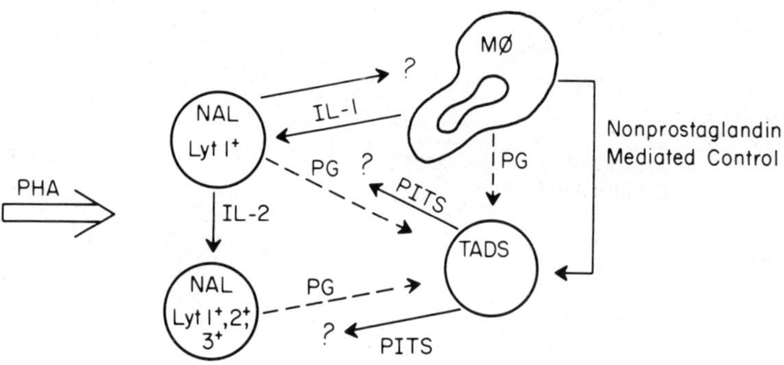

FIG. 3   Interaction of nonadherent lymphocytes, macrophages, and adherent suppressor T cells. NAL = nonadherent lymphocytes, MØ = macrophages, TADS = T-adherent suppressor cells.

Nowowiejski, Ref. 46. These experiments show that (1) macrophages can activate the adherent T suppressor cell via a PG-mediated mechanism and (2) macrophages and nonadherent T cells together may act synergistically to activate the adherent T suppressor cell. These data may be used to formulate a model of the control of lymphocyte activation as shown in Figure 3. As may be seen, there remain several possibilities. For example it is possible that the T cell which induces the suppressor cell is not the direct target of the suppressor cell product. Instead, the product PITS (prostaglandin-induced T suppressor) (21) may be directed against IL-2-sensitive cells. Consistent with this is the observation that PITS binds only to cells which have been activated (Webb and Nowowiejski, unpublished observations). On the other hand, it is possible that PITS could block IL-2 production, allowing IL-1-activated cells to proliferate and preventing the activation of IL-2-sensitive cells. It is not clear from the data of Parker's laboratory or from Goodman and Weigle whether products of the thromboxane synthetase or the lipoxidase can serve as intercellular signals or whether they operate only on the cells which synthesize these products.

One approach to addressing these problems is to use antigen-stimulated experimental models rather than mitogen-stimulated systems. The principal difficulty is that a fewer number of cells are activated by antigen as compared with mitogen (23). This makes analyses of biochemical parameters more difficult. A number of investigators have presented evidence suggesting that PG may be involved in antigen-induced lymphocyte activation. For example, Muscoplat and his associates (24) have shown that the period of maximum sensitivity of antigen-sensitive bovine peripheral blood lymphocytes to PG is within the first few hours following exposure to antigen. These workers found

TABLE 2   The Effect of Glass-adherent T Suppressor Cells on the Response of Spleen Cells to Sheep Erythrocytes

Cells	Drug	PFC per culture
Control whole spleen	None	80
Whole spleen + sRBC	None	900
T cells + B cells + sRBC	None	499
T cells + B cells (minus T suppressors) + sRBC	None	1499
T cells + B cells (minus T suppressors) + sRBC	Indomethacin $(10^{-6}$ M)	640

Note: Spleen cells were removed from 6-8-week-old male C57B1/6 mice and separated on glass wool columns into B and T cell populations. The various groups were then incubated with sRBC ± indomethacin for 5 days. Cultures were then assayed for the number of direct (19S) antibody-forming cells present.

evidence for an adherent suppressor cell participating in antigen-stimulated responses which seemed to either produce or be sensitive to PG. In a series of studies, Morley and his associates (25-27) have shown that PG released from antigen-stimulated macrophages can regulate production of lymphokines (such as IL-2 and MIF) which can regulate the further activation of macrophages and lymphocytes.

In our laboratory, we have carried out experiments designed to explore whether the PG-dependent feedback loop observed in our mitogen studies may also function when antigen-sensitive cells are used. Using the Mishell-Dutton culture system and sheep red blood cell (SRBC) as antigen, we have been able to show that removal of glass-adherent T cells enhances the 19S antibody-forming cell response to the same degree observed if a PG synthetase inhibitor is added to unseparated cells. Furthermore, after removal of the glass-adherent T cells, subsequent addition of a PG synthetase inhibitor has no enhancing effect (see Table 2). Similar results have been obtained by Orme et al., using a different culture system (28) but separating cell populations by glass adherence. In a more direct series of experiments, K. Wieder (in press) in this laboratory has used spleen cell subpopulations obtained from mice which had previously been primed to protein antigens such as BSA. These experiments showed clearly that antigen priming alters the nature of the adherent suppressor T cell population. Adherent suppressor T cells from primed

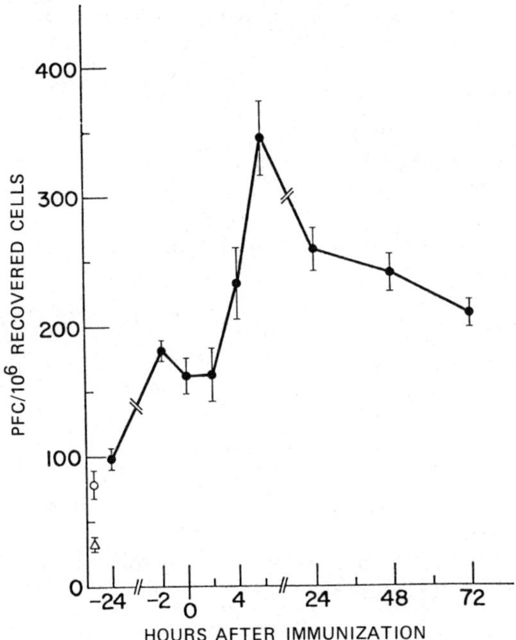

FIG. 4   The effect of delayed addition of PG synthetase inhibitors on
the primary response of purified "B" cultures from athymic mice exposed to PVP. B cell cultures were exposed to PVP (10^{-4} µg) and
Ro-20-5720 (10^{-6} M) was added at varying times. All cultures were
done in quadruplicate and the data are reported with standard errors.
o = PVP alone, △ = control cultures, ● = PVP + Ro-20-5720 added at
varying times. (From Ref. 29, ©1976 The Williams & Wilkins Co.,
Baltimore.)

mice were quite suppressive but were not activated via a PG-dependent mechanism. However, the nonadherent inducer T cell population
still produced PG; when primed nonadherent T cells were incubated
with antigen in the presence of unprimed, adherent T suppressor
cells, the ensuing suppression could be reversed by inhibiting PG
synthesis. These data suggest that the role of PG during T lymphocyte activation by antigen is to regulate blastogenesis only during the
primary response. Thus, once T lymphocytes have been primed, subsequent exposure to PG has only a minimal effect on their capacity to
transform into functional cells. As will become apparent later, this
appears to be generally the case with T cells; early stages of development are PG sensitive, whereas later stages are not.

Studies with B cells stimulated with either antigen or mitogen have been less extensive (29,30). In the mitogen studies it has been shown that human peripheral blood lymphocytes or mouse spleen cells stimulated with pokeweed mitogen or lipopolysaccharide (LPS), respectively, will not exhibit reduced blastogenesis if PGE_1 or PGE_2 is added at the beginning of culture. Further analysis of the pokeweed mitogen studies by Goodwin et al. (31) has suggested that any PGE_1-induced inhibition of blastogenesis was limited to T cells.

Our own experience with the effects of prostaglandin on mitogen-induced B cell activation confirms the studies mentioned above. In addition we have used PG synthetase inhibitors to show that the endogenous synthesis of PG by LPS-stimulated spleen cells also has no effect on B cell activation, as measured by either blastogenesis or antibody-forming cell response to sheep erythrocytes. Thus in terms of nonspecific activation by mitogens, B cells appear not to be sensitive to PG.

There are, however, two instances under which B cells may be influenced by PG-mediated control mechanisms. Under conditions in which the T-adherent suppressor cell is activated to make PITS, the activation of B cells is also inhibited by this product (21). Such conditions may exist during primary immune responses. The second instance concerns B cells which can respond to antigens in the absence of T cell help. In a series of studies conducted by M. Zimecki on the response of B cells to the T-independent antigens polyvinyl pyrrolidone (PVP) and dinitrophenol-ficoll (DNP-ficoll) (29), it was apparent that endogenous PG synthesis played a role during both the early and later stages of the response, depending on the experimental protocol. When whole spleen cell cultures were exposed to PVP and the PG synthetase inhibitor D,L-6-chloro-α-methylcarbazole-2-acetic acid (Ro-20-5720) was added at varying times after PVP addition, an enhanced response to PVP was observed. This enhancement was maximal when Ro-20-5720 was added 6 hr after the antigen (see Fig. 4). A delay of 24 hr in the addition of Ro-20-5720 resulted in no enhancement. When purified B cells were used instead of whole spleen cells, maximum enhancement of the response to PVP by Ro-20-5720 was still observed when the drug was added 6 hr after PVP. However additional enhancement is also observed when Ro-20-5720 is added 24-72 hr after antigen. This is true in purified normal B cell cultures and also true for B cells obtained from athymic mice. These data suggest that B cell activation by T cell-independent antigens may involve an autoregulatory B cell control which is mediated by PG and which functions early after exposure to antigen. Once the response machinery progresses, T cell-mediated control takes over and either masks or blocks any subsequent PG-mediated B cell control of B cell function.

Thus only under circumstances where B cells respond to T-independent antigens is there any evidence for PG control of B cell activation.

III. The Role of PG in Humoral Immune Responses

Several reports in the literature suggested that PGE_1 or PGE_2 can influence the development and/or outcome of antigenic challenge (31-35). In the late 1960s and early 1970s, investigations involving exogenous PGE_1 or PGE_2 showed that PGE in general inhibited the development of humoral responses in vitro with variable effects when used in vivo (35). Following our experiments showing that SRBC challenge in vivo led to rapid increases in splenic PG and cyclic nucleotide levels (36), we conducted a series of investigations on the effects of endogenous PG synthesis on humoral immune responses (37). For these studies we used a variety of PG synthetase inhibitors, including indomethacin, D,L-6-chloro-α-methylcarbazole-2-acetic acid, octadeca-9,12-diynoic acid (Ro-3-1314), and eicosatetraenoic acid (Ro-3-1428). The purpose of using such a variety of inhibitors (all of which block conversion of arachidonic acid by cyclooxygenase to endoperoxide) was to minimize possible artifacts resulting from the use of only one inhibitor (1).

The general conclusion reached from these studies was that blocking endogenous PG synthesis, both in tissue culture and in vivo, led to an enhanced 19S antibody response to antigen challenge. The degree of enhancement was dependent on the base response observed from experiment to experiment. As shown in Figure 5, if the response to antigen alone was low, the addition of a PG synthetase inhibitor enhanced the appearance of antibody-forming cells; on the other hand a very substantial antibody response was not notably enhanced when PG synthetase inhibitors were used. The same result was observed whether T-dependent or T-independent antigens were used, suggesting that PG effects were not at the level of T-B cell cooperation (29, 37). This left open the possibility of the effects being limited to B cells, T helper-T suppressor cells, or macrophages.

Results from the work of Zimecki (29) in our laboratory strongly pointed to an effect on B cells. As mentioned earlier, purified B cells responding to T-independent antigens showed increased numbers of antibody-forming cells when PG synthesis was inhibited. In another study, Zimecki investigated the effects of PG synthetase inhibitors on the autoimmune response to an antigen, -Hb-, exposed on autologous mouse red blood cells following treatment with bromylase. The investigation showed that when DNA synthesis was blocked, the addition of PG synthetase inhibitors resulted in increased numbers of anti-HB antibody-forming cells. These data correlated well with observations made in the early 1970s by Melmon et al. (34), and later we confirmed that antibody-forming B cells bear PG receptors and are sensitive to changes in PG (37). Both Melmon et al. and ourselves found that the addition of PGE_2 led to a reduction in the number of antibody-forming cells. This reduction could be induced when PGE_2 was added up to 4 hr prior to the assay of the antibody-forming cells. Since Melmon et al.

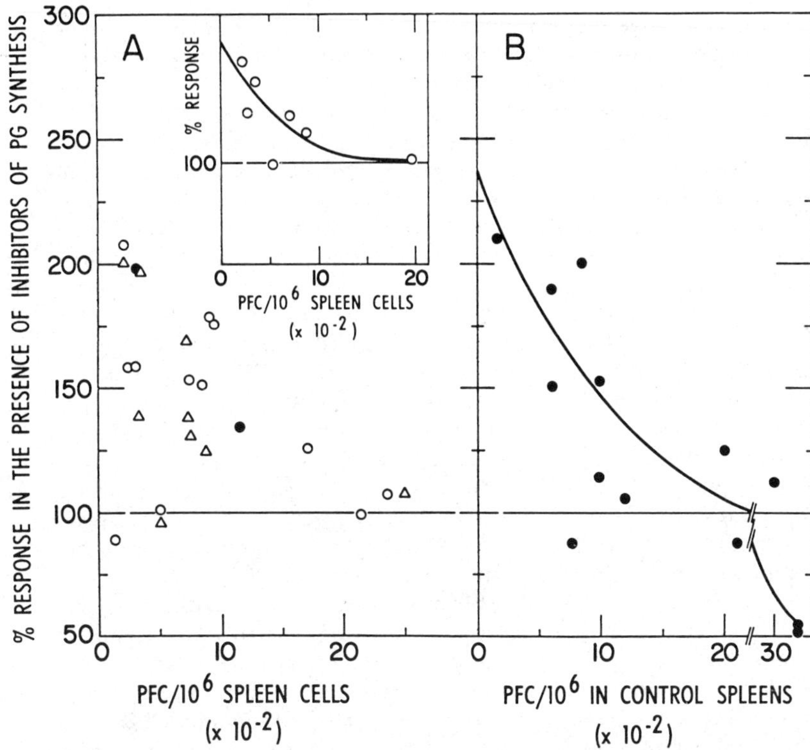

FIG. 5   The effects of inhibitors of PG synthetase on the primary 19S immune response to sRBC in vivo and in vitro. A: In vitro spleen cell cultures exposed to 1% sRBC (0.05 ml/ml of culture). Cultures were assayed for PFC on day 4. The values represent the mean percentage of control in triplicate cultures receiving PGSI + sRBC/sRBC. ○ = sRBC + Ro-20-5720 (10^{-7} M), △ = sRBC + Ro-3-1314 (10^{-7} M). The inset represents the average of those points between 0 and 1000 PFC/ 10^6 cells, 1000 and 2000 PFC/10^6 cells, etc. B: In vivo stimulation of the immune response in mice exposed to 2 × 10^7 sRBC intravenously with or without indomethacin (0.1 mg/mouse, i.p.) or Ro-20-5720 (0.6 mg/mouse, i.p.) given 24 and 2 hr, respectively, prior to antigen challenge. Mice were sacrificed and the spleens were assayed for PFC 5 days after challenge. The points represent the mean percentage of control using three mice per group given sRBC or PGSI + sRBC. No differentiation is made in this graph between mice receiving indomethacin or Ro-20-5720. (From Ref. 37.)

had shown that antibody-forming cells could be physically removed on
PGE_1-Sepharose columns, it appeared possible that PGE_2 could influence production or release of antibody.

To explore further the effects of PG on antibody-producing cells,
studies of the effects of PG on secondary immune responses were undertaken by K. Wieder in our laboratory (47,48). A number of other
investigators had presented evidence that the effects of PG on secondary responses might be different than that observed in primary responses. Stavitsky and his associates, as well as Ishizaka's laboratory
(38-40), showed that the response of antigen-primed rabbit lymph node
cells to antigen challenge could be enhanced by the addition of E type
PG. Mozes et al. (41) had earlier reported that exposure of murine
spleen cells to antigen in vitro in the presence of PGE_1 prevented a
reduction of the specific immune response on adoptive transfer. P. L.
Osheroff, in a related study performed in this laboratory (42), showed
that antigen challenge of mice primed previously resulted in large increases in splenic PG levels. These increases were shown to be hapten-
specific and dependent on the presence of specific antibody. In continuing these studies, Wieder has shown that antigen challenge of
primed spleen cells, in vitro, in the presence of PGE_2 leads to enhanced synthesis of total IgM (both antigen-specific and nonspecific
IgM). Conversely, the antigenic challenge of primed spleen cells in
the presence of a PG synthetase inhibitor induces a reduction of the
total IgM response. When these data are considered in light of the
studies discussed earlier showing no effect of endogenous PG on antigen-induced suppressor function, it is reasonable to conclude that
the target of PG in secondary immune responses may be limited to
either B cells or macrophages.

IV. The Role of PG in Cellular Immune Responses

Studies on the role of PG in cell-mediated cytotoxicity (K cells),
antibody-dependent cellular cytotoxicity (ADCC), and control of
natural killer (NK) cell function have been done by a number of
workers (43-45). In our laboratory, we have carried out limited experiments on mixed lymphocyte responses (MLR). These experiments
measure the activation of lymphocytes by allogeneic antigens present
on other lymphocytes using increases in DNA synthesis as a marker
for activation. We observed that the presence of PG synthetase inhibitors leads to enhanced incorporation of thymidine into DNA in both
a one-way and a two-way MLR (37). Since the MLR precedes the development of cytotoxic cells, it is not surprising that other studies
have shown that PG appears to play a role during both induction and
at the effector stage of cytotoxic killer cell function. Other workers
investigating the regulation of ADCC have shown that PG may regulate
the effector function in a fashion similar to that observed with K cells.

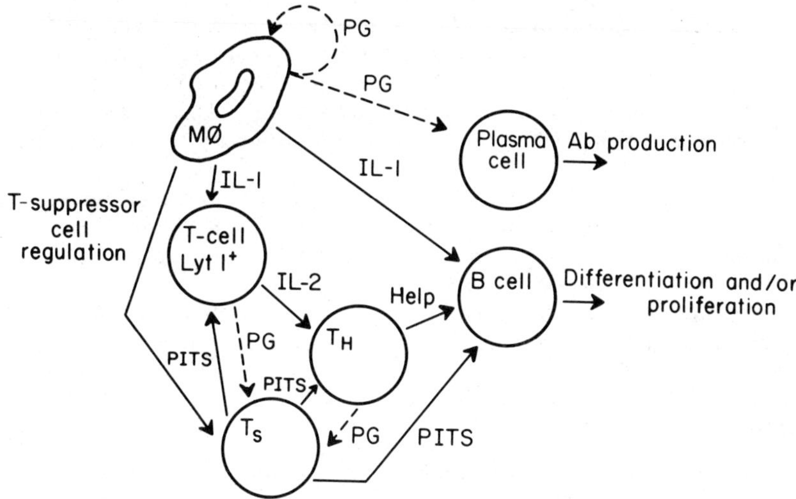

FIG. 6   Model of PG regulation of immunocompetent cell function.

V. Conclusion

The products of arachidonic acid metabolism, prostaglandins, thromboxanes, and hydroxy fatty acids influence immunocompetent cell
function. Our experiments, as well as those of other workers, suggest that PG may play a role in regulating the quality of the immune
response. The PG affect both the growth of T cells in response to
antigens or mitogens as well as the synthesis and release of antibody
by B cells. The mechanism of action of PG on lymphocytes is not
understood. The PG may act by inducing or blocking the production
of other mediators by T cells. These compounds may also act directly
on either T cells or B cells to alter cellular metabolism. The diagram
shown in Figure 6 represents an attempt to show how PG regulation
may function at the cellular level. With the apparent single exception
of antibody synthesis and release by plasma cells, all PG effects result in inhibition of cell function. In the diagram, the production of
PG either by macrophages or by Ly-1[+] T cells may have multiple
effects. Focusing on T cell regulation, PG production may lead to the
activation of a T suppressor cell (Ts), which by the production of a
soluble mediator (PITS) can regulate T cell differentiation and function. It may be that this is carried out by altering either the synthesis of other mediators (such as IL-2) or by blocking the further development of T cells (such as T_H) which are the targets of other
mediators. Our evidence suggests that PG affects only the early
stages of T cell development so that once functional, mature T cells
develop, all T cell interactions occur independently of PG regulation.

In the differentiation of B cells, PG may have a limited role either by the effects of PITS on blastogenesis or by directly affecting the subpopulation of B cells which can be stimulated by antigens in the absence of T cell help. Mature antibody-producing plasma cells are the only cell population of the lymphoid series in which function seems to be enhanced by PG.

The PG are among those mediators which seem to be involved in fine tuning the early stages of the immune response in order to maintain homeostasis. Once antigen-specific regulatory cells mature, these seem to override nonspecific controls. Thus the immune response includes a balance of nonspecific regulators which set the stage for subsequent regulation by antigen-specific cells and their products.

References

1. J. S. Goodwin and D. R. Webb, *Clin. Immunol. Immunopathol.* *15*:106 (1980).
2. H. Cantor and E. A. Boyse, *J. Exp. Med.* *141*:1376 (1975).
3. M. H. Julius, E. Simpson, and L. A. Herzenberg, *Eur. J. Immunol.* *3*:645 (1973).
4. H. Folch and B. Waksman, *Cell. Immunol.* *9*:12 (1973).
5. M. Loken and L. A. Herzenberg, *Ann. N.Y. Acad. Sci.* *254*:163 (1975).
6. L. Moretta, S. R. Webb, C. E. Grossi, P. M. Lydyard, and M. D. Cooper, *J. Exp. Med.* *146*:184 (1977).
7. M. Loken and L. A. Herzenberg, *Ann. N.Y. Acad. Sci.* *254*:163 (1975).
8. D. R. Webb and A. T. Jameison, *Cell. Immunol.* *24*:45 (1976).
9. D. R. Webb and I. Nowowiejski, *Cell. Immunol.* *41*:72 (1978).
10. S. Bauminger, *Prostaglandins* *16*:351 (1978).
11. J. P. Kelley, M. C. Johnson, and C. W. Parker, *J. Immunol.* *122*:1563 (1979).
12. C. W. Parker, W. F. Stenson, M. G. Huber, and J. P. Kelly, *J. Immunol.* *122*:1572 (1979).
13. J. L. Humes, R. J. Bonney, L. Pelus, M. E. Dahlgren, S. J. Sadowski, F. A. Kuehl, and P. Davies, *Nature (Lond.)* *269*:149 (1977).
14. W. Grimm, M. Seitz, H. Kirchner, and D. E. Gemsa, *Cell. Immunol.* *40*:419 (1978).
15. R. Murphy, S. Hammarstrom, and B. Samuelsson, *Proc. Natl. Acad. Sci. U.S.A.* *76*:4275 (1979).
16. C. A. Rouzer, W. A. Scott, Z. A. Cohn, P. Blackburn, and J. M. Manning, *Proc. Natl. Acad. Sci. U.S.A.* *77*:4928 (1980).
17. H. R. Bourne, L. M. Lichtenstein, K. L. Melmon, C. S. Henney, Y. Weinstein, and G. M. Shearer, *Science* *184*:19 (1974).

18.   M. G. Goodman and W. O. Weigle, *J. Immunol.* *125*:593 (1980).
19.   K. A. Smith, P. E. Baker, S. Gillis, and F. W. Ruscetti, *Mol. Immunol.* *17*:579 (1980).
20.   S. B. Mizel and J. J. Farrar, *Cell. Immunol.* *48*:433 (1979).
21.   T. J. Rogers, I. Nowowiejski, and D. R. Webb, *Cell. Immunol.* *50*:82 (1980).
22.   D. R. Webb, T. J. Rogers, and I. Nowowiejski, *Ann. N.Y. Acad. Sci.* *332*:262 (1979).
23.   M. Greaves and G. Janossy, *Transplant. Rev.* *11*:97 (1972).
24.   C. C. Muscoplat, T. M. Setcavage, and Y. B. Kim, *Am. J. Vet. Res.* *39*:129 (1978).
25.   M. A. Bray, D. Gordon, and J. Morley, *Br. J. Pharmacol.* *52*:453P (1974).
26.   D. Gordon, M. A. Bray, and J. Morley, *Nature (Lond.) 262*: 401 (1976).
27.   M. A. Bray, D. Gordon and J. Morley, *Prostagl. Med.* *1*:183 (1978).
28.   Orme et al. (personal communcation).
29.   M. Zimecki and D. R. Webb, *J. Immunol.* *117*:2158 (1976).
30.   F. Quagliata, V. J. W. Laurence, and J. M. P. Quagliata, *Cell. Immunol.* *6*:457 (1973).
31.   J. S. Goodwin, A. D. Bankhurst, and R. P. Messner, *J. Exp. Med.* *146*:1719 (1977).
32.   L. D. Loose and W. R. Diluzio, *J. Reticuloendothel. Soc.* *13*: 70 (1973).
33.   W. Braun and M. Ishizuka, *Proc. Natl. Acad. Sci., U.S.A.* *68*:1114 (1971).
34.   K. Melmon, H. R. Bourne, Y. Weinstein, G. M. Shearer, J. Kram, and S. Bauminger, *J. Clin. Invest.* *53*:13 (1974).
35.   H. R. Bourne, L. M. Lichtenstein, K. L. Melmon, C. S. Henney, Y. Weinstein, and G. M. Shearer, *Science 184*:19 (1974).
36.   P. L. Osheroff and D. R. Webb, *Proc. Natl. Acad. Sci. U.S.A.* *73*:1300 (1976).
37.   D. R. Webb and I. Nowowiejski, *Cell. Immunol.* *33*:1 (1977).
38.   R. G. Cook, A. B. Stavitsky, and W. W. Harold, *Cell. Immunol.* *40*:128 (1978).
39.   L. P. Sanford, A. B. Stavitsky, and R. G. Cook, *Cell. Immunol.* *48*:182 (1979).
40.   T. Kishimoto and K. Ishizaka, *J. Immunol.* *116*:534 (1976).
41.   E. Mozes, G. M. Shearer, K. L. Melmon, and H. R. Bourne, *Cell. Immunol.* *9*:226 (1973).
42.   P. L. Osheroff and D. R. Webb, *Cell. Immunol.* *38*:319 (1978).
43.   M. J. Droller, P. Perlmann, and M. U. Schneider, *Cell. Immunol.* *39*:154 (1978).

44. M. J. Droller, M. U. Schneider, and P. Perlmann, *Cell.
     Immunol.* *39*:165 (1978).
45. F. Wisloff and T. Christoffersen, *Int. Arch. Allergy Appl.
     Immunol.* *53*:42 (1977).
46. D. R. Webb and I. Nowowiejski, *Cell Immunol.* *63*:321 (1981).
47. K. J. Wieder and D. R. Webb, *Prost. and Med.* *7*:79 (1981).
48. K. J. Wieder and D. R. Webb, *Prost. and Med.* *7*:483 (1981).

8

Immunopharmacological Activities of MDP

LOUIS CHEDID, MONIQUE PARANT, and GILLES RIVEAU   Institut
Pasteur, Paris, France

Soon after the recognition of N-acetyl-muramyl-L-alanyl-D-isogluta-
mine (hereafter referred to as MDP for muramyl dipeptide) as being
the minimal subunit responsible for the activity of Freund's complete
adjuvant (FCA) (1,2), a great number of derivatives were synthe-
tized (3-5). Some were shown capable of enhancing nonspecific
resistance to infection (3,6-9). Because of its very low molecular
weight, it was hoped that MDP would retain selectively certain of
the numerous effects produced by the administration of mycobacterial organisms. Ideally, one could even envision that certain
activities would be strictly related to different derivatives according
to their affinity for a given type of immunocyte or even to a subset
of cell populations. It soon appeared, however, that the activity of
MDP was multifocal: evidence was gathered showing its *direct* effect
on B cells (10,11) and on macrophages (12-14) and, for certain
derivatives, on T cells (15). Moreover, the same molecule, according
to its time of administration, the dosage, or the system used, could
produce stimulation or inhibition of immune responses (16) reminis-
cent of what is unfortunately also observed with complex and heterogeneous agents such as BCG. During the ensuing studies, certain
other immunological and pharmacological facets were revealed. Since
the adjuvant and immunostimulating activities have been abundantly
reviewed elsewhere (3-5,17), the first part of the present report
will deal with modulation of immune or nonimmune responses by
chemical modification or by conjugation. The second part will review
pharmacological aspects which have been reported, excluding those
dealing with pyrogenicity. The last part will deal with the pyrogenic
activity of certain MDP derivatives administered alone or in association with indomethacin.

I. Modulation of Immune and Nonimmune Responses by Chemical Modification

It was first shown that when administered in Freund's incomplete adjuvant (FIA), MDP could elicit increased antibody response and delayed hypersensitivity (1,2). It was later shown that, in the absence of FIA, MDP could enhance humoral antibody responses and also nonspecific resistance to infection (6,18). In these first studies, all derivatives which increased nonspecific immunity were shown to be adjuvant active, but the reverse was not true, i.e., certain adjuvant-active molecules did not protect mice against infectious challenge (3). Because of the major importance of cell-mediated immunity (CMI), efforts were made in view of enhancing CMI responses with glycopeptides in the absence of FIA. Progress was made in this direction by synthesizing new lipophilic derivatives (19-21) and by injecting them either in saline or even in liposomes (22,23). Synergistic effects were also found by administering MDP with cord factor (24). Pyrogenicity of MDP was first described by Kotani et al., who related it to its adjuvant activity, since all inactive derivatives which were tested were devoid of pyrogenicity (25). In the course of these studies, the chemical structures responsible for these various activities were in certain cases recognized and mastered, at least partially. It is now possible to find derivatives which increase nonspecific resistance and have adjuvant activity, yet are no longer pyrogenic. Nonpyrogenic molecules which increase resistance to infection, only without enhancing the specific immune responses, or vice versa, have also been obtained.

A. Dissociation of Immunostimulant Activities of MDP by Linking Amino Acids or Peptides to the Glutaminyl Residue

As previously stated, MDP was shown to be adjuvant active and to protect mice nonspecifically against infection. By comparing several derivatives, it was shown that the linking of L-Lys, L-Ala, D-Ala, L-Lys-D-Ala, or L-Lys-L-Ala to MDP permits the dissociation of anti-infectious activity from adjuvant activity (26). The optical configuration of the added residues played the major role in this dissociation. It was noted that the muramyl tetrapeptide which mimicked the natural structure of the cell wall was devoid of anti-infectious activity. Previous investigation had shown that the two carboxyl groups of the glutamic acid residue and the stereochemistry of the peptide moiety were essential (2,18,27). As can be seen in Table 1, adjuvant activities were measured in guinea pigs [by administering MDP derivatives in a water-in-oil (w/o) emulsion with ovalbumin (OA)] and in mice (by administering MDP derivatives in saline with BSA). However, all adjuvant-active analogues did not protect mice against a *Klebsiella* infection. Such is the case of the pyrogenic derivative [6]. It is

therefore possible to dissociate adjuvant activity from anti-infectious
activity of synthetic glycopeptides by modifying their glutamyl residue.
By other chemical modifications, nonpyrogenic derivatives which enhance only antibody responses can also be obtained (derivative [4]).
The reverse situation can also be observed with certain lipophilic analogs not containing N-acetyl-muramic acid which retain their anti-
infectious activity although they are no longer adjuvant active (21).

B. Immunostimulant Activities of Lipophilic MDP Derivatives and of Des-muramyl Peptidolipid Analogs

Various fatty acid derivatives such as 6-O-mycoloyl were shown to
have new biological activities (19,28). Other MDP lipophilic analogs
having a fatty acid chain on the C terminal end of the peptide chain
were also studied. It was shown in particular that 1,O-(MDP-L-Ala)-
glycerol-3-mycolate had increased immunostimulant activity in comparison with MDP since it could induce hypersensitivity even in the absence of FIA (21). As can be seen in Table 1, this compound ([9])
gave higher protection against bacterial infection than did MDP. A
quite unexpected finding was obtained with the corresponding des-
muramyl compound 1,O-(L-Ala-D-isoGln-L-Ala)-glycerol-3-mycolate
([11]) which had no activity in producing humoral antibodies but was
just as active as the muramic acid-containing compound in stimulating
nonspecific resistance to bacterial infections. Moreover, this derivative was not pyrogenic. Modifications of the peptide moiety or the
lipid moiety of this peptidolipid led to decrease, or even loss, of protective activity (21).

C. Enhancement of Certain Biological Activities of MDP After Conjugation to a Multipoly(DL-alanine)-poly(L-lysine) Carrier

Previous studies had shown that most responses of MDP were abolished
upon the formation of glycosidic linkage with the paraaminophenyl
group. However, after cross-linking of the inactive β-D-*p*-aminophenyl
glycoside [12] with glutaraldehyde, several biological activities of MDP
were recovered. Moreover, the crosslinked oligomer [13] (∿6000 mol
wt) was more active than MDP in protecting mice nonspecifically against
bacterial challenge by *Klebsiella* or *Listeria* (29).

In another study MDP and some of its derivatives were conjugated
to a synthetic carrier, multipoly(DL-Ala)-poly(L-Lys), hereafter ab-
breviated as A--L. The branched polymers have been extensively used
as carriers to various synthetic haptens. The ability of these various
conjugates to enhance nonspecific resistance against infectious chal-
lenges was measured. Their activity was evaluated in two other biological test systems: pyrogenicity in rabbits and sensitization and elicitation of delayed hypersensitivity in guinea pigs (30).

TABLE 1 Examples of Dissociation between Various Biologic Activities of MDP Derivatives

Compound	Adjuvant effect[a] (in w/o emulsion)		Adjuvant effect[b] (in saline)	Anti-infectious effect[c]	Pyrogenic effect[d]
	Ab	DTH	Ab		
[1] AcMur–L–Ala–D–Glu–NH$_2$ = MDP	+++	+++	+++	+++	++
[2] AcMur–D–Ala–D–Glu–NH$_2$ = MDP(DD)	–	–	–	–	–[e]
[3] AcMur–L–Pro–D–Glu–NH$_2$	–	+++	+	–	–
[4] AcMur–NMe–L–Ala–D–Glu–NH$_2$	+++	+++	++	–	–[e]
[5] AcMur–L–Ala–D–Glu(L–Lys)NH$_2$	+++	+++	+++	+++	++
[6] AcMur–L–Ala–D–Glu(L–Lys–D–Ala)NH$_2$	+++	+++	+++	–	++
[7] AcMur–L–Ala–D–Glu(OCH$_3$)OC$_4$H$_9$	–	–	+++	+++	–
[8] AcMur–L–Ala–D–Glu(OC$_{10}$H$_{21}$)OCH$_3$	++	–	+++	+++	–
[9] MDP–(L–Ala–glycerol–3–mycolate)	+++	+++	++	++++	+
[10] MDP(DD)–(L–Ala–glycerol–3–mycolate)	–	–	–	+++	–[e]

[11] DP-(L-Ala-glycerol-3-mycolate)	-	-	-	++++	-[e]
[12] β-D-p-aminophenyl-MDP = PAP-MDP	+++	+++	-	-	-
[13] (PAP-MDP)$_n$	+++	+++	+	++++	++
[14] MDP-multi-poly(DL-Ala)poly(L-Lys) = MDP-A--L	+++	+++	+++	+++++	++++
[15] MDP(DD)-A--L	+	-	+	++++	+
[16] DP-A--L	-	-	-	-	-

[a]In guinea pigs; Ab, antibody titer; DTH, delayed-type hypersensitivity.

[b]In mice.

[c]Protective activity in mice infected with *Klebsiella*.

[d]Pyrogenicity in the rabbit by the intravenous route.

[e]Nonpyrogenic at 10 mg/kg.

Note: -, nonpyrogenic at 1 mg/kg; +, pyrogenic at 1 mg/kg; ++, pyrogenic at 100 µg/kg; +++, pyrogenic at 1 µg/kg.

Results can be summarized as follows. These studies demonstrated
that macromolecularization of muramyl dipeptide by attachment of several units to a multipoly (DL-Ala)-poly(L-Lys) carrier potentiates
both its pyrogenic and its immunostimulant activity [14]. After covalent linkage to MDP-A--L of a synthetic hapten (31) or of a synthetic
viral antigen (32), antibody responses were markedly enhanced.
Therefore, a completely synthetic vaccine was obtained by this procedure. Surprisingly, inactive N-acetylmuramyl-D-Ala-D-isoGln
[MDP (D-D)], after conjugation to A--L becomes capable of increasing
nonspecific immunity, although its lack of pyrogenicity is not greatly
modified. Moreover, MDP (D-D)-A--L conjugate remains devoid of adjuvant, sensitizing, or eliciting activity [15]. The influence of these
conjugates on the production of leukocytic pyrogen in vivo and in vitro
will be discussed in more detail in the last part of this review.

II. Pharmacological Aspects, Excluding Fever

A relatively small number of studies relating the pharmacological or
immunopathological activities of muramyl dipeptides have been pub-
lished. As previously stated, results dealing with pyrogenicity of MDP
will be excluded from this part of our review.

The "nec plus ultra" potency of an adjuvant is demonstrated by
the induction of autoimmune diseases, since it is generally assumed
that autoantigens are the "ultimate" in the hierarchy of antigen recognition. It was therefore paradoxically rewarding to find that several
autoimmune diseases could be established by administering MDP in FIA
with the appropriate antigen (33-37). Several models were used such
as orchitis (33) or uveoretinitis (34) and experimental allergic ence-
phalomyelitis (EAE) (35-37). In EAE, an interesting model of cell-
mediated immunity was provided by administering a synthetic encephalitogen with MDP. Thus, whereas the shortest active encephalitogen
in FCA was a tryptophannonapeptide, a shorter heptapeptide was capable of inducing the disease without producing antibodies if MDP was
injected instead of FCA (35). Nevertheless, in spite of its strong adjuvant activity, could the low molecular weight synthetic glycopeptide
be devoid of several of the "side effects" observed after administration
of BCG or *C. parvum* (adjuvant arthritis, sensitization to tuberculin,
increased susceptibility to endotoxin, granuloma formation, and lymphoid hyperplasia)?

Such indeed appeared to be the case during the first period of
investigations. 1. Even when administered in FIA, MDP alone did not
induce adjuvant arthritis (38) or elicit sensitization to tuberculin (10)
or to itself (3). 2. After administration in saline, muramyl dipeptides
did not render mice more susceptible to endotoxin, nor did they induce hepatosplenomegaly, lymphoid hyperplasia, or granuloma

formation (3). Further studies showed, however, that things were not
as clear.

Initial reports indicated that adjuvant-induced polyarthritis seemed
to require some additional structure—longer glycan chains—beyond that
of the muramyl dipeptide (38,39). Another study confirmed that a di-
mer of peptidoglycan (PG) represented the minimal essential structure
necessary for development of arthritis and that disaccharide peptides
(monomers of PG) or N-acetyl-muramyl peptides were inactive by
themselves unless they had been mixed in the water-in-oil emulsion
with poly(I:C) (40). However, in two recent papers, the same Japanese
authors described experiments showing that MDP produced moderate to
severe polyarthritis when administered alone in Difco oil (but not in
other mineral oils), whereas disaccharide peptides were less potent in
this vehicle (41,42). MDP-induced polyarthritis remains controversial,
however, since, in several other investigations using similar if not
identical conditions, this effect was not reproducible. A possible explanation may be offered by the following experiments. Under conditions in which MDP alone revealed essentially no arthritogenicity,
collagen-induced arthritis was definitely increased by its use (36).
These findings led the authors to postulate that, besides its adjuvant
activity, MDP exerts a synergistic effect with collagen.

Water-soluble peptidoglycan fragments are able to elicit a delayed-
type hypersensitivity (DTH)-like skin reaction in rats immunized with
M. tuberculosis cell walls in w/o emulsion. This reaction revealed a
close similarity to a typical DTH reaction with a predominant infiltration of mononuclear cells at 48 hr (43). It was suggested that the
putative cross-reactive antigenic determinant(s) might include both
the glycan chain and part of the peptide moiety of the peptidoglycan.
Synthetic muramyl dipeptide elicited only a marginal skin reaction and
showed a mild but significant mononuclear infiltration in immunized
animals, indicating a weak antigenicity of MDP to elicit the DTH-like
reaction (43). Even clearer results can be obtained in the guinea pig.
In guinea pigs sensitized by FCA, positive skin test reactions can be
obtained vis-à-vis tuberculin, but not MDP. Conversely in these first
experiments, when guinea pigs received MDP in FIA, they failed to
become sensitized to tuberculin or even to MDP (3). Later studies
showed, however, that such was not the case if sensitization was made
with the glycopeptide conjugated to a synthetic carrier and that the
use of the conjugate was also critical for elicitation of the reaction.
Thus, positive skin tests can be elicited with MDP-A--L in guinea
pigs which have been previously sensitized with MDP-A--L administered in FIA (30).

Previous treatment by BCG has been shown to lower the resistance
of mice to gram-negative lipopolysaccharide (LPS). Cord factor or
trehalose dimycolate was identified as being the mycobacterial component responsible for this effect (44). When administered instead of BCG
and under the same conditions (2 weeks before endotoxin challenge),

MDP did not modify the susceptibility of mice (unpublished results).
However it was later reported that, in guinea pigs of inbred strain 2,
simultaneous administration of MDP and endotoxin or *Pseudomonas*
vaccine exerted a strong toxic synergism (45). Such a synergism can
be observed in mice but only if both agents are administered simultaneously at high dosages (unpublished results).

In contrast to Wax D, MDP administered in saline does not elicit
the epithelioid granuloma formation evoked by the whole tubercle
bacilli (46). However, when incorporated in a water-in-oil emulsion,
its granulomagenic capacity was found stronger than that of killed
bacteria (47). An MDP derivative with a branched fatty acid chain also
produced granuloma formation in the draining lymph node of guinea
pig even when injected as a suspension in PBS (47).

The typical increase in phagocytic tissue mass consecutive to administration of mycobacteria has never been reported to occur following
MDP treatment. However, MDP and adjuvant-active analogues can stimulate the phagocytic function of mice in vivo (48-50). There was good
correlation between RES stimulation and adjuvant activity of MDP analogues, although the minimum effective doses were higher than those
required to obtain an effect on immune responses. In contrast to mice,
guinea pigs did not show stimulation of phagocytosis after MDP treatment, although their immune responses were also strongly increased by
this adjuvant (50). In vitro, peritoneal cells of several animal species,
including guinea pigs, can be directly activated by MDP. MDP causes
enhancement of attachment and spreading and inhibition of macrophage
migration (51-53). Inhibition of growth of tumor target cells was produced by mouse macrophages activated by free (54) or conjugated derivative (55). MDP also increased the cytolytic activity of macrophage
cell lines, showing a direct action without the participation of any
other cell type (56). Adjuvant-active glycopeptides were also shown
to stimulate the production of several monokines such as lymphocyte-
activating factor (LAF), colony-stimulating activity (CSA), leukocytic
pyrogen (LP), and fibroblast-activating factor (57-61). Several other
parameters have been studied such as glucose oxidation, prostaglandin
synthesis, enhanced levels of intracellular cAMP, collagenase production, and enhanced H_2O_2 release (61-64).

Besides their effects on macrophages, other pharmacological activities were observed such as complement activation, or serotonin release from blood platelets. In contrast to mycobacteria or cord factor,
which are capable of activating in vitro the alternate pathway of complement, MDP was found inactive when tested with normal human serum
or normal and C4-deficient guinea pig sera (65). Lack of activity of
MDP and of several 6-O-acyl muramyl peptides was confirmed by Kotani
et al., who also found that [B30]-MDP and [BH48]-MDP-L-Lys-D-Ala
could activate human complement through the alternate pathway (66).

Natural peptidoglycans display a lytic activity and can release serotonin when incubated with rabbit blood platelets. Comparable submicroscopic changes of blood platelets can be observed with MDP but only at an extremely high dose (67). In subsequent assays in which several synthetic compounds were tested, MDP and a large number of 6-O-acyl muramyl dipeptides did not release serotonin from rabbit blood platelets. However, the same 6-O-acyl muramyl tetrapeptide, ([BH48]-MDP-L-Lys-D-Ala), was shown to have a definite serotonin-liberating activity under the same conditions (68). The same authors reported an even more direct pharmacological activity of this glycopeptide: MDP and some of its acyl derivatives caused the contraction of a strip of guinea pig ileum, whereas [BH48]-MDP produced relaxation. Analogues devoid of adjuvant activity showed no such effect (68).

Although several of the side effects inherent to the administration of whole microorganisms can be partially reproduced by MDP, these effects are much weaker and often absent, particularly if MDP is administered in saline. Moreover, it is sometimes possible to avoid them by the proper choice of a derivative, or even to reverse them by procedures such as conjugation to an antigen. A notable point was made in the case of IgE production. In mice immunized with a suboptimal dose of BSA, MDP favored the induction of anaphylactic reactions: shortly after the intravenous administration of the BSA booster dose, some of the animals died, and a high level of IgG_1 was found (69). Production of reaginic (IgE) antibodies, in the primary or secondary response to ovalbumin was also increased in mice by the simultaneous administration of a large dose of MDP or of several adjuvant-active analogues, whereas stereoisomers were inactive (70). In contrast, IgE antibody response could be suppressed by a preadministration of allergen conjugated to a fatty acid derivative of MDP. In this study, 6-O-mycoloyl-MDP was mixed or conjugated to DNP. When mixed, both strong IgG and IgE responses to the antigen were observed, whereas the conjugate suppressed the IgE response even though the IgG was fully maintained (71).

III. Studies Related to the Pyrogenic Activity of MDP

As will be discussed in our concluding remarks, fever can be produced by innumerable agents and more particularly by viruses, bacteria, fungi, and parasites (72). Lipopolysaccharides of gram-negative organisms have constituted the most representative class of bacterial pyrogens (72). However, peptidoglycans, and especially those extracted from the streptococcal cell wall, can also induce a marked fever in rabbits (73). It is generally assumed that for such agents a high molecular weight material is required, and that during enzymatic degradation, decrease or complete loss of pyrogenicity is uniformly observed (74). It was therefore quite surprising that MDP (<500 daltons) could elicit fever in rabbits. In this first study, it was also assumed that adjuvant activity was strictly related to pyrogenicity since all the inactive stereoisomers tested were devoid of pyrogenicity (25). This conclusion, fortunately, is no longer warranted (see the results summarized in Table 1).

A. *In Vivo Studies of MDP and Certain of its Derivatives*

1. Comparison of Pyrogenicity by the Intravenous and by the Intracerebroventricular Route MDP and various derivatives were administered intravenously to groups of rabbits at dosage levels varying between 10 µg/kg and 10 mg/kg. Intracisternal injections of MDP were made at 10-fold dilutions varying between 1 and 10^{-4} µg/kg. Figure 1 represents the comparative activity of MDP by both routes and of LPS by intravenous route only. Results shown in Figure 1 are expressed at Δt_{max} (°C) and calculated as the log of the injected dose per kilogram. As can be seen, a good dose-response relationship was found for MDP by both routes. When administered intravenously, a good dose-response relationship was also observed with MDP-A--L, and the activity of the conjugate was greater (0.85 µg/kg). In contrast, the inactive MDP(D-D) stereoisomer was found to be nonpyrogenic at the dose of 10 mg/kg administered intravenously. Several adjuvant active derivatives were also nonpyrogenic at the same dose and by the same route (see Table 1). Time studies showed that, in the case of MDP, biphasic curves having a pattern similar to that obtained with LPS were elicited (60). However, the minimal pyrogenic dose for free or conjugated MDP is, respectively, about 10,000-fold and 500-fold greater than in the case of LPS. The effects on leukopenia of MDP were comparable to those observed after LPS administration.

After intracerebroventricular (i.c.v.) administration, a good dose-response curve was also obtained with a very marked increase in susceptibility, since the minimal pyrogenic dose was 0.13 ng/kg. Administered by this route, the D-D stereoisomer is found to be pyrogenic at the dose of 1-2 µg. This amount by intracerebroventricular route represents a dose which is 10,000-fold greater than for MDP, whereas by intravenous route the difference between 10 mg/kg and 30 µg/kg is only 300-fold. Surprisingly, MDP-A--L was found to be somewhat *less* pyrogenic than free MDP (0.5 ng/kg). In contrast, and notwithstanding the extreme sensitivity of this test, 50 µg of free or conjugated muramic acid or dipeptide did not elicit fever, showing that the glycopeptide represents the minimal pyrogenic structure (75).

2. Influence of Indomethacin (IM) and Nitrogen Mustard (NM) on the Production of Circulating Pyrogens Transferable circulating endogenous pyrogen can be demonstrated after an intravenous injection of MDP

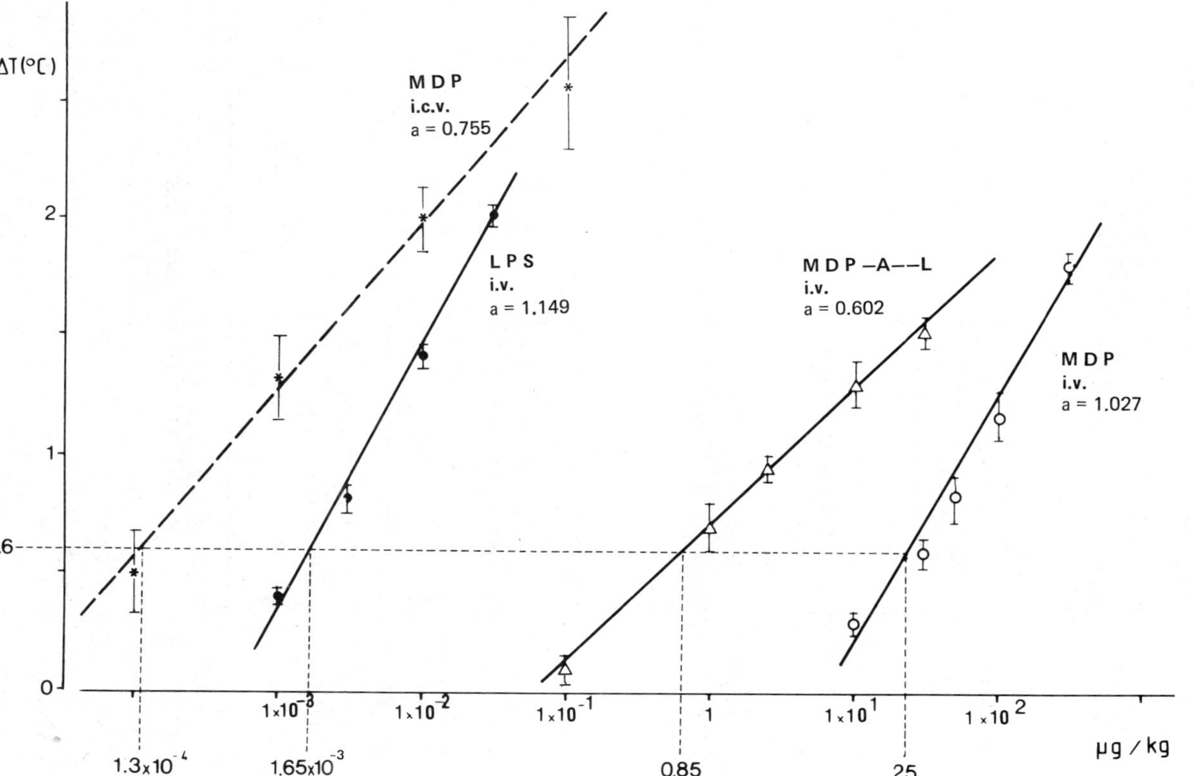

FIG. 1   Comparative pyrogenicity of MDP, MDP-A--L, and LPS in the rabbit. i.v. = intravenous route, i.c.v. = intracerebroventricular route, a = slope.

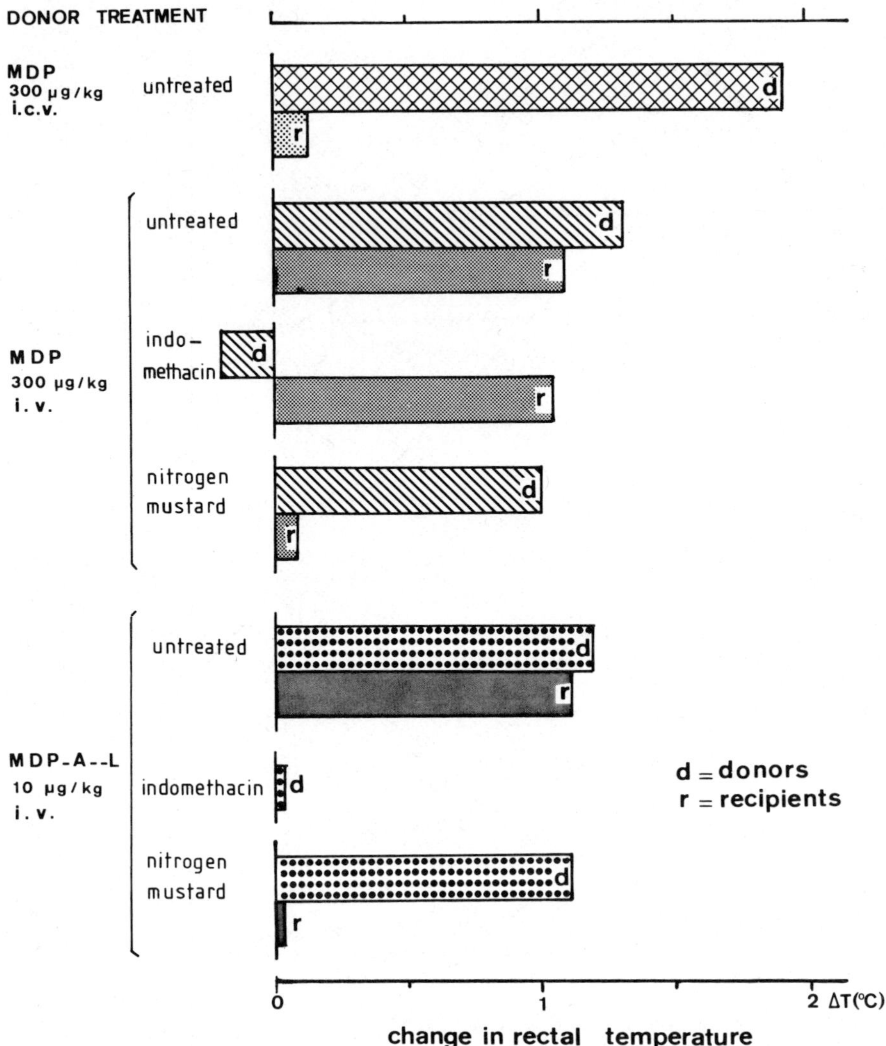

FIG. 2 Passive transfer experiments of plasma from febrile or afebrile rabbits into untreated animals. Maximal rise of temperature in donors (d) and in normal recipients (r) given 10 ml/kg of dialyzed plasma intravenously.

similar to what has been observed with lipopolysaccharides (76,77).
This serum factor which seems to be identical to leukocytic pyrogen
elicits a monophasic fever of short latency and duration. In the following experiments, donor rabbits received either 300 µg/kg, i.c.v.
or i.v., of MDP or 10 µg/kg, i.v., of MDP-A--L. Certain groups received either NM or IM before receiving free or conjugated MDP intravenously. NM (2.5 mg/kg, i.v.) was administered 3 days before and
IM (40 mg/kg, i.p.) 1 hr before the pyrogen. At the time of the fever
peak, blood was collected and 10 ml/kg of dialyzed plasma was injected
intravenously to normal recipients. The following results are illustrated
in Figure 2 which represents the cumulative data concerning 3-5
rabbits per group. When MDP was administered by the intracerebroventricular route, although a high and persistent fever was observed
in the donors, no endogenous pyrogen was detected in the plasma. In
certain experiments, the cerebrospinal fluid from donors which had
also received 300 µg/kg MDP was collected, dialyzed, and administered
by the extremely sensitive intracerebroventricular route to normal
recipients without eliciting fever (not shown in Fig. 2). In contrast,
endogenous pyrogen release in plasma can be observed after the intravenous administration of MDP or of smaller doses of MDP-A--L.

The release of circulating endogenous pyrogen is inhibited, however, if an intense leukopenia is produced by prior treatment with nitrogen mustard (Fig. 2). After such a treatment, the average blood
count was less than 10^3 cells/mm^3 instead of around 10^4 cells/mm^3, and
although a normal febrile response was observed in the MDP or MDP-
A--L-treated donors, the transferred plasma elicited no fever in the
recipients. In contrast, endogenous pyrogen can be elicited in the
blood of indomethacin-treated donors in the absence of febrile responses. Rabbits received indomethacin 1 hr before [^{14}C]MDP, and
blood was collected by cardiac puncture 150 min later. The plasma was
dialyzed to remove residual indomethacin and radioactive MDP before
being injected to recipient rabbits under the same conditions as previously. Although no fever was detectable in the donors, a significant
elevation of the temperature was observed in the recipients (Fig. 2).
Therefore, indomethacin treatment does not inhibit the production of
LP in vivo or, as will be shown later, in vitro.

Because of the nitrogen mustard results, and because of MDP's
great activity after administration by intracerebroventricular route,
it was assumed that MDP could elicit fever by at least two mechanisms:
direct activity on the thermoregulating centers and release of leukocytic pyrogen through its peripheral effect.

B. Influence of Indomethacin on the In Vitro Production of Leukocytic Pyrogens by MDP and Certain of Its Derivatives

When rabbit peritoneal exudate cells or human circulating monocytes
are incubated with MDP, the supernatants of these incubates injected

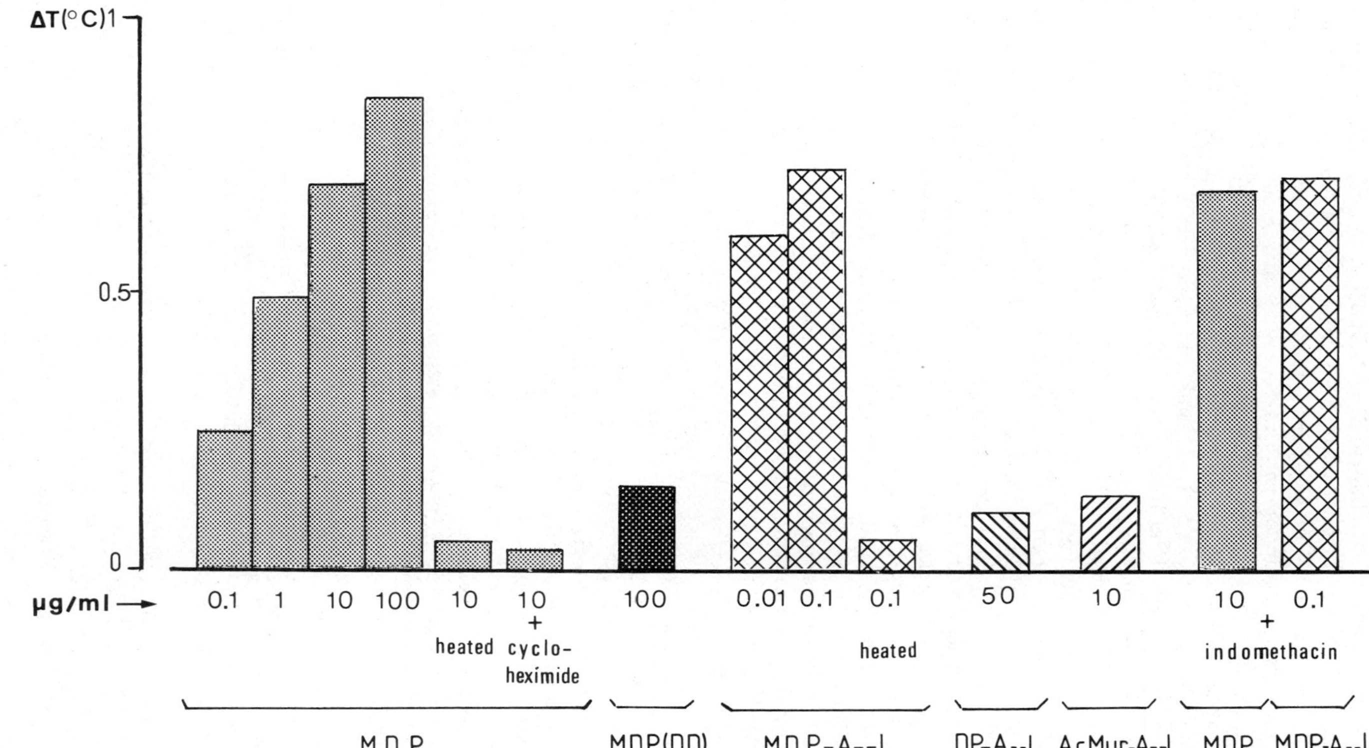

FIG. 3 Production of leukocytic pyrogen in vitro by rabbit peritoneal cells (10^7 cells/ml) incubated with MDP or derivatives. Supernatant (0.5 ml/kg) was injected in untreated rabbits (3 per group).

intravenously or by the much more sensitive intracerebroventricular
route produce a brief monophasic fever in rabbits. As can be seen in
Figure 3 there exists a dose-response relationship between the amount
of LP released and the amount of MDP incubated with the rabbit cells.
In contrast, the supernatant of cells incubated with 100 µg of the inactive MDP(D-D) stereoisomer does not induce fever. Much smaller
amounts of conjugated MDP can release endogenous pyrogens in vitro,
since 0.01 µg of MDP-A--L produces the same effect as 3 µg of free
glycopeptide. On the same figure, one can also observe that the conjugates containing only the dipeptide or the sugar moiety of MDP were
inactive. Finally, indomethacin at doses which inhibited the increase
of prostaglandins did not interfere with the in vitro production of
leukocytic pyrogen by either 10 µg of MDP or 0.1 µg of MDP-A--L
(78). In some control experiments, the supernatants of cells incubated
with MDP in the presence of IM were tested for both their LAF and
their LP content. Both activities were demonstrable despite the absence of PG elevation. These results are in conformity with what has
been found with MDP (61) or other LAF activators. In contrast, MDP-
induced production of LP can be abolished if cells are incubated with
cycloheximide, a protein synthesis inhibitor. This experiment was performed under conditions in which the number of viable cells remained
approximately the same as in control cell cultures incubated with MDP.
These results were therefore in agreement with what was observed in
vivo (see Fig. 2). In all cases the production of fever was related to a
thermolabile factor, since heating at 56°C for 30 min destroyed the
pyrogenic activity of the supernatants.

However, it must be emphasized that, according to the test system used, the compared activities of free or conjugated MDP are different. As can be seen in Table 2, the minimal pyrogenic dose by
intracerebroventricular route is 0.00013 µg/kg for MDP versus
0.00055 µg/kg for MDP-A--L (since the molecular size of the MDP-
A--L preparation is not absolutely homogeneous, one should not rule
out the possibility that this conjugate could be even less pyrogenic in
situ. Paradoxically, by intravenous route MDP-A--L is more pyrogenic
than the monomer, 0.85 µg/kg versus 25 µg/kg. Interestingly, it must
be noted that an even smaller dose, 0.01 µg/ml of the conjugate produces in vitro the same effect as 10 µg/ml MDP. Therefore, after intravenous injection, fever could be triggered in the case of conjugated
MDP mainly by the release of leukocytic pyrogens, especially if one
considers that free MDP could cross the brain barrier more easily.
Table 2 also shows that free or conjugated dipeptide, DP (L-Ala-D-
isoGln), without the sugar moiety was devoid of pyrogencity in vivo
even after intracisternal injection and did not release LP in vitro.

TABLE 2 Pyrogenic Effects of MDP and MDP Components after Conjugation to a Carrier

	Minimal effective dose		
	In vivo febrile response[a]		In vitro production[b]
Compound	i.v. (μg/kg)	i.c.v. (μg/kg)	(μg/ml)
MDP	25	0.00013	10
MDP-A--L	0.85	0.00055	0.01
DP	>1000	>100	>100
DP-A--L	>100	>100	>100
AcMur	>100	>100	>100
AcMur-A--L	NT	>10	>10
AcMur + DP-A--L	NT	NT	>100

[a]In rabbit by the intravenous (i.v.) route or by the intracerebro-ventricular (i.c.v.) route.

[b]By rabbit peritoneal cells.

C. Influence of Indomethacin on In Vivo Immunostimulant Effects of MDP and Certain of Its Derivatives

The adjuvant activity of MDP administered with a protein antigen is not decreased by previous administration of a high dose of indometha-cin: neither primary nor secondary responses were affected in mice and in guinea pig experiments (performed with FIA and adjuvant), elevated antibody titers and delayed hypersensitivity were both found as in controls (unpublished results). Enhancement of nonspecific re-sistance to infectious challenge by MDP was not antagonized by the anti-inflammatory drug but rather was even increased. Synergistic effects could be observed both with MDP and with conjugated MDP-A--L (78). One can therefore summarize the in vivo and in vitro results by saying that neither pyrogenicity nor increased prostaglandin levels appeared to be prerequisites for immunopotentiation by synthetic gly-copeptides. The synergistic effects are in agreement with Webb's findings indicating that prostaglandin elevation could exert a negative feedback mechanism via T suppressor cells (79,80).

Conclusions

Although the effects of MDP seem to be less selective than what was at
first assumed, and although this molecule can retain partially certain
of the unwanted activities of whole microorganisms, the following remarks must be strongly stressed:

1. Administered in saline, MDP is rapidly cleared through the
    kidney (81), and several of the "side effects" of BCG are
    weaker or even absent.
2. Moreover, these unwanted activities can be avoided by the
    choice of certain derivatives or of certain procedures.

Thus, serotonin release or adverse effects on blood platelets are produced by certain derivatives but are not detectable when other
adjuvant-active glycopeptides are used (68). Certain pharmacological
activities such as contraction or relaxation of guinea pig ileum have
also been reported to be dependent on the chemical structure of the
derivative. Conjugation procedures—such as polymerization with glutaraldehyde (29) or covalent coupling to synthetic carriers (30-32)—
have been shown to increase or even to produce new biological activities. Coupling of fatty acid derivatives of MDP to allergens can suppress the IgE response without inhibiting the production of other
classes of antibody (71). Last, but not least, it is now clearly demonstrable that derivatives of MDP can retain selectively their capacity to
increase specific or nonspecific immunity (or both) without being pyrogenic. Moreover, an antipyretic drug can abolish the febrile reaction
induced by MDP itself without inhibiting its in vitro effect on LAF
production or its in vivo immunopotentiating activities.

Should the elevation of body temperature be considered only as an
adverse reaction or primarily as one of the host's most primitive and
potent nonspecific immune responses? The beneficial role of fever has
been advocated constantly since the dawn of medicine and stated repeatedly during the 2400 years which have elpased between
Hippocrates* and Wagner-Jauregg, who received the Nobel Prize in
1927 because of the therapeutic use of malarial pyrexia.

As mentioned by Kluger in his excellent review (82), it was probably most unfortunate that aspirin, besides being antipyretic, re-
lieves discomfort and headache, leading people to believe that its use
is more beneficial than it really is during infectious diseases. Nevertheless, and although the fortunes of fever have waned in recent
years, a renewed interest in the field has lately developed.

---

*"Those who have quartan fever [malaria] rarely have convulsions;
those who have convulsions and later catch quartan fever are cured of
their convulsions," *Aphorisms* V, 70, Hippocrates (460-375 BC).

Theoretically, fever could enhance resistance by three possible mechanisms: (1) general increase of metabolism, (2) inhibition of proliferation of thermosensitive organisms, and (3) production by exogenous pyrogen of both fever and of monokines or other mediators which stimulate more directly the immune system. Until recently, the first argument has been generally assumed, although it seems rather paradoxical that selection should have retained such a costly process. (It is calculated that a rise in body temperature of 3°C will result in approximately 25% of increased energy expenditure.) More interesting is the second explanation: temperature increase may help the host to get rid of thermosensitive bacterial and viral agents. In harmony with this view are the insistent warnings of A. Lwoff against antipyretic drugs and their paradoxical use and abuse in certain viral infections (83). One hundred years previously, Louis Pasteur had recognized the role of fever during his memorable experiments on *Anthrax*, assuming that birds' resistance to *Anthrax* was related to their higher temperature which checked the proliferation of this bacillus. He showed by heating rabbits that they became more resistant, whereas fowls became more susceptible if their temperature was lowered. He did not hesitate to write in his report that "if this discovery is fully substantiated we could hope to cure a man infected by *Anthrax* . . . by elevating his temperature" (84). Several decades later similar experiments with various animal species have shown that pyrexia does enhance resistance to infection. It has been repeatedly found in recent years that, following inoculation of microbial organisms, ectotherms would select a warmer environmental temperature and fever could be developed by this process in many nonmammalian vertebrates. Thus, goldfish whose lower temperature preferendum is 28°C will survive after being infected by *Aeromonas hydrophila* if they maintain themselves at 33°C, whereas they will all die at 25.5°C (85). Similar experiments have been made in several nonmammalian vertebrates and even in mammals. When rabbits were infected with *Pasteurella multocida*, a beneficial effect was observed when their temperature was increased about 2°C, whereas a statistically higher mortality rate was observed when it was lowered by administration of sodium salicylate (86).

More recently a third explanation has been offered, postulating that a macrophage factor could be responsible for fever production and also for lymphocyte activation. As a matter of fact, a consensus has recently developed stating that several monokines previously identified as being separate entities represented different facets of the same molecule. In view of the numerous biological and biochemical similitudes with LAF of these various agents (such as mitogenic protein, T cell-replacing factors, B cell-activating factor, and B cell differentiation factor), the term interleukin 1 was coined to indicate that they were only different names of the same agent (87). As already mentioned, fever can be produced by viruses, bacteria, parasites, and fungi. In all cases the febrile response is mediated by the production of the leukocytic pyrogen (88). This endogenous agent is not H_2 restricted and can even cross the species barrier. Because of the similarities existing between the leukocytic pyrogen and lymphocyte-activating factor, investigators have suggested that leuko-cytic pyrogen should also belong to the class of interleukin 1. They showed by a series of experimental arguments that purified endogen-ous pyrogen obtained from stimulated rabbit peritoneal exudate cells had the same physicochemical and immunological properties as LAF which was produced in a separate laboratory from stimulated rabbit alveolar macrophages (89). Very similar results were observed also with human leukocytic pyrogen and human LAF (90).

Besides interleukin 1, the production of several other monokines playing an important role in the host's natural resistance, such as interferon or tumor necrotizing factor, is markedly increased by in-cubating cells with bacteria or viruses. These last two agents are clearly different from LAF or LP, although under certain conditions they can be produced simultaneously by immunostimulants such as LPS (91-93). In contrast, it is possible to induce both LAF and LP without interferon by incubating cells with MDP. It also seems possible to induce separately LAF or LP by incubating rabbit peritoneal cells with certain MDP derivatives (unpublished results). Phylogenetic studies have shown that febrile responses can be observed in most classes of vertebrates, and even in arthropods, and that endogenous pyrogens can be produced when their phagocytic cells are incubated with bacteria (94,95). To our knowledge the presence of LAF activity has not been investigated under the same conditions. Whether these two activities are supported by the same or by two different molecules, they clearly have been maintained in close relationship, at least in mammals, by strong selective processes. Fortunately the end responses can be modulated separately (immunostimulation without fever) by the use of chemically modified synthetic adjuvants administered alone or in association with pharmacologically active drugs.

Acknowledgments

The authors' work is supported in part by the Centre National de la Recherche Scientifique and by grant No. 79.7.0673 from the Délégation Générale à la Recherche Scientifique et Technique.

We are grateful to Drs. J. Choay and P. Lefrancier for the samples of synthetic MDP derivatives. The MDP used was MDP-Pasteur (Institut Pasteur Production, Paris).

The authors thank B. Cosmao Dumanoir for typing and layout of this manuscript.

References

1. F. Ellouz, A. Adam, R. Ciorbaru, and E. Lederer, *Biochem.
    Biophys. Res. Commun. 59*:1317 (1974).
2. S. Kotani, Y. Watanabe, T. Shimono, T. Narita, K. Kato,
    D. E. S. Stewart-Tull, F. Kinoshita, K. Yokogawa, S. Kawata,
    T. Shiba, S. Kusumoto, and Y. Tarumi, *Z. Immun.-Forsch.
    149*:302 (1975).
3. L. Chedid, F. Audibert and A. G. Johnson, *Prog. Allergy
    25*:63 (1978).
4. I. Azuma, M. Yemiya, I. Saiki, M. Yamawaki, Y. Tanio, S.
    Kusumoto, T. Shiba, T. Kusama, and K. Tobe, *Dev. Immunol.
    6*:311 (1979).
5. E. Lederer, *J. Med. Chem. 23*:819 (1980).
6. L. Chedid, M. Parant, F. Parant, P. Lefrancier, J. Choay,
    and E. Lederer, *Proc. Natl. Acad. Sci. U.S.A. 74*:2089 (1977).
7. F. Kierszenbaum and R. W. Ferraresi, *Inf. Immun. 25*:273
    (1979).
8. J. Tribouley, J. Tribouley-Duret, and M. Appriou, *CR Soc.
    Biol. (Paris) 173*:1046 (1979).
9. R. C. Humphres, P. R. Henika, R. W. Ferraresi, and J. L.
    Krahenbuhl, *Inf. Immun. 30*:462 (1980).
10. C. Damais, M. Parant, and L. Chedid, *Cell. Immunol. 34*:49
    (1977).
11. J. Watson and C. Whitlock, *J. Immunol. 121*:383 (1978).
12. D. Juy and L. Chedid, *Proc. Natl. Acad. Sci. U.S.A. 72*:4105
    (1975).
13. Y. Yamamoto, S. Nagao, A. Tanaka, T. Koga, and K. Onoue,
    Biochem. Biophys. Res. Commun. 80:923 (1978).
14. M. Fevrier, J. L. Birrien, C. Leclerc, L. Chedid, and P.
    Liacopoulos, *Eur. J. Immunol. 8*:558 (1978).
15. H. Takada, M. Tsujyimoto, S. Kotani, S. Kusumoto, M. Inage,
    T. Shiba, S. Nagao, I. Yano, S. Kawata, and K. Yokogawa,
    Inf. Immun. 25:645 (1979).
16. C. Leclerc, D. Juy and L. Chedid, *Cell. Immunol. 42*:336
    (1979).
17. P. Dukor, L. Tarcsay, and G. Baschang, *Ann. Rep. Med.
    Chem. 14*:146 (1979).
18. F. Audibert, L. Chedid, P. Lefrancier, and J. Choay, *Cell.
    Immunol. 21*:243 (1976).
19. I. Azuma, K. Sugimura, M. Yamawaki, M. Yemiya, S. Kusumoto,
    S. Okada, T. Shiba, and Y. Yamamura, *Inf. Immun. 20*:600
    (1978).
20. I. Azuma, M. Yamawaki, M. Uemiya, I. Saiki, Y. Panio, S.
    Kobayashi, T. Fukuda, I. Imada, and Y. Yamamura, *GANN 76*:
    847 (1979).

21. M. A. Parant, F. M. Audibert, L. A. Chedid, M. R. Level, P. L. Lefrancier, J. P. Choay, and E. Lederer, *Inf. Immun.* *27*:825 (1980).

22. S. Kotani, M. Tsujimoto, T. Okunaga, T. Shiba, S. Kusumoto, M. Inage, A. Inoue, and S. Kano, *Int. J. Immunopharmacol.* *2*:212 (1980).

23. W. A. Siddiqui, D. W. Taylor, S. C. Kan, K. Kramer, S. M. Richmond-Crum, S. Kotani, T. Shiba, and S. Kusumoto, *Bull. W.H.O.* *57*:199 (1979).

24. C. A. McLaughlin, S. M. Schwartzman, B. L. Horner, G. H. Jones, J. C. Moffat, J. J. Nestor, and D. Tegg, *Science 208*: 415 (1980).

25. S. Kotani, Y. Watanabe, T. Shimono, K. Harada, T. Shiba, S. Kusumoto, K. Yokogawa, and M. Taniguchi, *Biken J. 19*:9 (1976).

26. F. Audibert, M. Parant, C. Damais, P. Lefrancier, M. Derrien, J. Choay, and L. Chedid, *Biochem. Biophys. Res. Commun.* *96*:915 (1980).

27. A. Adam, M. Devys, V. Souvannavong, P. Lefrancier, J. Choay, and E. Lederer, *Biochem. Biophys. Res. Commun. 72*: 339 (1976).

28. M. J. Pabst, N. P. Cummings, T. Shiba, S. Kusumoto, and S. Kotani, *Inf. Immun. 29*:617 (1980).

29. M. Parant, C. Damais, F. Audibert, F. Parant, L. Chedid, E. Sache, P. Lefrancier, J. Choay, and E. Lederer, *J. Infect. Dis. 138*:378 (1978).

30. L. Chedid, M. Parant, F. Parant, F. Audibert, P. Lefrancier, J. Choay, and M. Sela, *Proc. Natl. Acad. Sci. U.S.A. 76*: 6557 (1979).

31. E. Mozes, M. Sela, and L. Chedid, *Proc. Natl. Acad. Sci. U.S.A. 77*:4933 (1980).

32. R. Arnon, M. Sela, M. Parant, and L. Chedid, *Proc. Natl. Acad. Sci. U.S.A. 77*:6769 (1980).

33. F. Toullet, F. Audibert, G. A. Voisin, and L. Chedid, *Ann. Immunol. (Inst. Pasteur) 128C*:267 (1977).

34. Y. de Kozak, F. Audibert, B. Thillaye, L. Chedid, and J. P. Faure, *Ann. Immunol. (Inst. Pasteur) 130C*:29 (1979).

35. Y. Nagai, K. Akiyama, K. Suzuki, S. Kotani, Y. Watanabe, T. Shimono, T. Shiba, K. Kusumoto, F. Ikuta, and S. Takeda, *Cell. Immunol. 35*:158 (1978).

36. T. Koga, S. Sakamoto, K. Onoue, S. Kotani, and A. Sumiyoshi, *Arthritis Rheum. 23*:993 (1980).

37. J. Colover, *Br. J. Exp. Pathol. 61*:390 (1980).

38. O. Kohashi, C. M. Pearson, Y. Watanabe, S. Kotani, and T. Koga, *J. Immunol. 116*:1635 (1976).

39. T. Koga, K. Maeda, K. Onoue, K. Kato, and S. Kotani, *Mol. Immunol. 16*:153 (1979).

40. O. Kohashi, S. Kotani, T. Shiba, and A. Ozawa, *Inf. Immun. 26*:690 (1979).

41. S. Nagao and A. Tanaka, *Inf. Immun. 26*:624 (1980).

42. O. Kohashi, A. Tanaka, S. Kotani, T. Shiba, S. Kusumoto, K. Yokogawa, S. Kawata, and A. Ozawa, *Inf. Immun. 29*:70 (1980).

43. K. Maeda, T. Koga, K. Onoue, S. Kotani, and A. Sumiyoshi, *Microbiol. Immunol. 24*:335 (1980).

44. M. Parant, F. Parant, L. Chedid, J. C. Drapier, J. F. Petit, J. Wietzerbin, and E. Lederer, *J. Infect. Dis. 135*:771 (1977).

45. E. E. Ribi, J. L. Cantrell, K. B. Von Eschen, and S. M. Schwartzman, *Cancer Res. 39*:4756 (1979).

46. K. Emori and A. Tanaka, *Inf. Immun. 19*:613 (1978).

47. A. Tanaka and K. Emori, *Am. J. Pathol. 98*:733 (1980).

48. A. Tanaka, S. Nagao, R. Saito, S. Kotani, S. Kusumoto, and T. Shiba, *Biochem. Biophys. Res. Commun. 77*:621 (1977).

49. M. Parant, F. Parant, and L. Chedid, *Proc. Natl. Acad. Sci. U.S.A. 75*:3359 (1978).

50. R. V. Waters and R. W. Ferraresi, *J. Reticuloendothel. Soc. 28*:457 (1980).

51. Y. Yamamoto, S. Nagao, A. Tanaka, T. Koga, and K. Onoue, *Biochem. Biophys. Res. Commun. 80*:923 (1978).

52. A. Adam, V. Souvanavong, and E. Lederer, *Biochem. Biophys. Res. Commun. 85*:684 (1978).

53. A. Tanaka, S. Nagao, K. Imai, and R. Mori, *Microbiol. Immunol. 24*:547 (1980).

54. D. Juy and L. Chedid, *Proc. Natl. Acad. Sci. U.S.A. 72*:4105 (1975).

55. A. Galelli, Y. Le Garrec, L. Chedid, P. Lefrancier, M. Derrien, and M. Level, *Inf. Immun. 28*:1 (1980).

56. T. Taniyama and H. T. Holden, *Cell. Immunol. 48*:369 (1979).

57. J. J. Oppenheim, A. Togawa, L. Chedid, and S. Mizel, *Cell. Immunol. 50*:71 (1980).

58. J. P. Tenu, E. Lederer, and J. F. Petit, *Eur. J. Immunol. 10*:654 (1980).

59. F. G. Staber, R. H. Gisler, G. Schumann, L. Tarcsay, E. Schläfli, and P. Dukor, *Cell. Immunol. 37*:174 (1978).

60. C. A. Dinarello, R. J. Elin, L. Chedid, and S. M. Wolff, *J. Infect. Dis. 138*:760 (1978).

61. S. M. Wahl, L. M. Wahl, J. R. McCarthy, L. Chedid, and S. E. Mergenhagen, *J. Immunol. 122*:2226 (1979).

62. K. Imai, M. Tomioka, S. Nagao, K. Kushima, and A. Tanaka, *Biomed. Res. 1*:300 (1980).

63. J. Hadden, A. Englard, J. R. Sadlik, and E. M. Hadden, *Int. J. Immunopharmacol.* *1*:17 (1979).

64. M. J. Pabst and R. B. Johnston, *J. Exp. Med.* *151*:101 (1980).

65. V. D. Ramanathan, J. Curtis and J. L. Turk, *Inf. Immun.* *29*:30 (1980).

66. S. Kotani, A. Kawasaki, S. Inai, K. Nagaki, M. Matsumoto, T. Shiba, S. Kusumoto, M. Inage, K. Yokogawa, S. Kawata, and A. Inoue, *Int. J. Immunopharmacol.* *2*:213 (1980).

67. J. Rotta, M. Rýc, K. Mašek, and M. Zaoral, *Exp. Cell. Biol.* *47*:258 (1979).

68. S. Kotani, K. Harada, T. Kitaura, T. Shiba, S. Kusumoto, M. Inage, K. Yokogawa, S. Kawata, and A. Inoue, *Int. J. Immunopharmacol.* *2*:213 (1980).

69. B. Heymer, H. Finger, and C. H. Wirsing, *Zeit. Immunität-Forsch.* *155*:87 (1978).

70. H. Ohkuni, Y. Norose, M. Ohta, M. Hayama, Y. Kimura, M. Tsujimoto, S. Kotani, T. Shiba, S. Kusumoto, K. Yokogawa, and S. Kawata, *Inf. Immun.* *24*:313 (1979).

71. T. Kishimoto, Y. Hirai, K. Nakanishi, I. Azuma, A. Nagamatsu, and Y. Yamamura, *J. Immunol.* *123*:2709 (1979).

72. E. Atkins and E. S. Snell, in *The Inflammatory Process* (B. W. Zweifach, L. Grant, and R. T. McCluskey, eds.), Academic, New York, 1965, p. 495.

73. J. Rotta, *Zeit. Immunitätforsch.* *149S*:230 (1975).

74. S. Hamada, T. Narita, S. Kotani, and K. Kato, *Biken J.* *14*:217 (1971).

75. G. Riveau, K. Mašek, M. Parant, and L. Chedid, *J. Exp. Med.* *152*:869 (1980).

76. E. Atkins and W. B. Wood, *J. Exp. Med.* *102*:499 (1955).

77. C. A. Dinarello and S. M. Wolff, *N. Engl. J. Med.* *298*:607 (1978).

78. M. Parant, G. Riveau, F. Parant, C. A. Dinarello, S. M. Wolff, and L. Chedid, *J. Infect. Dis.* *142*:708 (1980).

79. M. Zimecki and D. R. Webb, *J. Immunol.* *117*:2158 (1976).

80. D. R. Webb and I. Nowowiejski, *Cell. Immunol.* *33*:1 (1977).

81. M. Parant, F. Parant, L. Chedid, A. Yapo, J. F. Petit, and E. Lederer, *Int. J. Immunopharmacol.* *1*:35 (1979).

82. M. J. Kluger, in *Thermoregulatory Mechanisms and Their Therapeutic Implications* (B. Cox, P. Lomax, A. S. Milton, and E. Schönbaum, eds.), S. Karger, Basel, 1980, p. 65.

83. A. Lwoff, *Bact. Rev.* *23*:109 (1959).

84. L. Pasteur, *Bull. Soc. Agriculture (France)* *38*:127 (1878).

85. W. W. Reynolds and M. E. Casterlin, in *Thermoregulatory Mechanisms and Their Therapeutic Implications* (B. Cox, P. Lomax, A. S. Milton, and E. Schönbaum, eds.), S. Karger, Basel, 1980, p. 148.

86. L. K. Vaughn, W. L. Veale, and K. E. Cooper, in *Thermo-regulatory Mechanisms and Their Therapeutic Implications* (B. Cox, P. Lomax, A. S. Milton, and E. Schönbaum, eds.), S. Karger, Basel, 1980, p. 115.

87. Letter to the Editor, *Cell. Immunol.* **48**:433 (1979).

88. C. A. Dinarello, *Fed. Proc.* **39**:52 (1979).

89. P. A. Murphy, P. L. Simon, and W. F. Willoughby, *J. Immunol.* **124**:2498 (1980).

90. C. A. Dinarello and L. J. Rosenwasser, in *Advances in Immuno-pharmacology* (J. Hadden, L. Chedid, S. Mullen, and F. Spredfico, eds.), Pergamon, Oxford, 1981, p. 419.

91. D. N. Männel, R. N. Moore, and S. E. Mergenhagen, *Inf. Immun.* **30**:523 (1980).

92. N. Matthews, *Br. J. Cancer* **40**:534 (1979).

93. D. S. Elfenbein, P. A. Murphy, P. J. Chesney, D. S. Y. Seto, and D. H. Carver, *J. Gen. Virol.* **42**:185 (1979).

94. M. J. Kluger, *Fed. Proc.* **39**:30 (1979).

95. M. E. Casterlin and W. W. Reynolds, in *Thermoregulatory Mechanisms and Their Therapeutic Implications* (B. Cox, P. Lomax, A. S. Milton, and E. Schönbaum, eds.), S. Karger, Basel, 1980, p. 152.

9

The Chemistry and Biology of Lipopolysaccharides and Their Lipid A Component

ERNST TH. RIETSCHEL,* CHRIS GALANOS, OTTO LÜDERITZ, and OTTO WESTPHAL   Max-Planck-Institut für Immunbiologie, Freiburg, Federal Republic of Germany

I. Introduction

Lipopolysaccharides (LPS) are characteristic components of the cell envelope of gram-negative bacteria. They are unique to these organisms and have been detected in such phylogenetically remote groups as Enterobacteriaceae, photosynthetic bacteria, and anaerobes (1,2). LPS can be isolated from bacteria in an essentially protein-free and phospholipid-free, i.e., highly pure, form (3,4). With purified LPS preparations it was recognized that LPS represented the *O-antigens* and the *endotoxins* of gram-negative bacteria, and that they are amphipathic molecules endowed with an overwhelming spectrum of biological activities expressed both in vivo and in vitro (5-25). Although individually distinct in their chemical fine structure, LPS derived from distinct groups of gram-negative bacteria are built up according to a common architecture. For an increasing number of LPS the sugar composition and partial structures have been evaluated (summarized in Ref. 26), a prerequisite for investigations concerning mechanisms of their biological effects. Since the lipid component of LPS, i.e., lipid A, has been identified as the endotoxic principle of the molecule (18), recent chemical investigations have concentrated on the structure of lipid A in an attempt to reveal active substructures.

The role of LPS (lipid A) in bacterial virulence and infection (27-32,44), their interaction with humoral and cellular components of the host, and mechanisms of induction of mediators (6,7,9,10,12,16, 18,20-23,25,26,32) represent some of the current fields in endotoxin

---

*Present affiliation: Forschungsinstitut Borstel, Borstel, Federal Republic of Germany.

183

research. Other major topics concern special aspects of biosynthesis
and genetics (33,34), LPS as phage receptors (35,36), the assembly
and organization of the cell wall (24,37,38,246), and others.

The present article will concentrate mainly on some newer aspects
of the chemical structure, physiological function, and biological activity of LPS, with special reference to their lipid A component.

II. Structure and Function of Lipopolysaccharides

Lipopolysaccharides are components of the outer membrane of gram-
negative bacteria. In this membrane they are present exclusively in
the external leaflet (24). Thus, LPS are located on the surface of the
bacterial cell. This exposed position allows the gentle isolation of LPS
from bacteria, and various extraction methods have been developed
(18). Among these, the phenol-water procedure has received wide application for the isolation of purified S form LPS (3). For the isolation
of LPS from R mutants the phenol-chloroform-petroleum ether method
has proven to yield pure and water-soluble preparations (4). It is
emphasized that purified LPS represents an artifact not occurring in
nature as such. Disintegration of bacteria probably leads to water
soluble or insoluble complexes of LPS, proteins, phospholipids, and
other components of the bacterial cell. Such noncovalently bound complexes would represent natural endotoxin. It is obvious, however, that
for compositional and structural investigations the isolation and purification of the individual components of these complexes is a prerequisite.

Chemical analysis on purified preparations reveals that LPS from
different groups of gram-negative bacteria conform to a common structural principle: they consist of a polysaccharide and a covalently
bound lipid component, termed lipid A. The LPS molecule is anchored
to the bacterial cell through its lipid A component. The general architecture of a *Salmonella* LPS is shown in Figure 1. As this schematic
representation shows, the polysaccharide portion is divided into two
subregions, i.e., the O-specific chain and the core oligosaccharide.
These components are under separate genetic control, and distinct
biosynthetic pathways are involved in their assembly (summarized in
Refs. 5, 8, 26, 33, and 34).

III. Polysaccharide Component

A. *O-Specific Chain*

The O-specific chain represents a polymer of oligosaccharide molecules,
the so-called repeating units. The average number of repeating units
(n) in the O-specific chain appears to be on the order of n = 20-35
(Refs. 39-41). However, larger (up to n = 40) and smaller oligomers

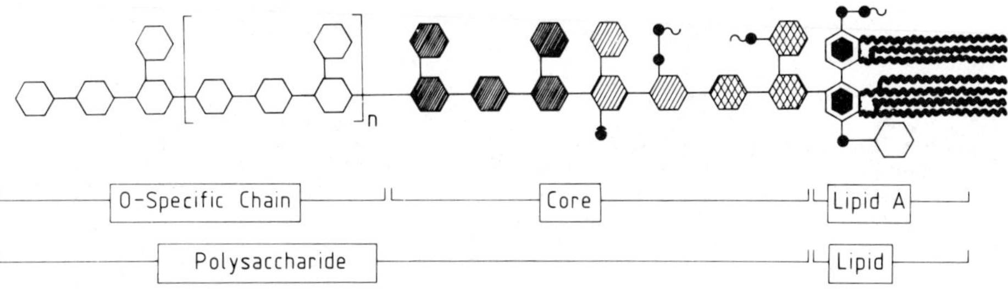

FIG. 1   Schematic structure of a *Salmonella* lipopolysaccharide (32).

also occur. This illustrates that in a given preparation a family of LPS molecules exists which differ in the length of their O-specific chain. The fact that the degree of polymerization of repeating units is not a defined number represents one of the reasons for the intrinsic hetero- geneity of LPS (227). Heterogeneity results also from the fact that, in a given S form preparation, larger amounts of LPS are present which lack the O-specific chain (40,41,227).

A large diversity of the constituent components of repeating units has been revealed within different gram-negative bacteria. These in- clude neutral sugars (hexoses, pentoses, and deoxy- and O-methyl derivatives) and charged sugars (aminohexoses and aminopentoses, hexuronic acids, and hexosaminuronic acids) which may carry a var- iety of substituents such as amino acids, phosphoryl, glyceryl, lactyl, and acetyl groups (reviewed in Refs. 17-19 and 26). Therefore, an immense compositional variability is revealed if the O-specific chains of distinct bacterial origin are compared. However, the nature, sequence, and type of linkage (and type of substitution) of the individual mono- saccharide residues within a repeating unit is characteristic and unique for a given LPS and the parental bacterial strain.

Today a large number of structures of O-specific chains are known in detail (reviewed in Ref. 26). As an example, Figure 2 shows the chemical structure of the O-specific chain of LPS from *Salmonella typhimurium*. It is made up of a branched pentasaccharide consisting of 2-O-acetyl-D-abequose, D-mannose, L-rhamnose, D-galactose, and D-glucose in the linkages indicated.

In nonencapsulated gram-negative bacteria such as *Salmonella*, the O-specific chain represents one of the exposed surface structures of the bacterial cell. In this position the O-specific chain plays an

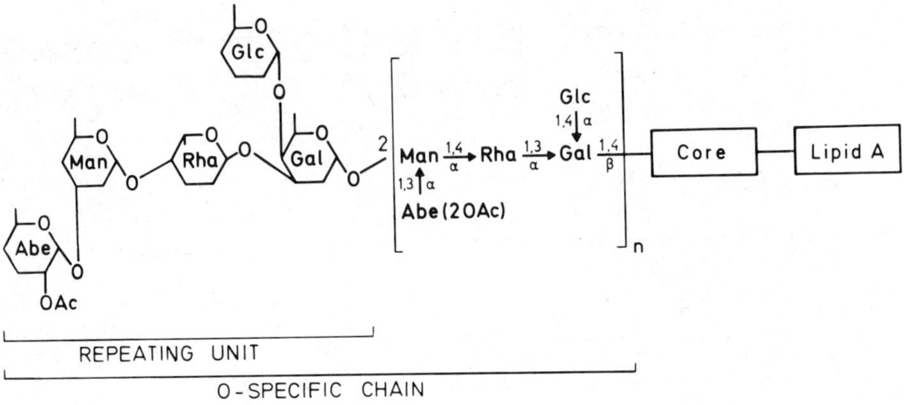

FIG. 2   Structure of the repeating unit (O-specific chain) of lipopolysaccharide from *Salmonella typhimurium* (80,205-207). Abe = D-abe-
quose, Man = D-mannose, Rha = L-rhamnose, Glc = D-glucose, Gal =
D-galactose, Ac = acetyl.

essential role in the interaction of bacteria with their environment.
Thus, it is likely that the O-specific chain protects gram-negative
bacteria from phagocytosis and killing (30,43,242). This is suggested
by the fact that R mutants have rarely been isolated from natural
sources (for exceptions, see Refs. 2, 235, and 236), indicating that in
a natural environment they are eliminated, i.e., that they cannot re-
pulse the attack of amoebae and that of cells of the host's immune system (42,43). Hence, the O-specific chain is important for the survival
of bacteria in vivo and has been considered a significant determinant
in bacterial virulence (27,44,241). It is not necessary, however, for
the survival, i.e., for the growth and division of gram-negative bacteria in vitro. This is indicated by the isolation in the laboratory of
R mutants which synthesize LPS lacking the O-specific chain.

On the other hand the O-specific chain has been recognized as the
carrier of immunodominant structures (O factors) against which the
host's immune system produces specific antibodies. In the O-specific
chain, therefore, determinants are embedded for immunoglobulins
which may promote the elimination of bacteria by phagocytes of the
host's defense system. It is the O-specific chain which is responsible
for the O-antigenic properties of LPS (26).

Furthermore, the O-specific chain represents the receptor for
certain (lysogenic) bacteriophages—a topic excellently reviewed in
Refs. 35 and 36.

A number of other biological activities of LPS are believed to be
mediated by the polysaccharide component. Since in these cases the
contribution of both the O-specific chain and the core, respectively,

have not yet been determined, these activities will be only briefly
discussed below (see Sec. VIII).

B. Core Oligosaccharide

The chemical structure of the *Salmonella* core oligosaccharide (Ra
core) is shown in Figure 3. It is made up of a branched undecasaccha-
ride which in its outer region (O chain proximal portion) contains a
hexose pentasaccharide. The lipid A proximal region (inner core) consists of branched trisaccharides of L-glycero-D-mannoheptose [L,D-
heptose (Hep)] and 3-deoxy-D-mannooctulosonic acid [dOclA, formerly
termed KDO (2-keto-3-deoxyoctonate)]. These trisaccharides are substituted by ionic groups such as phosphoryl, phosphorylethanolamine,
and pyrophosphorylethanolamine residues. These charged substituents
are not always present in molar amounts and, thus, a certain structural microheterogeneity of the core oligosaccharide is generated. The
genetics and biosynthesis of the *Salmonella* core has been elucidated
and reviewed (26,34,45). For the role of the core oligosaccharide as an
R-antigen and as a receptor for bacteriophages, see Refs. 14, 18, 19,
26, 35, and 36.

In LPS of all *Salmonella* species studied, the core oligosaccharides
are either identical or closely related in structure (18). In other enterobacterial genera, however, structurally distinct core types exist
(*Shigella, Citrobacter, Arizona,* and *Proteus*; for literature see Refs.
14, 17-19, and 26). Furthermore, several core types may be present
within one genus. This is the case, for example, in *Escherichia coli,*
where up to five different core structures (R_1 to R_4 and K-12) have
now been identified (Fig. 4). Although these core types differ from
each other (and from the *Salmonella* core) in their fine structure, they
nevertheless exhibit a common general architecture. In all cases, the
outer core region consists of a branched hexose pentasaccharide and
the inner core region contains phosphorylated Hep and dOclA.

In other bacterial groups (e.g., *Pseudomonas, Bacteroides,* and
Xanthomonas) structurally distinct core types are present which may
lack either heptose, or dOclA or both of these monosaccharides (for
literature see Refs. 17, 18, and 26). Evidently also a certain structural variability in the core oligosaccharides is recognized if LPS of different origin are compared. In contrast to the excessive structural
diversity of O-specific chains, however, the variability of the core
oligosaccharide appears to be much more limited.

Since R mutants are known which form LPS lacking the hexose pentasaccharide and heptose (Re mutants), the outer core region is dispensable for growth and division of the bacterial cell. Viable enterobacterial R mutants, the LPS of which is devoid of dOclA, have not
been isolated, and it appears that the innermost portion of the core

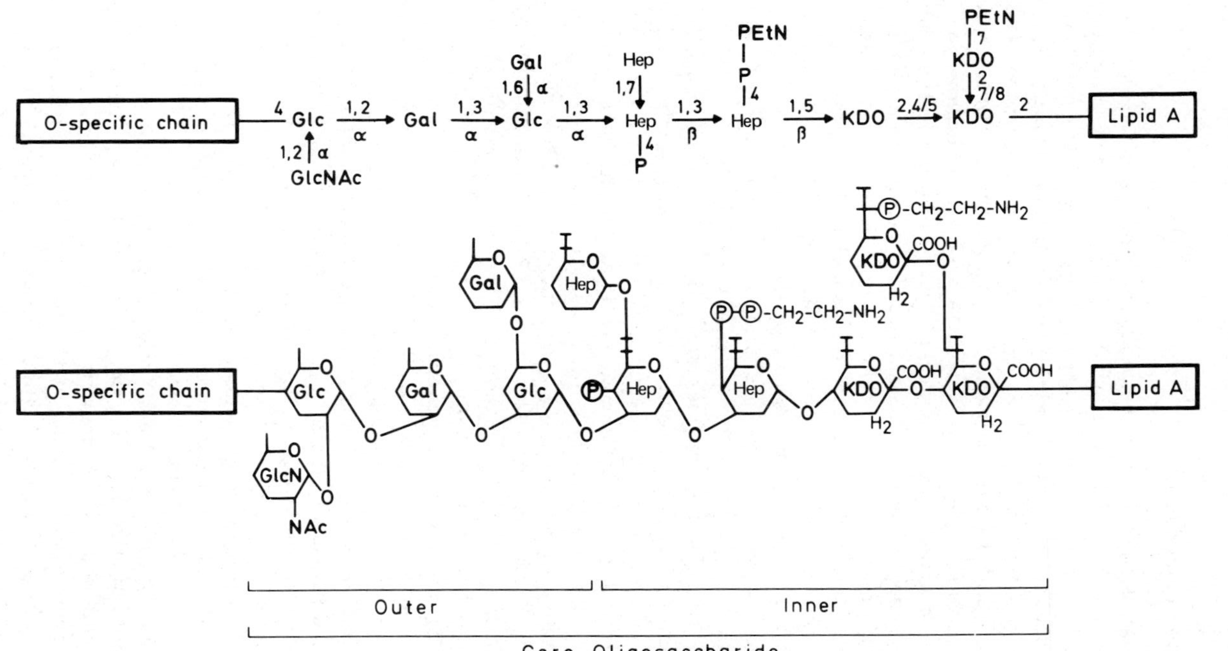

FIG. 3 Structure of the core oligosaccharide of lipopolysaccharides from *Salmonella* (18,26, 205,208,209). GlcN = D-glucosamine, β-Hep = β-L-D-Hep = L-α-D-Hep (L-glycero-α-D-mannoheptose, KDO = 2-keto-3-deoxyoctonate (dOclA), P = phosphate.

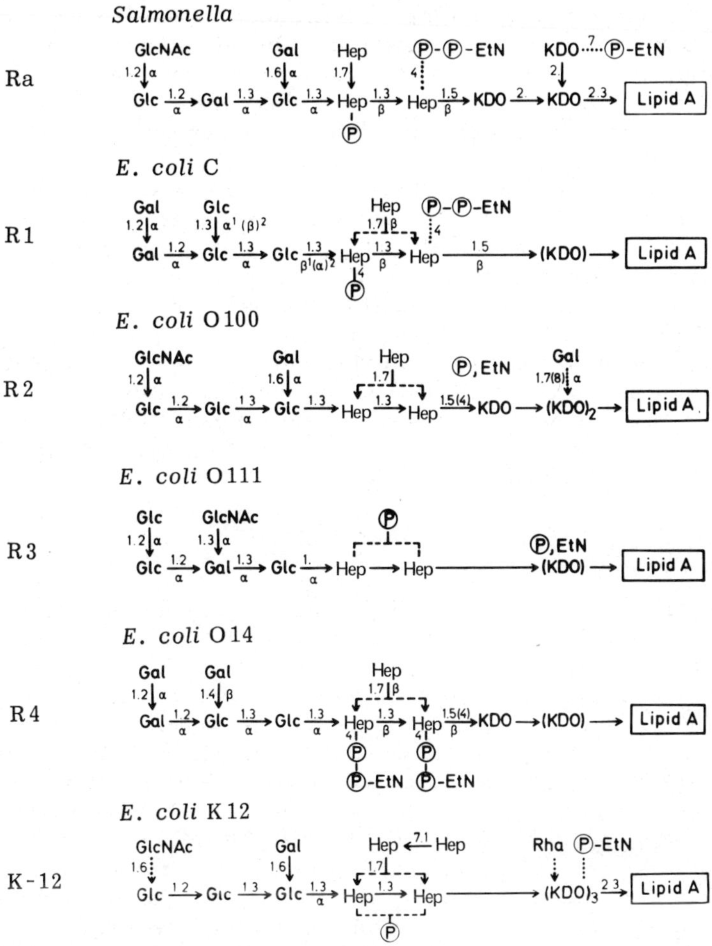

Salmonella

Ra

    GlcNAc   Gal   Hep P-P-EtN   KDO···^{7}···P-EtN
    1.2↓α   1.6↓α 1.7↓   4┊   2↓
    Glc $\xrightarrow[\alpha]{1.2}$ Gal $\xrightarrow[\alpha]{1.3}$ Glc $\xrightarrow[\alpha]{1.3}$ Hep $\xrightarrow[\beta]{1.3}$ Hep $\xrightarrow[\beta]{1.5}$ KDO $\xrightarrow{2}$ KDO $\xrightarrow{2.3}$ | Lipid A |
                                     ┊
                                     P

E. coli C

R1

    Gal   Glc   Hep P-P-EtN
    1.2↓α   1.3↓α^1 (β)^2 1.7↓β   ┊4
    Gal $\xrightarrow[\alpha]{1.2}$ Glc $\xrightarrow[\alpha]{1.3}$ Glc $\xrightarrow[\beta^1(\alpha)^2]{1.3}$ Hep $\xrightarrow[\beta]{1.3}$ Hep $\xrightarrow[\beta]{1.5}$ (KDO) → | Lipid A |
                                     ┊4
                                     P

E. coli O100

R2

    GlcNAc   Gal   Hep P,EtN   Gal
    1.2↓α   1.6↓α   1.7↓   1.7(8)↓α
    Glc $\xrightarrow[\alpha]{1.2}$ Glc $\xrightarrow[\alpha]{1.3}$ Glc $\xrightarrow{1.3}$ Hep $\xrightarrow{1.3}$ Hep $\xrightarrow{1.5(4)}$ KDO → (KDO)$_2$ → | Lipid A |

E. coli O111

R3

    Glc   GlcNAc P
    1.2↓α   1.3↓α   ┊
    Glc $\xrightarrow[\alpha]{1.2}$ Gal $\xrightarrow[\alpha]{1.3}$ Glc $\xrightarrow{1.}$ Hep → Hep P,EtN
                                                                                            → (KDO) → | Lipid A |

E. coli O14

R4

    Gal   Gal   Hep
    1.2↓α   1.4↓β   1.7↓β
    Gal $\xrightarrow[\alpha]{1.2}$ Glc $\xrightarrow[\alpha]{1.3}$ Glc $\xrightarrow[\alpha]{1.3}$ Hep $\xrightarrow[\beta]{1.3}$ Hep $\xrightarrow[\beta]{1.5(4)}$ KDO → (KDO) → | Lipid A |
                                     4↓   4↓
                                     P P
                                     P-EtN P-EtN

E. coli K12

K-12

    GlcNAc   Gal   Hep ←$^{7.1}$ Hep   Rha P-EtN
    1.6┊   1.6↓   1.7↓   ┊   ┊
    Glc $\xrightarrow{1.2}$ Glc $\xrightarrow{1.3}$ Glc $\xrightarrow[\alpha]{1.3}$ Hep $\xrightarrow{1.3}$ Hep   → (KDO)$_3$ $\xrightarrow{2.3}$ | Lipid A |
                                     ┊
                                     P

FIG. 4 Structure of core oligosaccharides of enterobacterial lipopolysaccharides (261). For designations of sugars, see Figs. 2 and 3.
References: Ra (18,26,205,208,209), R$_1$ (210,211 linkages[1], 212 linkages[2], R$_2$ (213), R$_3$ (214,215), R$_4$ (216), K-12 (217,218).

(together with lipid A) plays a vital role in the structural and functional integrity of the bacterial cell (see also Sec. VI).

The innermost core region of enterobacterial LPS is characterized
by an accumulation of charged groups (phosphoryl, carboxyl, and
amino groups), and there is evidence that some of the physiological
functions of LPS are mediated through polar residues of the core region. Thus, it has been demonstrated that in *S. typhimurium* LPS the

dOclA trisaccharide represents a high affinity binding site for Ca^{2+} and Mg^{2+}. Phosphoryl residues were shown to be an additional, low affinity binding site for these ions (46). Bivalent cations are known to be essential for the optimal function of several enzymes and for the structural organization of membranes. It therefore appears that the innermost core region, by interacting with Ca^{2+} and Mg^{2+} and thereby disposing a high concentration of bivalent cations in the close environment of the cell surface, plays an essential role in the assembly as well as the structural and functional integrity of the outer membrane.

LPS from a number of different gram-negative bacteria, however, lack dOclA (18). In LPS of **Vibrio cholerae** strains, probably fructose (47,100) or D-seduheptulose [D-altro-2-heptulose (48)] provide the connecting link between the polysaccharide and the lipid A component. Unfortunately, structural details of the core oligosaccharide of these **Vibrio** strains have not yet been revealed, and further studies are required to elucidate the physiological significance of the replacement of dOclA by noncharged ketoses.

IV. Lipid A Component

In enterobacterial and most other LPS studied so far, the polysaccharide portion is bound to lipid A through a ketosidic linkage. Ketosidic bonds are known to be highly susceptible to acid hydrolysis and, hence, free lipid A may be obtained by treatment of LPS with mild acid (18). Acid hydrolysis must be used, since enzymes which cleave this linkage (but see Ref. 238) or mutants which synthesize polysaccharide-free lipid A are so far unknown. (For the genetics, biosynthesis of lipid A and its role as a carrier in the biosynthesis of the core oligosaccharide, see Refs. 5, 8, 18, 26, 33, 34, 226, 246).

In the present paper the bound lipid moiety of LPS from gram-negative bacteria is called lipid A. On the other hand, the lipoidal precipitate obtained after treatment of LPS with acid is termed free lipid A (49,50). As will be shown below, lipid A of different bacterial origin are chemically related but also exhibit compositional and structural differences among each other. Therefore, the term lipid A is used in a similar fashion as the term phospholipid: it designates a family of gram-negative bacterial lipids which are similar in their general architecture but which show differences in their fine structure.

A. *Salmonella Lipid A*

Previous structural studies performed on both lipid A (as it is present in LPS) as well as on free (isolated) lipid A revealed that lipid A represents an unusual phospholipid which, in general, consists of D-glucosamine, phosphate, and long chain nonhydroxylated as well as hydroxylated fatty acids (51). The lipid A component of **Salmonella** has

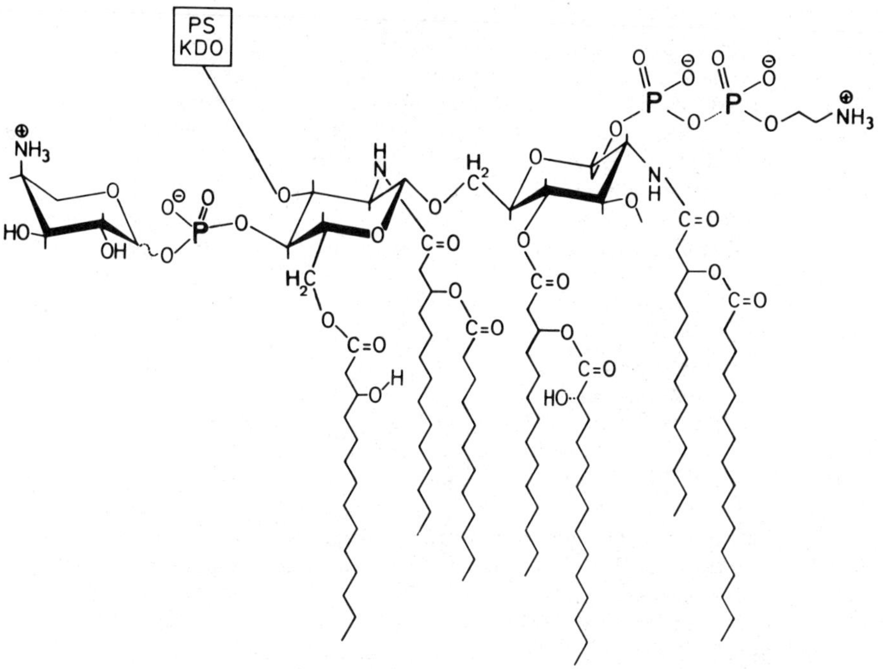

FIG. 5   Proposed structure of lipid A of *Salmonella* lipopolysaccharides. Shown is the tentative *Salmonella* lipid A structure with the
attached polysaccharide (PS) component. The exact position of the
two ester-bound 3-hydroxytetradecanoic acid residues has not yet
been determined. Also unknown is the distribution of dodecanoic and
hexadecanoic acids over the 3-hydroxyl groups of amide-bound 3-
hydroxytetradecanoic acid (56,97). For other details, see Section 4.1.

been studied in some detail, and Figure 5 shows the chemical structure
of *Salmonella* lipid A according to our present knowledge. This structure will serve as a basis relative to which structural features of other
lipid A's will be discussed.

The saccharide backbone of *Salmonella* lipid A consists of a β1.6-
linked D-glucosamine disaccharide (Refs. 52 and 53 and Fig. 5). The
pyranose form of the nonreducing D-glucosamine residue (GlcN II) has
been established; that of the reducing glucosaminyl group (GlcN I),
however, is not proven. The glucosamine disaccharide carries phosphate residues in positions 1 and 4' (54). In the present paper the
diphosphorylated β1.6-linked D-glucosamine disaccharide is referred
to as the lipid A backbone. This hydrophilic lipid A backbone carries
a number of substituents.

The ester-bound phosphoryl residue at position 4' of GlcN II is partially (30-60%) substituted by a 4-amino-4-deoxy-L-arabinosyl residue (4-AraN) (50,55). At present it is not known whether 4-AraN is present in the pyranose (as shown) or in the furanose form. Since after deamination of *Salmonella* LPS, 4-AraN is no longer detectable, it is assumed that it possesses the pyranose ring structure (64). Furthermore, it is not known whether 4-AraN is bound as the α or β anomer. On treatment of LPS with alkali, 4-AraN-phosphate is released probably through the formation of a cyclic phosphate involving the 2 hydroxyl group of the aminopentose. If L-4-AraN is present as the C1 conformer (hydroxyl group at C_2 = equatorial), both the α and β form of the 4-aminoarabinosyl-1-phosphoryl residue would be expected to form a five-membered 4-AraN cyclic phosphate [methyl α(or β)-L-arabinopyranoside possesses the C1 ring conformation (57,257)]. If L-4-AraN-1-P would have the 1C conformation (hydroxyl group at C_2 = axial) only the β anomer would undergo phosphate cyclisation (58). Since, however, the conformation of LPS-bound L-4-AraN is unknown, its anomeric form remains to be established. The hydroxyl and amino functions of 4-AraN appear to be nonsubstituted, although L-4-AraN as present in LPS is, for unknown reasons, resistant to periodate oxidation (62,63,64,98).

The glycosidic hydroxyl group of the glucosamine disaccharide of lipid A carries a phosphate residue, and also here it is not known whether the reducing D-glucosaminyl residue (GlcN I) is present as the α or β anomer. Other naturally occurring D-hexosamine-1-phosphates always possess the α configuration, and it appears likely that this is also the case in lipid A. Proof for this assumption however, is lacking. The C_1-phosphate group is partially (40-50%) substituted by a phosphorylethanolamine residue, the amino group of which is not substituted (55).

Lipid A of a polymyxin-resistant *S. typhimurium* mutant (*pmrA*) has been shown to be altered in the substitution of phosphate group(s) (34,244). Recently, these substituents could be identified as phosphorylethanolamine and 4-aminoarabinose, the latter being bound to the phosphate group of GlcN II (252).

In free lipid A the hydroxyl group at position 3' (GlcN II) of the disaccharide is free since it represents the attachment site of the polysaccharide portion (dOclA) in intact LPS (54).

Each of the two amino groups of the central glucosamine disaccharide is acylated with a D-3-hydroxytetradecanoic [(R)-3-hydroxytetradecanoic, β-hydroxymyristic, 3-OH-14:0)] acid residue. Furthermore, approximately 1 mol (per GlcN disaccharide) of dodecanoic (12:0), hexadecanoic (16:0), and D-3-hydroxytetradecanoic acid are present in ester linkage (56). In addition, 1 mol of D-3-hydroxytetradecanoic acid which is 3-0-acylated with tetradecanoic (14:0) and, to a smaller extent, with L-2-hydroxytetradecanoic acid (α-hydroxymyristic,

2-OH-14:0), is ester bound. In most preparations tested, the sum of 14:0 and 2-OH-14:0 equals 1 mol eq (78). Thus, approximately 5 mol of ester-bound and 2 mol of amide-bound fatty acids are present (per 2 mol GlcN). *Salmonella* lipid A (Fig. 5), therefore, contains a total of 7 mol of fatty acids [and not 6 as described previously (56)].

Little is known about the exact location of ester-bound fatty acids in *Salmonella* lipid A. It had previously been assumed that these fatty acids are bound to available hydroxyl groups of the backbone disaccharide (56). Recently, however, it was found that the 3-hydroxyl groups of amide-bound 3-hydroxytetradecanoic acids are acylated (50,96). Therefore, ester-bound fatty acids in lipid A may be linked to hydroxyl groups present on the glucosamine disaccharide and on the amide-bound 3-hydroxy fatty acids. Very recent experiments performed in our laboratory revealed that 12:0 and 16:0 are linked to hydroxyl groups of amide-bound 3-hydroxytetradecanoic acid (97). It is presently unknown whether 12:0 and 16:0 are each linked to a defined amide-bound 3-hydroxytetradecanoyl group or whether they are distributed randomly over the two available hydroxyl functions of the N-acyl residues. Furthermore, it has yet to be determined whether only a part or the total amount of 12:0 and 16:0 present in *Salmonella* lipid A is involved in this type of linkage. If the 3-hydroxyl groups of amide bound 3-hydroxytetradecanoic acids would be quantitatively acylated by 12:0 and 16:0, it would follow that the lipid A glucosamine backbone is exclusively acylated by 4 mol of 3-hydroxytetradecanoic acid residues: 2 mol in amide linkage and 2 mol bound to hydroxyl groups. Since, according to our present knowledge, 3 hydroxyl groups are available (at C_3 and C_4 of GlcN I and at C'_6 of GlcN II), it would further follow that 1 hydroxyl function of the lipid A backbone is not acylated.

In *Salmonella* lipid A, three structural elements can be defined: (1) the phosphorylated glucosamine backbone, (2) the substituents of the backbone phosphate residues (polar head groups), and (3) the fatty acids. In the following, our present knowledge on these structural parts in lipid A of other gram-negative bacteria will be summarized.

B. Lipid A Backbone

1. Salmonella-like lipid A's   Sequential chemical degradation of *Salmonella* LPS and free lipid A allows the isolation of the lipid A backbone. By enzymatic, physicochemical, and chemical analysis, notably, combined gas-liquid chromatography-mass spectrometry (53,59), it was shown to consist of a diphosphorylated β1,6-linked D-glucosamine disaccharide. The degradation procedure combined with methylation analysis was applied to LPS of a range of gram-negative bacteria, and in all strains investigated (Fig. 6), a β1,6-linked D-glucosamine disaccharide which carries an ester-bound phosphate group (in

Salmonella (54) and *E. coli* K-12 (60) at C'_4 of GlcN II) and a glycosidic phosphate residue (C_1 of GlcN I) were identified. Other laboratories showed this structural principle to be present in lipid A of
Pseudomonas aeruginosa, Shigella sonnei, Serratia marcescens, Sele-
nomonas ruminantium, and *Rhodospirillum tenue* (for literature, see
the legend of Fig. 6). In the latter strain, an additional (nonacylated)
glucosaminyl residue is bound to C_4 of GlcN I (61).

These results show that the diphosphorylated β1,6-linked D-
glucosamine disaccharide is found in lipid A of bacterial families and
orders which are taxonomically quite remote. Hence, this structure
represents a common, ubiquitous, and nonvariable structural element
in lipid A of different origin. D-glucosamine disaccharides (N-acetyl
derivatives) with a β-glycosidic linkage are present in other natural
molecules such as glycoproteins (76), the bacterial murein (229), and
chitin. In these cases, however, the disaccharide linkage is 1,4. To
our knowledge, β1,6-linked glucosamine units have not been found in
other natural substances, and consequently, this structure appears to
be a unique and characteristic component of lipid A.

2. **Other Lipid A's**   Some groups of bacteria have, however, been encountered where the lipid A structure is distinct from that found in
Salmonella. These groups include *Rhodopseudomonas viridis, Rhodo-*
pseudomonas palustris, Rhodopseudomonas sulfoviridis (2), *Pseudo-*
monas diminuta, and *Pseudomonas vesicularis* (62). In these cases, a
phosphorylated GlcN disaccharide is absent from lipid A. Instead, a
(N-acylated)2,3-diamino-2,3-dideoxy-D-glucose (3-amino-D-glucosa-
mine) which is not phosphorylated is present. Very recently, the lipid
A component of *Chromatium vinosum, Thiocapsa roseopersicina,* and
Rhodomicrobium vaniellii was shown to be devoid of phosphate residues
(2).

C. *Substituents of the Phosphate Groups of the Lipid A Backbone*

Studies on the lipid A component of *Chromobacterium violaceum* had revealed that both the nonglycosidic (of GlcN II) and the glycosidic (of
GlcN I) phosphoryl groups of the backbone are substituted (63). Subsequent investigations in our and other laboratories showed that phosphate substitution may also occur in the lipid A of other gram-negative
bacteria. In Table 1 the nature of substituents identified so far is
shown. The ester-bound phosphate group (at C'_4 in *Salmonella* and *E.*
coli) carries a 4-amino-4-deoxy-L-arabinosyl residue in lipid A of *C.*
violaceum (63), *Proteus mirabilis* (64), *Rhodospirillum tenue* (61),
Yersinia enterocolitica (65), and *Salmonella minnesota* (50,55). In the
latter two cases, 4-AraN is not present in molar amounts. No substitution of the ester phosphate was found in *E. coli* (60) and *V. cholerae*
(66). Up to now, therefore, only one type of group (4-AraN) has been
identified as a substituent of the phosphate group at GlcN II.

Salmonella spp	S,Re
Escherichia coli	S,Ra,Re
Shigella flexneri (sonnei)	S,Re
Serratia marcescens	S
Proteus mirabilis	S,Re
Yersinia enterocolitica	S,Re
Pseudomonas alcaligenes	S
Pseudomonas aeruginosa	S
Xanthomonas sinensis	S
Chromobacterium violaceum	S
Rhodopseudomonas gelatinosa	S
Rhodospirillum tenue	S
Fusobacterium nucleatum	S
Selenomonas ruminantium	S
Aeromonas liquefaciens	S
Rhizobium trifolii	S
Vibrio cholerae	R

FIG. 6   Bacteria containing a diphosphorylated β1.6-linked D-gluco-
samin disaccharide as the lipid a backbone. The position of the ester-
bound phosphoryl residue has only been established in *Salmonella
minnesota* (54) and *E. coli* K-12 (60). S = LPS of wild type bacteria
(S form); Ra, Re = LPS of rough mutant bacteria (R form). References:
Salmonella (52,53,251), *E. coli* (53,60), *S. flexneri* (53), *S. sonnei*
(202), *S. marcescens* (219), *P. mirabilis* (64), *Y. enterocolitica* (65),
P. aeruginosa (220), *X. sinensis* (53), *C. violaceum* (63), *R. gelatinosa* (53), *R. tenue* (61), *F. nucleatum* (203), *S. ruminantium* (221),
A. liquefaciens (222), *R. trifolii* (85), *V. cholerae* (66).

Different types of residues, however, were found to be linked to
the phosphoryl group in the glycosidic position. These include phosphate [*E. coli* K-12 (60)], phosphorylethanolamine [*S. minnesota* (55),
V. cholerae (66)], D-glucosamine [*C. violaceum* (63)], and furano-
sidic D-arabinose [*R. tenue* (61)]. In the two latter cases, D-GlcN and
D-Ara(f) are linked to phosphate through their glycosidic hydroxyl
function. Thus, nonreducing structures are formed. Also, the groups
substituting the C_1 phosphate may not be present in molar amounts as
is the case in *Salmonella* and *E. coli* K-12. No substitution of the glycosyl phosphate group was found, for example, in *P. mirabilis* (64)
and *Y. enterocolitica* (65).

Therefore, with regard to the presence and nature of phosphate
substituents, a certain variability is noted if lipid A structures of

TABLE 1   Nature of Substituents of Lipid A Phosphate Groups

| Lipid A | Substituent[a] of phosphate group at | | References |
	C'_4[b] (GlcN II)	C_1 (GlcN I)	
Escherichia coli K-12	—	P[a]	60
Vibrio cholerae	—	PETN	66
Yersinia entero- colitica	L-4-AraN[c]	—	65
Proteus mirabilis	L-4-AraN	—	64
Salmonella minnesota	L-4-AraN[c]	PETN[c]	50,55
Chromobacterium violaceum	L-4-AraN	D-GlcN	63
Rhodospirillum tenue	L-4-AraN	D-Ara$_{(f)}$	61

[a]L-4-AraN = 4-amino-4-deoxy-L-arabinose; P = phosphate; PETN = phosphorylethanolamine; D-GlcN = 2-amino-2-deoxy-D-glucose; D-Ara(f) = D-arabinofuranoside.

[b]The C'_4 position of this phosphate group is established only in *Salmonella* (54) and *E. coli* K-12 (60).

[c]Not present in molar amounts.

various origins are compared. It should be emphasized again that, in a number of cases, the substitution of phosphoryl residues is not quantitative. This shows that lipid A, as it is present in intact LPS, exhibits an intrinsic heterogeneity. Since the degree of substitution appears to be influenced by the growth conditions (67,68), it is possible that bacteria depending on their physiological demands are able to add (or omit) ionic headgroups and thereby regulate their surface charge (55).

It has occasionally been postulated that lipid A units (as shown in Fig. 5) are interlinked by phosphodiester or pyrophosphate linkages to form polymeric structures. In recent studies involving ^{31}P nuclear magnetic resonance, however, such phosphate bridges could be ruled out for lipid A of *Salmonella* (55) and *E. coli* K-12 (69). Furthermore, polymer formation involving (pyro) phosphate linkages is not possible

in lipid A's where one or both of the backbone's phosphate groups are
quantitatively substituted (*C. violaceum, R. tenue, P. mirabilis,*
and *V. cholerae*). It is, therefore, concluded that in the lipid A preparations studied, (pyro)phosphate bridges interlinking lipid A units
do not exist.

D. Fatty Acids

Long chain (C10-C18) nonhydroxylated and (2- and 3-) hydroxylated
fatty acids confer to lipid A its hydrophobic character. Among these,
unsaturated and cyclopropane fatty acids have not been encountered
in significant quantities (but see Sec. IV.D.2). In lipid A's of distinct
origin, fatty acids are, in general, present in both ester and amide
linkage (237).

1. Amide (N) bound Fatty Acids Systematic studies performed on a
range of LPS and free lipid A preparations have shown that the amino
groups of the hexosamine backbone are acylated by D-3-hydroxy fatty
acids. This was previously concluded from fatty acid analyses of deesterified LPS and free lipid A (18). Direct evidence for an involvement of 3-hydroxy fatty acids in amide linkage was obtained by combined gas-liquid chromatography-mass spectrometry analysis of partially degraded and permethylated lipid A fractions of *C. violaceum*
(63) and *R. tenue* (61). The recent application of specific amidases
(isolated from *Dictyostelium discoideum*) to O-deacylated LPS of *E. coli*
K-12 (70) has confirmed the previous notion that in *E. coli,* as in other
Enterobacteriaceae, 3-hydroxytetradecanoic acid is linked to the amino
groups of the backbone.

   Table 2 shows examples of bacterial groups where the nature of
amide-linked 3-hydroxy fatty acids has been elucidated. It is obvious
that, depending on the bacterial strain, the chain length of amide
linked 3-hydroxy fatty acids may vary. Thus, the following groups
contain the following acids: *R. tenue* and *R. gelatinosa,* 3-hydroxy-
decanoic acid; *Pseudomonadaceae,* 3-hydroxydodecanoic acid / Enterobacteriaceae and *V. cholerae,* 3-hydroxytetradecanoic acid; *Fusobac-
terium nucleatum,* 3-hydroxyhexadecanoic acid. In contrast to these
bacteria which contain only one type of 3-hydroxy fatty acid in the
lipid A component, others, for example, *Xanthomonas sinensis* (71),
Myxococcus fulvus (72), and *Rhizobium trifolii* (73), contain two types
of N-3-hydroxyacyl residues. It is not known at present whether within one lipid A molecule each of these two 3-hydroxy fatty acids is bound
to a defined glucosaminyl residue, or whether they are distributed
statistically over the available amino groups. An even more complex
situation is found in lipid A of *Bacteroides fragilis* (74,107) and *Bru-
cella* (75,228), where three to four distinct D-3-hydroxy fatty acids
were found as N-acyl residues. A unique pattern of N-acyl residues
was identified in *Vibrio anguillarum* (99) and *Rhodopseudomonas*

TABLE 2   Amide-bound Fatty Acids in Lipid A of Various Gram-negative Bacteria

Lipid A	N-acyl Residue	References
Rhodospirillum tenue	D-3-OH-10:0	2
Rhodopseudomonas gelatinosa		2
Pseudomonas aeruginosa	D-3-OH-12:0	17
Chromobacterium violaceum		63
Escherichia coli		17,18,60
Salmonella spp.		17,18,56
Shigella flexneri		17,18
Shigella sonnei	D-3-OH-14:0	202
Klebsiella pneumoniae		17,18
Proteus mirabilis		64,82
Yersinia enterocolitica		65
Rhodopseudomonas viridis		2
Fusobacterium nucleatum	D-3-OH-16:0	203
Rhizobium trifolii	D-3-OH-16:0 D-3-OH-18:0	73
Xanthomonas sinensis	D-3-OH-12:0 D-3-OH-11-Me-12:0	71
Bacteroides fragilis	D-3-OH-16:0 D-3-OH-15-Me-16:0 D-3-OH-17:0	74

Source: Ref. 16.

sphaeroides ATCC 17023 (156). In the lipid A component of these strains, 3-oxotetradecanoic acid (besides 3-hydroxytetradecanoic acid) was found to be amide linked.

Among the lipid A acyl groups, D-3-hydroxy fatty acids are common and prominent (as a rule approximately 65% of total fatty acids). Since they are, in general, missing in other lipids of gram-negative bacteria (for exceptions, see Ref. 18), D-3-hydroxy fatty acids are characteristic for lipid A (123). Their estimation, therefore, represents a useful tool in the detection and quantitation of LPS (lipid A) in bacteria, physiological fluids, and other inorganic or organic material (77,256).

2. **Ester (O)bound Fatty Acids**   On comparison of lipid A's of different origin, a large diversity of ester-bound fatty acids is found. These include nonhydroxylated and D-3-hydroxy fatty acids (both

types saturated, even-numbered, iso- or anteisobranched). In some
bacteria L-2-hydroxy fatty acids are found (for a summary, see Ref.
78). In a LPS-associated lipid component of *Bordetella pertussis* (Ref.
79, "lipid X"), 2-methyl-3-hydroxy fatty acids were identified (for
summary see Refs. 17 and 18). It should be noted that the lipid A
fatty acid spectrum (O- and N-acyl groups) is a rather constant and
characteristic feature of a bacterial family or, in some cases, even of
a genus (80). Since the fatty acid composition of lipid A is largely independent of culture conditions and other external factors (but see
Ref. 221 and below) it appears that its analysis may provide important
information as to the taxonomic position of a bacterial strain (80,81).

Changes of the lipid A fatty acid pattern have, however, been
noted after cultivation of bacteria at low temperature. These changes
relate to O-acyl residues. In *P. mirabilis* it was found that LPS derived from cells grown at 15°C contained larger amounts of hexade-
cenoic acid (palmitoleic, 16:1) and smaller amounts of hexadecanoic
acid as compared with lipid A from bacteria cultivated at 37°C (82).
Also, in *E. coli* K-12 grown at 12°C, significant amounts of 16:1
(which is absent from LPS of cells grown at 37°C) were identified (83).
The same was recently found to be true for *Salmonella* R mutant bacteria (84). LPS from *S. typhimurium* R strains (Ra, Rb_2, and Rd)
which were grown at 12°C contained high amounts (1-2 µmol/mg) of
Δ^g-cis-hexadecenoic acid. As in *E. coli* K-12, this unsaturated fatty
acid was completely absent from LPS of *Salmonella* strains grown at
30, 37, and 43°C (34). In contrast to LPS from cells cultivated at
these higher temperatures, the LPS of bacteria grown at 12° was
largely devoid of 12:0. In all cases studied so far, the amount of 3-
OH-14:0 present in LPS was unaffected by the growth temperature.

The incorporation of unsaturated fatty acids into lipid A is believed to reflect the need of the bacterial cell to maintain a certain
fluidity of the outer membrane. This fluidity is, in general, regulated
by phospholipids, the fatty acid composition of which is greatly dependent on external factors such as growth temperature. At extremely
low temperatures (<15°C), lipid A also seems to participate in the
maintenance of correct membrane fluidity (83,253).

As was first noted in LPS of *Salmonella* (56), part of the ester-
bound 3-hydroxy fatty acids may be 3-O-acylated by other fatty acids.
In recent years, ester-bound 3-acyloxyacyl residues have been encountered in LPS of several bacterial groups. Figure 7 summarizes
some of the structures identified. But a number of bacterial strains are
known where an ester-bound 3-acyloxyacyl group is absent from lipid
A. The latter include *M. fulvus* (72), *C. violaceum* (63), *X. sinensis*
(71), *B. pertussis* (79), *R. trifolii* (85), and others.

The location of ester-bound fatty acids in lipid A has not been
studied systematically, i.e., it is not known whether one fatty acid is
bound to a defined hydroxyl group or whether ester-linked fatty acids

BACTERIA   **3-ACYLOXYACYL GROUP**

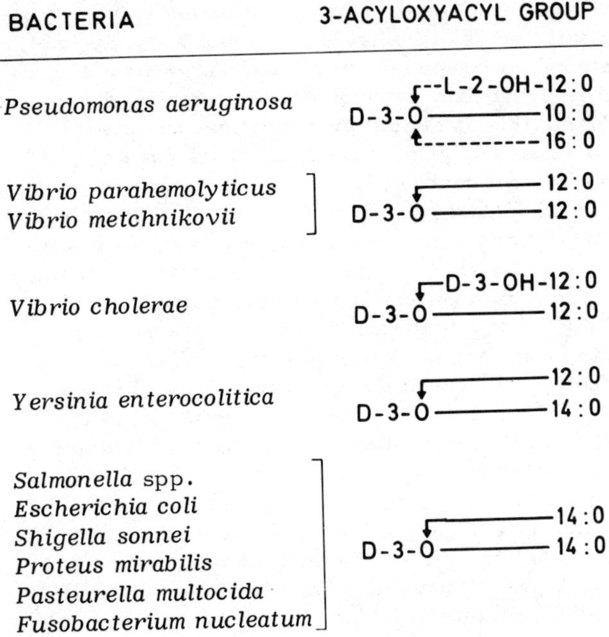

FIG. 7   Bacteria containing ester-bound 3-acyloxyacyl groups in their
lipid A component. In *Salmonella*, part of 14:0 is present in the α-
oxidized form (78). References: *P. aeruginosa* (220); *V. parahemoly-
ticus* and *metchnikovii* (224), *V. cholerae* (66), *Y. enterocolitica* (65),
Salmonella (56), *E. coli* (97), *S. sonnei* (202), *P. mirabilis* (64), *P.
multocida* (225), *F. nucleatum* (203).

are distributed statistically over available hydroxyl groups. In *Salmonella* lipid A (compare Sec. IV.A) the nonhydroxylated fatty acids
(12:0, 14:0, and 16:0) are linked to 3-hydroxyl groups of ester- and
amide-bound 3-hydroxytetradecanoic acids (97). Such a distribution
of nonhydroxylated fatty acids is also present in lipid A's of other
gram-negative bacteria (115).

V. Conformation of Lipid A

It is evident from the foregoing discussion that our present knowledge
on the primary structure of lipid A is still limited. Several laboratories
have nevertheless performed physicochemical studies together with
computer calculations which have shed some light on the conformation
of certain regions of the lipid A molecule.

With the aid of computer calculations, according to Ramachandran it could be shown that in *S. minnesota* Re LPS (containing a dOclA trisaccharide and lipid A), due to considerable steric hindrance, unique positions exist for rotation around the axes of the ketosidic linkage of the lipid A proximal dOclA residue and C'_3 of GlcN II (86,233). Also, the rotation angles of the phosphate group linked to the nonreducing GlcN residue (position C'_4) is highly restricted.

No calculations have so far been performed on the rotation around the angles within the glucosamine disaccharide of the lipid A backbone. But empirical force field calculations on β1.6-linked D-glucopyranose disaccharides showed that β-gentiobiose exhibits an extreme flexibility which did not allow any conclusions as to the most probable conformation of lipid A to be drawn (87,231).

X-ray diffraction studies on dried preparations of *S. minnesota* Re LPS revealed a single strong reflection which corresponded to a lattice periodicity of about 4.1 Å (88). This reflex is similar to that known from x-ray studies on triglycerides, where it indicates a parallel orientation of fatty acid residues in possibly a hexagonal dense packing (89). This reflection had also been seen in x-ray diffraction patterns of outer membrane preparations of *S. typhimurium*, where it was interpreted to originate from both phospholipid and lipid A fatty acids (90). Although a less well-ordered conformation of fatty acids was postulated for *E. coli* LPS (91), it can tentatively be assumed that the fatty acids in lipid A are oriented in one direction and that they are arranged in a more or less parallel fashion (Fig. 8). In this arrangement, fatty acid motion at the carboxy terminal would be highly restricted. This conclusion was independently reached by electron spin resonance studies on outer membrane preparations of *E. coli* (92) and *S. typhimurium* (93).

Investigations into the physical shape of LPS by electron microscopy (94) and x-ray diffraction (88) indicate that LPS (in aqueous medium) forms a bilayer, the center of which consists of a lipid A leaflet with a width of approximately 40 Å. Thus, the lipid A monolayer would have a thickness of approximately 20 Å.

On the basis of our current knowledge on the primary structure and conformation of *Salmonella* lipid A, a three-dimensional atomic model has been constructed (Fig. 8). In this model, the long chain fatty acids (7 mol/2 mol GlcN) are oriented in a parallel fashion. They are anchored directly or through hydroxy fatty acids to the diphosphorylated β1.6-linked D-glucosamine disaccharide to which L-4-aminoarabinose (upper left) and phosphorylethanolamine (upper right) are attached. In addition, the model shows a dOclA trisaccharide in the calculated conformation (86) bound to lipid A at position 3' of the nonreducing GlcN II residue.

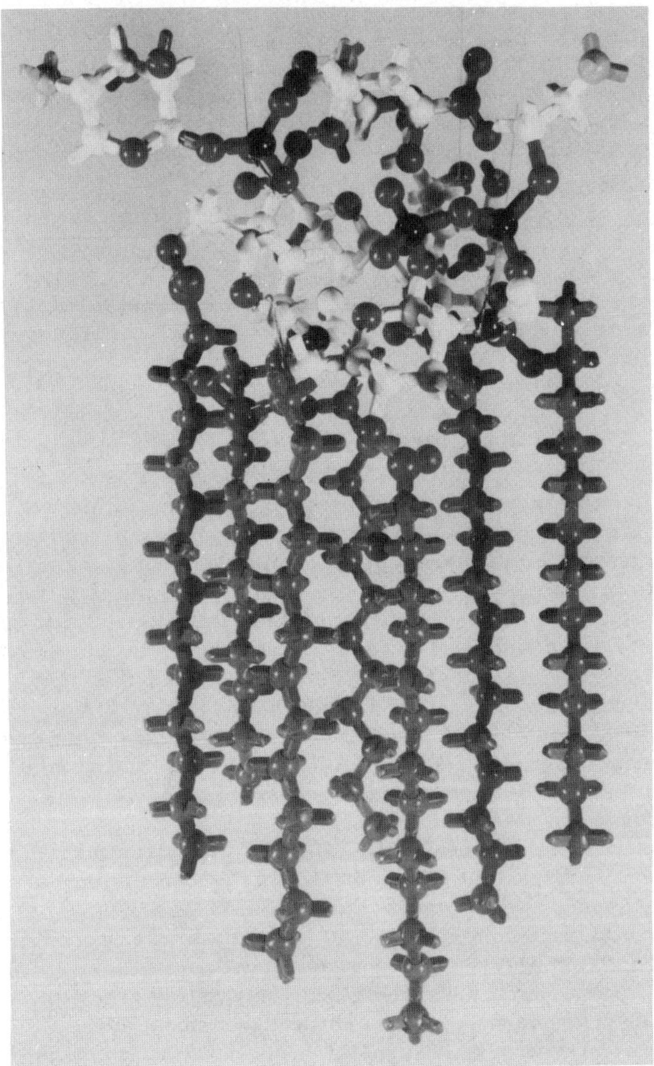

FIG. 8   Three-dimensional atomic model of *Salmonella* lipid A. The model was built according to the presently available structural (see Fig. 5) and conformational (88,233) data.

VI. Relation of Lipid A Structure to Function

The model shown in Figure 8 indicates that lipid A is an amphipathic
molecule with both hydrophobic (fatty acids) and hydrophilic regions
(substituted backbone). Moreover, it may be an amphoteric molecule
of zwitterionic character containing both negatively (phosphate) and
positively (in *Salmonella*, 4-AraN and ethanolamine) charged residues.

Its unique architecture endows lipid A with properties which make
it a vital constituent of the outer membrane of gram-negative bacteria.
Owing to their ordered arrangement, the lipid A fatty acids form a
comparatively rigid structure. Thus, lipid A (LPS) may be regarded as
a building block of the outer membrane, where it plays primarily a
structural role (24,243). In addition, the high viscosity of lipid A
fatty acids could be responsible for the limited permeability of the
outer membrane for hydrophobic molecules (24). Thus lipid A would
play an essential role in the function of the outer membrane as a per-
meation barrier (95).

Besides its passive functions, i.e., to serve as a structural and
passage-limiting membrane component, lipid A also participates in other
more dynamic functions of the outer membrane. Thus, it has been
shown that lipid A is required for the expression of bacteriophage receptor activity (phages K3 and Tu*II) of the outer membrane protein
d (83,101). This protein is also involved in bacterial conjugation, and
for this activity an association with lipid A is also a prerequisite.
These and other findings (Ref. 102, summarized in Ref. 24) indicate
that, in the external leaflet of the outer membrane where LPS (lipid A)
is exclusively located, lipid A interacts with certain proteins and it has
been postulated that lipid A (LPS) mediates the positional specificity
(103) and the ordered arrangement (104) of outer membrane matrix
proteins. Thus, lipid A appears to be involved in the proper assembly
and organization of the membrane as well as the maintenance of the
cell shape (246,24).

VII. Relation of Lipid A Structure to Biological Activity

A. *Antigenicity*

Free lipid A (adsorbed to suitable carriers) represents a potent immunogen capable of inducing the production of specific anti-lipid A
antibodies in a number of animal species (105,106,110,239,240). These
antibodies (e.g., induced by free lipid A from *Salmonella*) cross react
in vitro with free lipid A of a number of gram-negative bacteria
(Table 3). This shows that the free lipid A preparations investigated
share a common determinant(s). On the other hand, non-crossreacting lipid A systems have been identified (Table 3). Thus, free
lipid A of *Salmonella* does not cross-react with free lipid A from

TABLE 3 Serological Cross Reactivity of Free Lipid A Derived from LPS of Various Gram-negative Bacteria

Free lipid A	Cross reactivity[a]	References
Salmonella spp.	+	106
Escherichia coli spp.	+	106
Shigella sonnei	+	109
Proteus mirabilis	+	204
Yersinia enterocolitica	+	65,106
Vibrio cholerae	+	106
Chromobacterium violaceum	+	106
Pseudomonas fluorescens	+	106
Neisseria gonorrhoeae	+	106
Coxiella burnetii (phase I)	+	106
Rickettsia canada	+	106
Chlamydia psittaci	+	234
Rhodopseudomonas gelatinosa	+	108
Rhodospirillum tenue	+	108
Rhodopseudomonas viridis	−	108
Rhodopseudomonas palustris	−	108

[a]+, present, -, absent.

R. viridis or *R. palustris* strains (108). This finding corroborates the differences discussed here in the chemical structure of these molecules (compare Sec. IV.D.2).

The lipid A precursors (67,68,245) and O-deacylated free lipid A are strongly immunoreactive, indicating that the polar head groups (Table 1) and ester-bound fatty acids do not participate in the serological specificity of lipid A. According to the chemical investigations discussed (Sec. IV.B.1), deesterified lipid A's of distinct origin are structurally related in that they consist of a diphosphorylated β1.6-linked D-glucosamine disaccharide which carries amide-bound D-3-hydroxy fatty acids. In fact, 3-hydroxy acyl residues [hydroxamates (109), or bound to D-GlcN (110,111)] have been shown to inhibit the lipid A-anti-lipid A system. It was recently found, however, that N-tetradecanoyl-D-glucosamine-6-phosphate exhibited an inhibitory activity comparable to that of the racemic N-3-hydroxyacyl derivative. N-acetyl-D-glucosamine and D-glucosaminyl-6-phosphate were not active in this system. Although the inhibitory capacity of the synthetic samples was considerably lower than that of free lipid A, these data were interpreted to show that the 3-hydroxyl group of amide-linked acyl residues may not be an essential part of the lipid A immunoreactive determinant (110).

A lipid A-derived and largely phosphate-free (β1.6-linked) D-glucosamine disaccharide containing only one amide-linked D-3-hydroxytetradecanoyl residue showed full inhibitory activity comparable to that of intact free lipid A (111). This indicates that phosphate is probably not involved in the serological lipid A determinant. From the results of a recent study on the antigenic activity of subfractions of free lipid A incorporated into liposomes, the authors concluded that the immunoreactive group was embedded in the (N-acylated) glucosamine backbone of lipid A, and that ester-bound fatty acids where even inhibitory for the binding of antibody to lipid A (112).

The presently available data do not provide a final definition of the structural or conformational nature of the lipid A antigenic determinant. This very structure, however, seems to comprise the β1.6-linked D-glucosamine disaccharide, the amide linkage, and a certain region of the acyl residue(s). It should be emphasized that, in vitro, lipid A antibodies do not react to a significant extent with lipid A as it is present in LPS (for in vivo cross-reactivity see Ref. 113). Serological activity of lipid A is expressed only after the release of the polysaccharide component (or possibly other constituents) by mild acid hydrolysis (106). This indicates that part of the polysaccharide portion shields the immunoreactive site, and that the lipid A determinant may be located in the lipid A region proximal to the polysaccharide.

B. Endotoxicity

1. **Structural Requirements** The available evidence shows that the polysaccharide component does not play a direct role for the expression of biological activities of LPS (for possible exceptions, compare Sec. VIII). It is the lipid A component which represents the endotoxically active principle of bacterial LPS. The presence of the polysaccharide portion influences lipid A activity indirectly in that it serves as a solubilizing carrier because insoluble free lipid A preparations are not active in most endotoxin tests. A direct modifying influence of the polysaccharide portion on lipid A toxicity has been found in the case of LPS from *R. tenue* (108). Here, the intact LPS exhibited a low lethal toxicity in (adrenalectomized) mice (LD_{50} = 10 µg/mouse), whereas polysaccharide-free isolated lipid A was more toxic by a factor of approximately 140 (LD_{50} = 0.07 µg). These findings suggest that lipid A of *R. tenue* possesses an intrinsic toxicity which, however, is hidden in intact LPS, i.e., shielded by the polysaccharide portion (or some other LPS constituent present in acid labile linkage). In this connection it is worthwhile mentioning that phthalylation of LPS also masks lipid A activity (114).

Free lipid A (in a soluble form; see Sec. VII.B.2) has been demonstrated to be as active as intact LPS in inducing typical endotoxic
effects such as fever (rabbits), hypothermia, (mice), the local
Shwartzman reaction, changes in white cell counts, mitogenicity for
B lymphocytes, induction of prostaglandin synthesis in macrophages,
lethal toxicity, and others (for a summary, see Ref. 18). Although the
elucidation of the general architecture of lipid A has contributed to an
understanding of its physicochemical properties (see Sec. VII.B.2),
little is known of those groups, structures, or conformations which
confer biological activity to lipid A.

Attempts to define endotoxically essential lipid A regions are difficult since it has been recognized that a defined LPS preparation
(such as the triethylammonium salt of an S form LPS) may be highly
active in one endotoxin test (e.g., pyrogenicity) but completely inactive in another assay (e.g., complement activation), whereas with a
different LPS preparation (e.g., the LPS sodium salt), the reverse
may be true (see Sec. VII.B.2 and Fig. 9). This suggests that different features of the lipid A molecule may be important for the expression of distinct biological manifestations. Furthermore, the enormous inherited or acquired differences of various mammalian species in
their susceptibility to endotoxin raises the possibility that, in distinct
organisms, lipid A (LPS) is recognized and handled in different ways.
Thus, in defining toxic lipid A structures, host factors have to be
considered. And finally, the possibility exists that the lipid A "toxophore group" has so far escaped detection and chemical identification.
Although this possibility cannot be presently excluded, it appears
to be an unlikely one. Thus, the known components of endotoxically
highly active LPS from *S. abortus equi* (S form) and from a Re mutant
of *S. minnesota* amount to approximately 100% (Table 4). Although the
methodology for the estimation of some LPS components (such as dOclA)
may not be completely satisfactory, presently there is no basis to assume that a major lipid A component has escaped the many analytical
studies hitherto performed.

The results of several studies do nevertheless allow tentative conclusions to be drawn as to the nature of lipid A constituents which are
essential or not important for the expression of endotoxic activity.

LPS derived from *P. mirabilis* and *E. coli* are of comparable pyrogenicity in rabbits (MPD-3 = 0.002-0.005 µg/kg in both cases). The
former contains molar amounts of L-4-aminoarabinose in lipid A, whereas the latter is devoid of this sugar (see Table 1). This indicates that
the presence or absence of 4-AraN, or probably of any substituent at
the ester-bound phosphate group in general, has no demonstrable influence on lipid A pyrogenicity. Likewise, LPS derived from *V. cholerae* exhibits pyrogenic activity comparable to LPS from *Y. enterocolitica* (MPD-3 = 0.01 µg/kg in both cases). Since in the former LPS preparation the glycosyl phosphate group is substituted with phosphoryl-

S. abortus equi LPS	Sedimentation Coefficient	Solubility (Water)	Lethal Toxicity Mice Rats	Pyrogenicity (Rabbits)	Rate of clearance from the blood	Interaction with C' in vivo and in vitro	Affinity for cells	Mitogenic activity
Triethylamine (TEN)	9.3					(a)		(b)
Pyridine								
Ethanolamine								
Na								
K								
Putrescine	230							
Ca	partly insol.							

FIG. 9 Physicochemical properties and biological activities of the lipopolysaccharide of *Salmonella abortus equi* in different salt forms (140). Arrows show direction of increasing activity. (a): In the triethylammonium salt form the LPS is completely nonanticomplementary. (b): No significant difference within the above range of S values.

TABLE 4 Chemical Composition (percentage; wt/wt) of Salmonella S and Re Form Lipopolysaccharides

LPS Constituent[a]	*S. abortus equi* S-LPS[b]	*S. minnesota* Re-LPS[c]
D-Abequose	13.5	0
L-Rhamnose	15.2	0
D-Mannose	15.7	0
D-Galactose	17.8	0
D-Glucose	4.0	0
L,D-Heptose	5.0	0
D-Glucosamine	4.2	12.1
dOclA (KDO)	6.8	17.3
Fatty acids (12:0, 14:0, 16:0, L-2-OH-14:0, D-3-OH-14:0)	10.7	55.0
Phosphate	5.0	8.5
4-Amino-L-arabinose	0.3	2.8
Ethanolamine	0.2	0.8
Na^+	1.8	2.8
Ca^{2+}, Mg^{2+}	0.5	0.4
Amines (spermidine, putrescin, and others)	ND	ND
Protein	0.3	0.01
Total	101.0	99.7

[a]Calculated as anhydro compounds.

[b]Sodium salt (140, 191).

[c]PCP extract (4).

Note: ND = no data available.

ethanolamine (see Table 1), and in the latter one it is free, it can also be tentatively concluded that this substituent at the C_1-phosphate group does not modify the biological activity of lipid A to a significant extent. Collectively, these data indicate that polar head groups (phosphate substituents) do not play a direct role [but possibly do play an indirect role (232)] in the expression of LPS (lipid A) endotoxicity (232). This conclusion is corroborated by the

fact that free lipid A which is devoid of groups present in LPS in
acid labile linkage (e.g., 4-AraN) is biologically fully active. Therefore, the endotoxic principle must be embedded in the acylated backbone of lipid A.

Studies on the possible significance of the type of glycosidic
linkage in lipid A and the glucosamine residues (configuration,
anomeric form, etc.) have not been performed. The fact that free
lipid A from *C. violaceum* lacking the C_1-phosphoryl group is a potent
pyrogen (120) suggests that the glycosyl phosphate is not involved
in pyrogenic activity. Little is presently known on the role of the
ester-bound phosphate group. The finding, however, that the
phosphate-free lipid A from *C. vinosum* (2) is a potent pyrogen
(MPD-3 = 0.01 µg/kg) seems to exclude phosphoryl residues as important toxophore constituents. The biological analysis of synthetic
phosphate-free or phosphate-containing lipid A should greatly further our knowledge of its role (133,134,250).

A number of investigations have pointed to fatty acids as essential determinants of lipid A endotoxicity. Enzymic or chemical release
of O- and N-acyl residues from S or R form LPS yields preparations
which are biologically inactive (116,117,226,230). Also, selective
chemical deesterification leads to preparations which are of considerably lower endotoxic activity (factor 10^2 - 10^3) than intact LPS or
free lipid A in a number of in vivo tests (for literature, see Refs.
6, 118, and 119). These observations suggest that O-acyl residues
play a directly (e.g., as part of the toxophore) or indirectly (e.g.,
in generating or stabilizing a toxic conformation) essential role in
lipid A endotoxicity (6,119). The nature of nonhydroxylated ester-
linked fatty acids seems not to be a decisive factor for the expression of biological activity. This is indicated by the fact that, in LPS
of different bacterial origin, fatty acids of different chain length and
branched acyl residues occur; yet these preparations are of comparable biological activity. Furthermore, LPS derived from *Salmonella*
and *E. coli* cells grown at 12°C are of similar pyrogenicity as LPS
from bacteria grown at 37°C [MPD-3 = 0.005 µg/kg in both cases
(120)]. As discussed above (see Sec. IV.D.2), the former contain
ester-bound 16:1 and lack 12:0, while in the latter 16:1 is absent
and 12:0 represents one of the major lipid A components. For the
expression of lethal toxicity of lipid A, nonhydroxylated O-acyl residues are to a larger extent dispensable. This follows from the observation that the *Salmonella* lipid A precursor (67,68) which lacks
12:0, 14:0, and partly, 16:0 (but contains 2 mol of ester-bound
D-3-OH-14:0 in addition to N-acyl groups) is of comparable lethal
toxicity as LPS or free lipid A [LD_{50} = 0.03 µg/mouse, for all preparations, in adrenalectomized mice (121)]. The precursor, however,
is a less potent pyrogen (MPD-3 = approximately 0.2 µg/kg) than
LPS or free lipid A (121).

Little is known about the significance of amide-bound fatty acids for endotoxicity. In this context it is of interest that O-deacylated LPS from *E. coli, Salmonella typhosa,* and a *S. minnesota* Re mutant (R 595) is active as a B lymphocyte mitogen in vitro (18,122). Also, a (LPS-derived) D-glucosamine disaccharide, carrying only one D-3-hydroxytetradecanoyl residue in amide linkage exhibits residual B cell mitogenicity (111). Furthermore, synthetic N-acyl-D-glucosamine derivatives have been shown to be *Limulus* positive and mitogenic in vitro (124,260) and to possess (moderate) adjuvant and tumor cell growth inhibitory activity in vivo (125,260). These results suggest that N-acyl residues are of importance for some biological effects induced by lipid A. All so far known endotoxically active lipid A preparations contain, in addition to a range of O-acyl groups (see Sec. IV.D.2), amide-bound D-3-hydroxy fatty acids. Perhaps the presence of amide-linked D-3-hydroxyacyl groups is a necessary but not sufficient prerequisite for the expression of endotoxicity. Full biological activity may only be developed if O-acyl residues, notably D-3-hydroxy fatty acids, are simultaneously present.

An initial event in the sequence of reactions leading to the manifestation of endotoxic effects in vivo consists of the interaction of lipid A with certain humoral factors, including high density lipoprotein (HDL), the kinin, complement, and coagulation system, and particularly, cellular components such as macrophages, monocytes, platelets, endothelial cells, and lymphocytes of the host (7,9,10,12,16,18,20,21-23,25,32,126-130,161). If this interaction would be of hydrophobic nature, the importance of lipid A fatty acids for endotoxicity would be plausible. Since, however, O-deacylated LPS (lipid A) preparations which are, in general, biologically *less* active are known to possess an even *higher* affinity toward both artificial and natural membranes than does LPS, other factors such as specificity or selectivity of LPS binding must be of importance (21,131,132).

In summary, the results discussed suggest that both ester- and amide-bound fatty acids (notably 3-hydroxy fatty acids) play a role in the expression of biological activity of lipid A. Obviously, however, the exact molecular basis of their role for specific effects remains to be elucidated.

From this discussion it is evident that our present knowledge on those minimal structural and conformational requirements which confer biological activity to lipid A is still limited. Conclusions as to their nature have so far been predominantly drawn from comparative biological and structural studies on chemically degraded or modified LPS and free lipid A preparations as well as on natural lipid A's of different origin. Such studies have proven to be most valuable in that they have pointed to certain biologically important lipid A components and in that they have revealed lipid A's with unusual structures and very low endotoxic activity. The unequivocal identification of important determinants of endotoxicity, however, will probably be possible only by the conformational and biological analysis of chemically synthesized substructures and derivatives of lipid A and, ultimately, of complete lipid A. The chemical synthesis of lipid A has recently been initiated (133-135, 249,250,258,259), and presently, synthetic lipid A analoges are analyzed in various biological systems (259). It is our hope that these analyses will further our understanding on those minimal structural requirements which determine the physiological functions, serological specificity, and endotoxic activity of lipid A.

2. **Physicochemical Requirements**   Isolation of LPS from bacteria may be carried out by a variety of extraction procedures (18). Depending on such factors as growth conditions, bacterial strain, and method of extraction, LPS preparations exhibit large differences in their physicochemical properties.

Many of the factors influencing the physical state (e.g., particle size, aggregation, and solubility) of LPS are intrinsic and related to the chemical properties of the LPS. Thus, hydrophobic interactions exerted by the acyl moiety of lipid A participate in the formation of micelles and aggregates. However, extrinsic factors such as low and high molecular weight contaminants also influence the physical state of LPS and are primarily responsible for the difference in solubility seen with different preparations. Macromolecular contaminants most usually encountered in LPS preparations are proteins, lipoproteins, phospholipids, and glycans. Their amount may vary depending on the bacterial strain, the culture condition and the isolation procedure. Although they are associated only physically, their presence may significantly influence the biological activity of LPS. It is known that gram-negative cell wall components other than LPS possess intrinsic biological activities, some of which may resemble those of LPS. Thus, the lipoprotein and other cell wall proteins exhibit mitogenic activity for mouse B lymphocytes which, however (by the use of a LPS-nonresponder mouse strain), could be distinguished from that of LPS (136-138). Today, owing to the improvement of isolation and purification methodology, it is possible to prepare LPS completely free of phospholipids, proteins, nucleic acids, and saccharide polymers (18).

In addition to macromolecular contaminants, LPS regardless of the method of isolation always contain low molecular weight components, most common being metal cations like Na^+, Ca^{2+}, and Mg^{2+} and amines such as ethanolamine, putrescine, cadaverine, spermine, and spermidine (18). These ions are bound to negatively charged phosphoryl and carboxyl groups present in lipid A (LPS), and they influence not only the physicochemical but also the biological properties of free lipid A and LPS. Their removal by electrodialysis leads to acidic LPS which, by subsequent neutralization with a defined inorganic or organic base, can be converted into uniform salt forms (139).

Different salt forms of LPS exhibit characteristic and constant physicochemical properties. Thus, the triethylammonium salt of LPS is highly soluble, exhibiting a low degree of aggregation as determined by sedimentation coefficient measurements. Decreased solubility and an increased sedimentation coefficient is observed on comparison of the Na^+ and Ca^{2+} form of LPS, respectively (Fig. 9).

Biological studies with uniform LPS salt forms show that, e.g., lethal toxicity for mice and pyrogenicity for rabbits increase with decreasing sedimentation coefficient values of LPS and are highest in the triethylammonium salt form (18,106,140). On the other hand, lethal toxicity for rats (141), the rate of LPS clearance from the blood (141), cell surface affinity (142), and the property to interact with the complement system (141,143,144) increase with increasing sedimentation coefficient values as long as the LPS preparation remains soluble (Fig. 9). Thus, the triethylammonium salt of S form LPS is highly pyrogenic but does not inactivate complement. Likewise, the sodium salt is only moderately pyrogenic but interacts strongly with the complement system. Therefore, by converting a LPS preparation to a defined salt form, certain biological effects can be separated. It is remarkable that the various salt forms behave so differently also in vivo, which indicates that there is not a fast exchange of cations in the circulation or tissues of higher animals.

It follows that both the *spectrum* of effects induced by a given LPS preparation and the *degree* of its activity is greatly influenced by the physicochemical state. Solubility of LPS, however, is a general and essential prerequisite for the expression of acute endotoxicity.

This is also true for isolated free lipid A. It has been repeatedly demonstrated that free lipid A, as it is obtained after mild acid hydrolysis of LPS, is not soluble in water or physiological saline, and that it is, if injected in this form into experimental animals, not, or only moderately, endotoxically active. By subjecting free lipid A to electrodialysis and converting the free lipid A to the triethylammonium salt, however, highly water-soluble (10 mg/ml) free lipid A preparations are obtained (18). If the soluble free lipid A salt is analyzed biologically, it shows in several in vivo and in vitro systems (pyrogenicity, hypothermia, lethal toxicity, B cell mitogenicity, and others) endotoxic activity comparable or identical to that of (soluble) LPS (18). Therefore, in the case of free lipid A, solubility is also an indispensable prerequisite for the expression of full endotoxic activity.

VIII. Conclusion

Our laboratory started work on LPS about 30 years ago, dealing with the question of the chemical nature of *bacterial pyrogens* (51). Very soon it was realized that we were dealing with endotoxin, and that

toxicity and pyrogenicity were practically inseparable. Then protein-
free LPS became available by applying the phenol-water extraction procedure, and the lipid A component of LPS could be isolated almost
without protein or peptide contaminants. After many enterobacterial
LPS had been analyzed, it became clear that the water-insoluble precipitate, which formed after acid hydrolysis, was a hitherto unknown,
unusual phospholipid common to all then investigated LPS. Because
the lipid-free polysaccharide components were endotoxically completely
inactive and because lipid A appeared to be a *common* structure in the
many endotoxically (pyrogenically) active LPS, we proposed that lipid
A represented the LPS portion responsible for endotoxicity (51). But
at that time the most active free lipid A preparations retained only
about one-tenth to one-fifth of the biological activities of the respective LPS.

More than 20 years elapsed before final proof for our hypothesis
could be reached. After the manufacture of highly purified LPS from
a *Salmonella minnesota* Re mutant [which consists of only a dOclA
trisaccharide and lipid A (26,52,145,226)] the preparation of free lipid
A by mild acid hydrolysis and its transformation into uniform salt
forms could be achieved. With such preparations it was found that free
lipid A in high dispersion—for example in the form of its triethylammonium salt—is endotoxically as active as the parent S or R form
LPS (in some cases even more active; Ref. 18).

There seem to be only few exceptions to this general statement.
For example, the tumor-necrotizing activity of LPS appears to be dependent on the presence of parts of the carbohydrate chain. In experiments with transplantable mouse tumors (fibrosarcomas), we
originally found that free lipid A, complexed with dextran as a carrier,
was active (146); but later investigators found that free lipid A applied without carrier was not (147,148). Recently we have confirmed
that purified and standardized free lipid A, indeed, does not induce
tumor necrosis, but even causes enhancement (149). In this case it
appears that, for disturbing tumor cell metabolism followed by hem-
orrhage and necrosis, lipid A must be carried by polysaccharide. Also,
in other LPS activities the polysaccharide portion was shown to play an
important role. Thus, a LPS-derived nontoxic polysaccharide-rich
fraction (which was free of fatty acids) protected against lethal irradiation (150) and induced the production of colony-stimulating activity
(150 and 151, but see 152). Furthermore, the polysaccharide component of LPS has been postulated to determine the specificity of the
interaction of certain Rhizobiaceae with their legume host (153). Similarly, in the binding of gram-negative bacteria to macrophages, regions of the polysaccharide portion of LPS are involved (154). The
adherence of *S. minnesota* R mutants (Ra and Rb$_2$) to lectin-like receptors on T lymphocytes was also shown to be mediated by determinants of the polysaccharide portion of R form LPS (155). This latter

interaction is most likely to be of high physiological significance since it prevents the generation of killer T-lymphocytes (155). Finally, the mitogenic activity of **Proteus** and **Bordetella** LPS for spleen cells of C3H/HeJ mice is believed to be mediated by the polysaccharide component (154).

Free lipid A as it is obtained from S or R form LPS by acid hydrolysis probably represents an artifact. From studies on the biosynthesis of lipid A it is clear that oligosaccharide-free lipid A does not occur in bacteria as an intermediate (for literature, see Ref. 26). Also, in higher animals, lipid A, in its free form, has not been found so far. However, circulating anti-lipid A antibodies have been encountered in humans and experimental animals (18,26,106,197,247,248). Since the formation of anti-lipid A immunoglobulins is only inducible by free lipid A [and not by LPS or bacteria (105)], it is possible that higher animals have been in contact with polysaccharide-free lipid A. It could be speculated that, after lysis of gram-negative bacteria (derived from the digestive flora or infectious sites), in vivo active structures of lipid A, then probably bound to carrier material (126, 127), are being expressed as immunogens acting as biological signals in a similar manner as injected free lipid A.

Present knowledge about the structure of lipid A, especially from **Salmonella**, has been described in detail (Sec. IV). Not only the general type of this lipid is unusual, but also some of its details are peculiar. In particular the occurrence of long chain 3-acyloxyacyl-esters and -amides, which resemble β-branched fatty acids and which confer a high degree of lipophilic character should be noticed. In the same molecule two polar phosphate groups are located at distant ends of the disaccharide backbone, 4-phosphoryl-D-glucosaminyl-β-1.6-D-glucosamine-1-phosphate (in **Salmonella** and many others; see Fig. 5). Several structural questions are still open, but their clarification appears to be a matter of now available methodology.

Lipid A does not represent a single, chemically defined molecular entity. The lipid A components of LPS of strains remote from Enterobacteriaceae differ in the backbone, the phosphate content, and other features. But also lipid A's from closely related Enterobacteriaceae, although generally very similar in structure, may show certain variations, e.g., with regard to the type of fatty acids and head groups present (18,26,50).

Structural studies performed in several laboratories have revealed that (free) lipid A from one bacterial species exhibits a certain heterogeneity (18,26,49,50,52,55,60; Sec. IV.C). This intrinsic microheterogeneity does not, however, preclude investigations into the structure of lipid A (255). In fact, the detailed structural investigations performed on lipid A of **Salmonella** and **E. coli** K-12 have shed some light on the molecular basis of this heterogeneity which had been previously demonstrated by physicochemical studies (112,157-159).

LPS or free lipid A induce a series of biological activities (see Ref. 18), most of which are elicited by remarkably small amounts. Thus, the minimal pyrogenic dose (MPD) of LPS or free lipid A is on the order of 0.001 µg/kg in rabbits, horses, or humans. For many of these activities it has hitherto been impossible to dissociate them chemically. For example, all claims of having separated toxicity from any other typical endotoxic activity such as pyrogenicity by specific "detoxification" could not be confirmed: decrease in toxicity was practically always accompanied by a similar decrease in other endotoxic activities. The history of endotoxin research was often greatly influenced by investigators who started with an interest in a special biological effect exerted by bacterial extracts—an effect which later turned out to be exerted by LPS.

On the other hand endotoxin acts in very small amounts, and bacterial contamination on such dose levels cannot be easily avoided during the course of manufacture or handling of biological materials. Thus, the activity of many biologically effective principles later turned out to be due to a "micro"-contaminant, i.e., LPS.

Endotoxin represents a complex molecule which exerts not only lethal toxicity according to the original definition of Pfeiffer (160), but many so-called endotoxic activities. Subsequently the term "endotoxicity" has come into use to describe the totality of these activities of one and the same chemical entity which, thus, distinguishes itself from most other biologically active principles. Accordingly, many different tests have been developed to prove or disprove the presence of LPS in a given sample.

It might be reasonable to differentiate between *acute* (immediate) and *nonacute* (delayed) activities of LPS. The acute responses of the higher animal, such as changes of white cell counts, fever, or the activation of fibrinolysis are the more typical for endotoxin, as long as the very *low* doses which induce these changes are concerned. On the other hand, some long-term activities, like adjuvanticity or induction of nonspecific resistance to infection or to irradiation, are being induced by many chemically quite different materials. Hence, such activities are not typical for LPS only.

Many endotoxic activities are induced via mediators of host origin (25). LPS exert their actions in most instances because the higher animal reacts with the production of such mediators as endogenous pyrogen (168), tumor necrotizing factor (169,170), superoxide anion (171), colony stimulating factor (150-152), interferon (162), interleukin 1 (163,164), glucocorticoid antagonizing factor (165), plasminogen activator (166), prostaglandins (167), histamine and serotonin (128), activated hormonal and enzymatic systems, and others (for literature, see Refs. 20, 22, 23, and 25). Humoral systems and more or less specific receptors on target cells of the host make endotoxin such an active biological principle. LPS contains the very structures that act as biological signals for the subsequent activation or release of many endogenous mediators which are finally responsible for many effects of endotoxin in vivo.

This means that in a detailed analysis of LPS actions, starting from the mechanisms of primary attack, we must go on to an elaboration of secondary mechanisms in which endogenous mediators play the major role. Since these mediators act more *selectively*, this is one way of differentiating between the many endotoxic activities.

The functioning of these complex biological systems obviously depends on various factors, including general genetic and individual conditions. It is known that there are great species differences with regard to the sensitivity or resistance to one and the same LPS preparation. Rabbits, dogs, horses, or humans are highly sensitive; mice, rats, and guinea pigs are generally of medium sensitivity; and certain primates such as baboons or vervets are highly insensitive (172). The susceptibility of humans and baboons to LPS pyrogenicity differs by a factor of more than 1:100,000. A mouse mutant (C3H/HeJ) has been found which is largely resistant to LPS activities (129,130, 173,174). For experiments to be comparable and reproducible, the use of genetically controlled animal material is, therefore, indispensable. Species differences in the susceptibility may also allow a more detailed insight into the endogenous conditions that make LPS in certain species, like man, so highly active, and inactive in others. The fact that very small amounts of LPS are active in sensitive species is one of the reasons for the difficulty in following its fate in vivo by the usual radiolabeling techniques, making highly sensitive tests for endotoxin studies so urgent.

Further, it is known that the nutritional state (200) and environmental factors such as temperature (175,176) play a role in endotoxicity. In addition, animals or man may react to the same LPS preparation quite differently according to their hormonal state (177), to their past experience with endotoxin [LPS tolerance and LPS hyperreactivity (178-181)], or to their pharmacological conditioning (20,167, 179,223). For example, after pretreatment with BCG, *Corynebacterium parvum* (179) and galactosamine (183), or after adrenalectomy (182), animals have a greatly increased sensitivity to LPS. Nonsteroidal anti-inflammatory drugs such as acetylsalicylic acid and indomethacin, which are prostaglandin synthetase inhibitors (184), will generally suppress LPS-induced changes of body temperature (185) and often also acute toxicity (186), but have no influence in many other endotoxic activities, such as changes in white cell counts or fibrinolytic system activity (187,223).

These few comments emphasize that the standardization of experimental conditions, especially in endotoxin research, is of great importance. This is true for the genetic and individual (hormonal, pharma-

cological, and immunological) make-up of the "biological substract" of
LPS and for the LPS preparation as well.

We have shown that several conditions must be fulfilled to declare
a certain LPS preparation as standardized. Firstly, the choice of the
bacterial strain must be considered because in the whole kingdom of
gram-negatives there may be significant differences with regard to the
endotoxicity of the LPS (although many bacteria, especially Enterobacteriaceae, whether pathogenic or not, produce similar LPS). Secondly,
the state of purity, i.e., freedom from other components and the salt
form, which reflects on the particle size and solubility of the preparation, may play a crucial role, for which examples were given in Sec.
VII.B.2.

It should be noticed that standard LPS preparations are artifacts
in that they are unlikely to be released from disintegrating bacteria in
such form. After their injection they are likely to undergo metabolic
changes, and in this way LPS in vivo is in a dynamic state. It is not
known what chemical state of LPS would be the most active one with
regard to a given endotoxic reaction. It would be of importance to
follow endotoxin from the moment of its release or injection to its inactivation or detoxification and/or excretion. Work along these lines is
at present being performed with radio-double-labeled LPS in high
doses in LPS-insensitive animals [vervets and rats (201)].

Standard preparations are necessary for many bioanalytical procedures such as the quantitation of commercial *Limulus* lysates in the
Limulus test for endotoxin (188), or, generally, for a comparison of
different endotoxin preparations in the same test. They are also necessary for the evaluation of antiendotoxic drugs like antipyretics.
They would be in demand if any endotoxic preparation would be introduced into clinical trials for therapeutic or diagnostic application along
the lines of the traditional, but still often considered so-called, "nonspecific therapy" (189,190).

New therapeutic approaches appear to be reasonable under the as-
pect of (1) the availability of standardized preparations and (2) the
possible pharmacological conditioning of man for a more selective expression of wanted LPS effects in vivo and the suppression of harmful
or unwanted side effects (see Ref. 149).

Recently we described a procedure for the manufacture of a standard LPS from *Salmonella abortus equi* (191) with these considerations
in mind. Its constituents are known almost up to 100% (see Table 4),
and the structure of the large molecule, besides certain details, has
been elaborated. Other standard LPS or free lipid A's could also be
prepared in a similar way.

The history of the question as to the *nature of endotoxin* originated about 90 years ago when E. Centanni (192) prepared endotoxic
extracts from bacteria which he called "pirotoxina bacteria" (for the
history of pyrogen research, see Ref. 193). Then A. Boivin, W.T.J.

Morgan, and W. F. Goebel prepared the O-antigenic endotoxic complexes by applying various extraction procedures (194-196). These complexes were later shown to constitute an important part of the bacterial cell wall. They were further dissociated into protein and lipopolysaccharide, the latter one being the most active component. Using bacterial rough mutants with incomplete polysaccharides, it was shown that the respective LPS [glycolipids (198,199)] still retained full endotoxicity. Finally, free lipid A could be produced from LPS of R mutant strains, especially of Enterobacteriaceae, and its structure be clarified to a large extent. *Salmonella* lipid A with an approximate molecular weight of 2400 is at present the most reduced structure of the large endotoxic complex retaining endotoxicity.

For the chemist the formula of lipid A (from *Salmonella*) as the active nucleus of endotoxin is so far established that the synthetic approach to defined lipid A substructures and analogues is now open (125,133-135,250,258-259). These efforts of a sophisticated carbohydrate and lipid chemistry may lead to further standard preparations and to a deeper understanding about the structures necessary for signaling endotoxic actions in vivo.

Future research will especially focus on the elucidation of mechanisms of LPS action and its fate in defined biological systems. In this context the definition, purification and analysis of endogenous mediators involved in endotoxin action, on the one hand, and the possible application of refined natural or synthetic endotoxic preparations for clinical use, on the other, will certainly keep interest in LPS alive in the years to come.

Acknowledgments

We thank Drs. D. Shaw and H. Mayer for critically reading the manuscript and Mrs. Helga Kuttler and R. Schneider for typing it. The help of Dr. H. Formanek in constructing the lipid A model (Fig. 8) is gratefully acknowledged. We also thank Miss Helga Kochanowski and Mrs. Ingrid Himmelspach for preparing illustrations and photographs, respectively.

Part of the work described in this paper was supported by a grant from the Stiftung Volkswagenwerk.

References

1. G. Weinbaum, S. Kadis, and S. J. Ajl, eds., *Microbial Toxins*, vol. 4, Academic, New York, 1971, pp. 1-47.
2. J. Weckesser, G. Drews, and H. Mayer, *Ann. Rev. Microbiol.* *33*:215 (1979).

3.   O. Westphal, O. Luderitz, and F. Bister, *Z. Naturf.* *7b*:148 (1952).

4.   C. Galanos, O. Luderitz, and O. Westphal, *Eur. J. Biochem.* *9*:245 (1969).

5.   M. J. Osborn, *Ann. Rev. Biochem.* *38*:501 (1969).

6.   A. Nowotny, *Bacteriol. Rev.* *33*:72 (1969).

7.   S. E. Mergenhagen, R. Snyderman, H. Gewurz and H. S. Shin, in *Current Topics in Microbiology and Immunology*, vol. 50, Springer-Verlag, Berlin, 1969, pp. 38-77.

8.   A. Wright and S. Kanegasaki, *Physiol. Rev.* *51*:748 (1971).

9.   S. Kadis, G. Weinbaum, and S. J. Ail, eds., *Microbial Toxins*, vol. 5, 1-507, Academic, New York, 1971, pp. 1-507.

10. E. H. Kass and S. M. Wolff, eds., *Bacterial Lipopolysaccharides*, University of Chicago Press, 1973, pp. 1-304.

11. L. Leive, ed., *Bacterial Membranes and Walls*, Dekker, New York, 1973.

12. M. K. Agarwal, *Naturwissensch.* *62*:167 (1975).

13. F. Patocka, A. Soucek, and A. Ryc, eds., *J. Hyg. Epid. Microbiol. Immunol.* *18*:381 (1975).

14. K. Jann and O. Westphal, in *The Antigens*, Vol. III (M. Sela, ed.), Academic, New York, 1975, pp. 1-125.

15. I. Orskov, F. Orskov, B. Jann, and K. Jann, *Bacteriol. Rev.* *41*:667 (1977).

16. D. Schlessinger, ed., *Microbiology—1977*, Am. Soc. Microbiol., Washington, D.C., 1977, pp. 219-326.

17. S. G. Wilkinson, in *Surface Carbohydrates of the Prokaryotic cell* (I. W. Sutherland, ed.), Academic, New York, 1977, pp. 97-175.

18. C. Galanos, O. Luderitz, E.Th. Rietschel, and O. Westphal, in *International Review of Biochemistry, Biochemistry of Lipids II*, vol. 14 (T. W. Goodwin, ed.), 1977, pp. 239-335.

19. K. Jann and B. Jann, in *Surface Carbohydrates of the Prokaryotic Cell* (I. Sutherland, ed.), Academic, New York, 1977, pp. 247-287.

20. L. J. Berry, *Crit. Rev. Toxicol.* *5*:239 (1977).

21. S. Kabir, D. L. Rosenstreich, and S. E. Mergenhagen, in *Bacterial Toxins and Cell Membranes* (J. Jeljaszewicz and T. Wadstrom, eds.), Academic, New York, 1978, pp. 59-87.

22. D. C. Morrison and R. J. Ulevitch, *Am. J. Pathology* *93*:526 (1978).

23. S. G. Bradley, *Ann. Rev. Microbiol.* *33*:67 (1979).

24. H. Nikaido and T. Nakae, in *Adv. Microbiol. Physiology*, vol. 20 (A. H. Rose and J. G. Morris, eds), Academic, New York, pp. 163-250.

25. D. Schlessinger, (ed.), *Microbiology—1980*, Am. Soc. Microbiol., Washington, D.C., 1980.

26. O. Luderitz, M. A. Freudenberg, C. Galanos, V. Lehmann, E.Th. Rietschel, and D. W. Shaw, in *Microbial Membrane Lipids* (S. Razin and S. Rottem, eds.), Academic, New York, *17*:79-151 (1982).

27. R. J. Roantree, in *Microbial Toxins*, vol. 5 (S. Kadis, G. Weinbeim, and S. J. Ajl, eds.), Academic, New York, 1971, pp. 1-37.

28. J. W. Shands, in *Microbiology—1975* (D. Schlessinger, ed.), Am. Soc. Microbiol., Washington, D. C., 1975, pp. 330-335.

29. W. R. McCabe, *Bull. N.Y. Acad. Med. 51*:1085 (1975).

30. H. Smith, *Bact. Rev. 41*:475 (1977).

31. H. Smith, J. J. Skehel, and M. J. Turner, eds., *The Molecular Basis of Microbial Pathogenicity*, Verlag Chemie, Weinheim, 1980.

32. E.Th. Rietschel, U. Schade, M. Jensen, H. Wollenweber, O. Luderitz, and S. G. Greisman, *Scand. J. Infect. Dis. Suppl. 31*:8-21 (1982).

33. H. Nikaido, in *Bacterial Membranes and Walls* (L. Leive, ed.), Dekker, New York, 1973, pp. 131-208.

34. P. H. Makela and B. A. D. Stocker, in *Genetics as a Tool in Microbiology, 31* (S. Glover, ed.), Symp. Soc. Gen. Microbiol. (in press).

35. A. A. Lindberg, in *Surface Carbohydrates of the Prokaryotic Cell* (I.W. Sutherland, ed.), Academic, New York, 1977, pp. 289-356.

36. V. Braun and K. Hantke, in *Organization of Procaryotic Cell Membranes*, vol. 2, (Ghosh, B.K., ed.), CRC Press, 1981.

37. U. Henning, *Ann. Rev. Microbiol. 29*:46 (1975).

38. M. J. Osborn, P. D. Rick, and N. S. Rasmussen, *J. Biol. Chem. 255*:4246 (1980).

39. R. E. Hurlbert and I. M. Hurlbert, *Inf. Immun. 16*:983 (1977).

40. E. T. Palva and P. H. Makela, *Eur. J. Biochem. 107*:137 (1980).

41. R. C. Goldman and L. Leive, *Eur. J. Biochem. 107*:145 (1980).

42. G. Gerisch, O. Luderitz, and E. Ruschmann, *Z. Naturf. 22b*: 109 (1967).

43. C. J. Van Oss, *Ann. Rev. Microbiol. 32*:19 (1978).

44. P. H. Makela, V. V. Valtonen, and M. Valtonen, *J. Infect. Dis. 128* (Suppl.):73 (1973).

45. M. J. Osborn and L. I. Rothfield, in *Microbial Toxins*, vol. 4 (G. Weinbaum, S. Kadis, and S. J. Ajil, eds.), Academic, New York, 1971, pp. 331-350.

46. M. Schindler and M. J. Osborn, *Biochemistry 18*:4425 (1979).

47. J. W. Redmond, M. J. Korsch, and G. D. F. Jackson, *Austr. J. Exp. Biol. Med. 51*:229 (1973).

48. K. Broady, E.Th. Rietschel, G. D. F. Jackson, and O. Luderitz (in preparation).

49. O. Luderitz, in *Microbiology—1977* (D. Schlessinger, ed.), Am. Soc. Microbiol., Washington, D. C., 1977, pp. 239-246.

50. E.Th. Rietschel, S. Hase, M.-T. King, J. Redmond, and V. Lehmann, in *Microbiology—1977* (D. Schlessinger, ed.), Am. Soc. Microbiol., Washington, D.C., 1977, pp. 262-268.

51. O. Westphal and O. Luderitz, *Angew. Chem. 66*:407 (1954).

52. J. Gmeiner, O. Luderitz, and O. Westphal, *Eur. J. Biochem. 7*:370 (1969).

53. S. Hase and E.Th. Rietschel, *Eur. J. Biochem. 63*:101 (1976).

54. J. Gmeiner, M. Simon, and O. Luderitz, *Eur. J. Biochem. 21*:355 (1971).

55. P. F. Muhlradt, V. Wray, and V. Lehmann, *Eur. J. Biochem. 81*:193 (1977).

56. E.Th. Rietschel, H. Gottert, O. Luderitz, and O. Westphal, *Eur. J. Biochem. 28*:166 (1972).

57. R. E. Reeves, *J. Am. Chem. Soc. 72*:1499 (1950).

58. H. G. Khorana, G. M. Tener, R. S. Wright, and J. G. Moffat, *J. Am. Chem. Soc. 79*:430 (1957).

59. M. Jensen, D. Borowiak, H. Paulsen, and E.Th. Rietschel, *Biomed. Mass Spectrom. 6*:559 (1979).

60. M. R. Rosner, J. Y. Tang, I. Barzilay, and H. G. Khorana, *J. Biol. Chem. 254*:5906 (1979).

61. R. N.Tharanatan, J. Weckesser, and H. Mayer, *Eur. J. Biochem. 84*:385 (1978).

62. S. G. Wilkinson and D. P. Taylor, *J. Gen. Microbiol. 109*:367 (1978).

63. S. Hase and E.Th. Rietschel, *Eur. J. Biochem. 75*:23 (1977).

64. Z. Sidorczyk, M. Jensen, and E.Th. Rietschel, *Eur. J. Biochem.* (in preparation).

65. M. Jensen, Thesis, University of Freiburg, 1979.

66. K. Broady, E.Th. Rietschel, and O. Luderitz, *Eur. J. Biochem. 115*:463 (1981).

67. V. Lehmann and E. Rupprecht, *Eur. J. Biochem. 81*:443 (1977).

68. V. Lehmann, J. Redmond, A. Egan, and I. Minner, *Eur. J. Biochem. 86*:487 (1978).

69. M. T. Rosner, H. G. Khorana, and A. C. Satterthwait, *J. Biol. Chem. 254*:5918 (1979).

70. M. R. Rosner, R. C. Verret, and H. G. Khorana, *J. Biol. Chem. 254*:5926 (1979).

71. E.Th. Rietschel, O. Luderitz, and W. A. Volk, *J. Bacteriol. 122*:1180 (1975).

72. G. Rosenfelder, O. Luderitz, and O. Westphal, *Eur. J. Biochem. 44*:411 (1974).

73. R. Russa and Z. Lorkiewicz, *J. Bacteriol.* *119*:771 (1974).

74. H. W. Wollenweber, E.Th. Rietschel, T. Hofstad, A. Weintraub, and A. A. Lindberg, *J. Bacteriol.* *144*:898 (1980).

75. D. R. Kreutzer, C. S. Buller, and D. C. Robertson, *Inf. Immun.* *23*:811 (1979).

76. J. Montreuil, *Adv. Carb. Chem. Biochem.* *37*:157 (1980).

77. S. K. Maitra, M. C. Schotz, Th.T. Yoshikawa, and L. B. Guze, *Proc. Natl. Acad. Sci. U.S.A.* *75*:3993 (1978).

78. K. Bryn and E.Th. Rietschel, *Eur. J. Biochem.* *86*:311 (1978).

79. N. Haeffner, R. Chaby, and L. Szabo, *Eur. J. Biochem.* *77*:535 (1977).

80. E.Th. Rietschel and O. Luderitz, *Forum Mikrobiologie 1/80*:12 (1980).

81. H. Nikaido, *Int. J. System. Bacteriol.* *20*:383 (1970).

82. S. Rottem, O. Markowith, and S. Razin, *Eur. J. Biochem.* *85*:445 (1978).

83. L. van Alphen, B. Lugtenberg, E.Th. Rietschel, and Ch. Mombers, *Eur. J. Biochem.* *101*:571 (1979).

84. H.-W. Wollenwebe, S. Schlecht, and E.Th. Rietschel, *J. Bacteriol.* (to be submitted).

85. R. Russa and E.Th. Rietschel (in preparation).

86. H. Formanek and H. Weidner, *Z. Naturforsch.* *36c*:71 (1981).

87. S. Melberg and K. Rasmussen, *Carbohydr. Res.* *71*:25 (1979).

88. H. Wawra, H. Buschmann, H. Formanek, and S. Formanek, *Z. Naturforsch.* *34c*:171 (1979).

89. H. Hauser, I. Pascher, R. H. Pearson, and S. Sundell, *Biochim. Biophys. Acta 650*:21 (1981).

90. T. Ueki, T. Mitsui, and H. Nikaido, *J. Biochem.* *85*:173 (1979).

91. G. Emmerling, U. Henning, and T. Gulik-Krzywicki, *Eur. J. Biochem.* *78*:503 (1977).

92. S. Rottem and L. Leive, *J. Biol. Chem.* *252*:2077 (1977).

93. H. Nikaido, Y. Takeuchi, S. Ohnishi, and T. Nakae, *Biochim. Biophys. Acta 465*:152 (1977).

94. J. W. Shands, Jr., in *Microbial Toxins*, vol. 4, (G. Weinbaum, S. Kadis, and S. J. Ajl, eds.), Academic, New York, 1971, pp. 127-144.

95. H. Nikaido, *Angew. Chem.* *91*:394 (1979).

96. H.-W. Wollenweber, Diploma Thesis, University of Freiburg, 1979.

97. H.-W. Wollenweber, K. W. Broady, O. Luderitz, and E.Th. Rietschel, *Eur. J. Biochem. 124*:191 (1982).

98. W. A. Volk and O. Luderitz, in *Methods of Carbohydrate Chemistry*, vol. 9 (J. N. BeMiller, ed.), in press.

99. D. Shaw (unpublished data).

100. B. Jann, K. Jann, and G. O. Beyaert, *Eur. J. Biochem.* *37*:531 (1973).

101. D. B. Datta, B. Arden, and U. Henning, *J. Bacteriol. 131*:821 (1977).

102. U. Henning and K. Jann, *J. Bacteriol. 137*:664 (1979).

103. M. Schweizer, J. Hindennach, W. Garten, and U. Henning, *Eur. J. Biochem. 82*:211 (1978).

104. H. Yamada and S. Mizushima, *Eur. J. Biochem. 103*:209 (1980).

105. C. Galanos, O. Luderitz, and O. Westphal, *Eur. J. Biochem. 24*:116 (1971).

106. C. Galanos, M. Freudenberg, S. Hase, F. Jay, and E. Ruschmann, In *Microbiology—1977* (D. Schlessinger, ed.), Am. Soc. Microbiol., Washington, D.C., 1977, pp. 269-276.

107. W. R. Mayberry, *J. Bacteriol. 143*:582 (1980).

108. C. Galanos, J. Roppel, J. Weckesser, E.Th. Rietschel, and H. Mayer, *Inf. Immun. 16*:407 (1977).

109. C. Lugowski and E. Romanowska, *Eur. J. Biochem. 48*:81 (1974).

110. V. I. Gorbach, I. N. Krasikova, P. A. Lukyanov, O. Y. Razmakhnina, T. F. Soloveva, and Y. S. Ovodov, *Eur. J. Biochem. 98*:83 (1979).

111. F. Jay and C. Galanos (in preparation).

112. B. Banerji and C. R. Alving, *J. Immunol. 123*:2558 (1979).

113. E.Th. Rietschel and Ch. Galanos, *Inf. Immun. 15*:34 (1977).

114. F.C. McIntire, M. P. Hargie, J. R. Schenck, R. A. Finley, H. W. Sievert, E.Th. Rietschel, and D. L. Rosenstreich, *J. Immunol. 117*:674 (1976).

115. H.-W. Wollenweber, O. Luderitz, and E.Th. Rietschel, *Eur. J. Biochem.* (in preparation).

116. D. Malchow, O. Luderitz, B. Kickhofen, and O. Westphal, *Eur. J. Biochem. 7*:239 (1969).

117. A. M. Abdelnoor, Thesis, University of Michigan, 1969.

118. B. M. Sultzer, In *Microbial Toxins*, vol. 5 (S. Kadis, G. Weinbaum, and S. J. Ajl, eds.), Academic, New York, 1971, pp. 91-124.

119. D. Tripodi and A. Nowotny, *Ann. N.Y. Acad. Sci. 133*:604 (1966).

120. E.Th. Rietschel (unpublished data).

121. V. Lehmann, E. Ruschmann, and C. Galanos (unpublished data).

122. G. W. Goodman and B. M. Sultzer, *Inf. Immun. 17*:205 (1977).

123. E.Th. Rietschel, *Eur. J. Biochem. 64*:423 (1976).

124. D. L. Rosenstreich, J. Asselineau, S. E. Mergenhagen, and A. Nowotny, *J. Exp. Med. 140*:1404 (1974).

125. U. H. Behling, B. Campbell, Ch.-M. Chang, Ch. Rumpf, and A. Nowotny, *J. Immunol. 117*:847 (1976).

126. R. J. Ulevitch, A. R. Johnston, and D. V. Weinstein, *J. Clin. Invest. 64*:1516 (1979).

127. M. A. Freudenberg, T. C. Bøg-Hansen, U. Back, and C. Galanos, *Inf. Immun.* *28*:373 (1980).

128. B. Urbascheck and W. G. Forssmann, in *The Reticuloendothelial System and the Pathogenesis of Liver Disease* (H. Liehr and M. Grun, eds.), Elsevier North-Holland, 1980, pp. 401-407.

129. J. Watson, K. Kelly, and M. Largen, in *Microbiology—1977* (D. Schlessinger, ed.), Am. Soc. Microbiol., Washington D.C., 1977, pp. 298-309.

130. D. L. Rosenstreich, M. Glode, L. M. Wahl, A. L. Sandberg, and S. E. Mergenhagen, in *Microbiology—1977* (D. Schlessinger, ed.), Am. Soc. Microbiol., Washington, D.C., 1977, pp. 314-320.

131. J. W. Shands, Jr., *J. Infect. Dis. 128* (Suppl.):197-201 (1973).

132. G. F. Springer, J. C. Adye, S. E. Mergenhagen, and D. L. Rosenstreich, in *Microbiology—1977* (D. Schlessinger, ed.), Am. Soc. Microbiol., Washington, D.C., 1977, pp. 326-329.

133. M. Inage, H. Chaki, S. Kusumoto, and T. Shiba, *Tetrahedron Lett. 21*:3889 (1980).

134. M. Inage, H. Chaki, S. Kusumoto, T. Shiba, A. Tai, M. Nakahata, T. Harada, and Y. Jzumi, *Chem. Lett. (Japan)* p. 1373 (1980).

135. M. Kiso, H. Nishiguchi, and A. Hasegawa, *Carbohyd. Res. 81*: C13 (1980).

136. F. Melchers, V. Braun, and C. Galanos, *J. Exp. Med. 142*:473 (1975).

137. D. C. Morrison, S. J. Betz, and D. M. Jacobs, *J. Exp. Med. 144*:840 (1976).

138. B. M. Sultzer and G. W. Goodman, *J. Exp. Med. 144*:821 (1976).

139. C. Galanos and O. Luderitz, *Eur. J. Biochem. 54*:603 (1975).

140. C. Galanos, M. A. Freudenberg, O. Luderitz, E.Th. Rietschel, and O. Westphal, in *Biomedical Applications of the Horseshoe Crab (Limulidae)* (E. Cohen, ed.), Alan R. Liss, New York, pp. 1979, pp. 321-332.

141. M. A. Freudenberg and C. Galanos, *Inf. Immun. 19*:875 (1978).

142. M. D. Praino, C. Galanos, and E. Neter, *Immunol. Commun. 8*: 85 (1979).

143. C. Galanos, *Z. Immun.-Forsch. 149*:214 (1975).

144. C. Galanos and O. Luderitz, *Eur. J. Biochem. 65*:403 (1976).

145. O. Luderitz, C. Galanos, H. J. Risse, E. Ruschmann, S. Schlecht, G. Schmidt, H. Schulte-Holthausen, R. Wheat, O. Westphal, and J. Schlosshardt, *Ann. N.Y. Acad. Sci. 133*:349 (1966).

146. E. Mihich, O. Westphal, O. Luderitz, and E. Neter, *Proc. Soc. Exp. Biol. Med. 107*:816 (1961).

147. B. L. Wasilauskas and J. A. Cameron, *Cancer 27*:217 (1971).

148. K. Tanamoto, Ch. Abe, J. Y. Homma, and Y. Kojima, *Eur. J. Biochem.* **97**:623 (1979).

149. O. Westphal, U. Westphal, R. Andreesen, and P. G. Munder, *Pontif. Acad. Scient. Scripta Var.* **43**:373 (1979).

150. A. Nowotny, U. H. Behling, and H. L. Chang, *J. Immunol.* **115**:199 (1975).

151. R. M. Urbascheck, R. V. Shadduk, C. Bona, and S. E. Mergenhagen, in *Microbiology—1980* (D. Schlessinger, ed.), Am. Soc. Microbiol., Washington, D.C., 1980, pp. 115-119.

152. R. N. Apte, C. Galanos, and D. V. Pluznik, *J. Cell Physiol.* **87**:71 (1975).

153. J. S. Wolpert and P. Albersheim, *Bioch. Biophys, Res. Comm.* **70**:729 (1976).

154. D. M. Weir, *Immunol. Today* **1**:45 (1980).

155. V. Lehmann, H. Streck, I. Minner, P. H. Krammer, and E. Ruschmann, *Eur. J. Immunol.* **10**:685 (1980).

156. W. Strittmatter, H.-W. Wollenweber, J. Weckesser, C. Galanos, and E.Th. Rietschel (in preparation).

157. A. Nowotny, in *Microbial Toxins*, vol. 4 (G. Weinbaum, S. Kadis, and S. J. Ajl, eds.), Academic, New York, 1971, pp. 309-329.

158. C. H. Chen, A. G. Johnson, N. Kasai, B. A. Key, J. Levin, and A. Nowotny, *J. Infect. Dis.* **128** (Suppl):35 (1973).

159. C. M. Chang and A. Nowotny, *Immunochemistry* **12**:19 (1975).

160. R. Pfeiffer, *Z. Hyg. Infekt.* **11**:393 (1892).

161. P. A. Ward and K. J. Johnson, in *Microbiology—1977* (D. Schlessinger, ed.), Am. Soc. Microbiol., Washington, D.C., 1975, pp. 327-329.

162. J. S. Youngner, D. S. Feingold, and J. K. Chen, *J. Infect. Dis.* (Suppl) **128**:219 (1973).

163. D. L. Rosenstreich and J. M. Wilton, in *Proceedings of the 9th Leukocyte Culture Conference*, Academic, New York, 1975, pp. 113-132.

164. S. B. Mizel, J. J. Oppenheim, and D. L. Rosenstreich, *J. Immunol.* **120**:1504 (1978).

165. L. J. Berry, R. N. Moore, K. J. Goodrum, and Jr. R. E. Couch, in *Microbiology—1977* (D. Schlessinger, ed), Am. Soc. Microbiol., Washington, D.C., 1977, pp. 321-325.

166. S. Gordon, J. C. Unkeless, and Z. A. Cohn, *J. Exp. Med.* **140**:995 (1974).

167. E.Th. Rietschel, U. Schade, O. Luderitz, H. Fischer, and B. A. Peskar, in *Microbiology—1980* (D. Schlessinger, ed.), Am. Soc. Microbiol., Washington, D.C., 1980, pp. 66-72.

168. P. Murphy, D. F. Hanson, P. L. Simon, W. F. Willoughby, and B. E. Windle, in *Microbiology—1980* (D. Schlessinger, ed.), Am. Soc. Microbiol., Washington, D.C., 1980, pp. 158-161.

169. E. A. Carswell, L. J. Old, R. L. Kassel, S. Green, N. Fiore, and B. Williamson, *Proc. Natl. Acad. Sci. U.S.A.* **72**:3666 (1975).

170. D. N. Mannel, R. N. Moore, and S. E. Mergenhagen, in *Micro-biology—1980* (D. Schlessinger, ed.), Am. Soc. Microbiol., Washington, D.C., 1980, pp. 141-142.

171. M. J. Pabst and R. B. Johnston, Jr., *J. Exp. Med.* **151**:101 (1980).

172. O. Westphal, *Int. Arch. Allergy Appl. Immunol.* **40**:1 (1975).

173. B. M. Sultzer and G. W. Goodman, in *Microbiology—1977* (D. Schlessinger, ed.), Am. Soc. Microbiol., Washington, D.C., 1977, pp. 304-309.

174. J. Watson, M. Largen, and K. P. W. J. McAdam, *J. Exp. Med.* **147**:39 (1978).

175. L. J. Berry, *Fed. Proc.* **25**:1264 (1966).

176. R. P. Atwood and E. H. Kass, *J. Clin. Invest.* **43**:151 (1964).

177. E. Tonutti, *Dtsch. Z. Chirurg.* **264**:61 (1950).

178. D. W. Watson and Y. B. Kim, in *Bacterial Endotoxins* (M. Landy and W. Braun, eds.), Rutgers Univ. Press, New Brunswick, 1963, pp. 522-536.

179. L. Chedid and M. Parant, in *Microbial Toxins*, vol. 5 (S. Kadis, G. Weinbaum, and S. J. Ajl, eds.), Academic, New York, 1971, pp. 415-451.

180. S. E. Greisman and R. B. Hornick, *J. Infect. Dis. 128* (Suppl.): 157 (1973).

181. G. G. Greer and E.Th. Rietschel, *Inf. Immun.* **20**:366 (1978).

182. L. Chedid, F. Boyer, and M. Saviard, *Compt. Rend.* **233**:713 (1951).

183. C. Galanos, M. A. Freudenberg, and W. Reutter, *Proc. Natl. Acad. Sci. U.S.A.* **76**:5939 (1979).

184. J. R. Vane, *Nature (New Biol.) 231*:232 (1971).

185. W. Feldberg, *Proc. R. Soc. Lond. [Biol.] 191*:199 (1975).

186. J. R. Fletcher and P. W. Ramwell, in *Adv. Prostagl. Thrombox. Res.* vol. 3 (C. Galli, G. Galli, and G. Porcellati, eds.), Raven, New York, 1978, pp. 183-192.

187. O. Westphal (unpublished data).

188. E. Cohen (ed.), *Biomedical Applications of the Horseshoe Crab (Limulidae)*, Alan R. Liss, New York, 1979.

189. F. Hoff, Thieme-Verlag, Stuttgart 1957.

190. H. Fischer, in *XII Reinbecker Kollogium*, 1975, pp. 47-68.

191. C. Galanos, O. Luderitz, and O. Westphal, *Zbl. Bakt. Hyg. I. Abt. Orig. A 243*:226 (1979).

192. E. Centanni, *Dtsch. Med. Wochenschr.* **20**:148 (1894).

193. O. Westphal, U. Westphal, and Th. Sommer, in *Microbiology—1977* (D. Schlessinger, ed.), Am. Soc. Microbiol., Washington, D.C., 1977, pp. 221-238.

194. A. Boivin and L. Mesrobeanu, *C. R. Soc. Biol. 112*:611 (1933).
195. W. T. J. Morgan and S. M. Partridge, *Biochem. J. 35*:1140 (1941).
196. C. Tal and W. F. Goebel, *J. Exp. Med. 92*:25 (1950).
197. M. Westenfelder, C. Galanos, A. Withoft, and G. Lang, *Infection 5*:144 (1977).
198. A. Nowotny, N. Kasai, and D. Tripodi, in *Coll. Int. Cent. Nat. Rech. Sci.*, vol. 174 (L. Chedid, ed.), Ed. Cent. Nat. Rech. Sci., Paris, 1969, p. 79.
199. O. Luderitz, W. Droge, P. Muhlradt, E. Ruschmann, and O. Westphal, in *Coll. Int. Cent. Nat. Rech. Sci.*, vol. 174 (L. Chedid, ed.), Ed. Cent. Nat. Rech. Sci., Paris, 1969, p. 95.
200. J. A. Cook, W. C. Wise, and C. Callihan, *Fed. Proc. 38*:1261 (1979).
201. B. Kleine, C. Galanos, and O. Westphal (in preparation).
202. C. Lugowski and E. Romanowska, *Eur. J. Biochem. 48*:319 (1974).
203. S. Hase, T. Hofstad, and E.Th. Rietschel, *J. Bacteriol. 129*:9 (1977).
204. Z. Sidorczyk, A. Rozalski, and K. Kotelko, *Arch. Immun. Therap. Exp. 26*:239 (1978).
205. O. Luderitz, A. M. Staub, and O. Westphal, *Bact. Rev. 30*:192 (1966).
206. C. G. Hellerqvist, B. Lindberg, and S. Svensson, *Carbohydr. Res. 8*:43 (1968).
207. C. G. Hellerqvist, B. Lindberg, S. Svensson, T. Holme, and A. A. Lindberg, *Carbohydr. Res. 9*:237 (1969).
208. M. J. Osborn, *Ann. N.Y. Acad. Sci. 133*:375 (1966).
209. C. G. Hellerqvist and A. A. Lindberg, *Carbohydr. Res. 16*:39 (1971).
210. U. Feige and S. Stirm, *Biochim. Biophys. Res. Comm. 71*:566 (1976).
211. P.-E. Jansson and B. Lindberg, *Carbohydr. Res. 54*:261 (1977).
212. U. Feige, S. Stirm, and H. Mayer, *Carbohydr. Res.* (in preparation).
213. G. Hammerling, O. Luderitz, O. Westphal, and P. H. Makela, *Eur. J. Biochem. 22*:331 (1971).
214. J. H. Johnston, R. J. Johnston, and D. A. R. Simmons, *Biochem. J. 105*:79 (1967).
215. P.-E. Jansson, B. Lindberg, A. A. Lindberg, and R. Wollin, *Carbohydr. Res. 68*:385 (1979).
216. U. Feige, B. Jann, K. Jann, G. Schmidt, and S. Stirm, *Biochem. Biophys. Res. Comm. 79*:88 (1977).
217. H. Mayer, A. M. C. Rapin, G. Schmidt, and H. G. Boman, *Eur. J. Biochem. 66*:357 (1976).

218. P. Prehm, S. Stirm, B. Jann, K. Jann, and H. G. Boman, *Eur. J. Biochem.* *66*:369 (1976).

219. G. A. Adams and P. P. Singh, *Biochim. Biophys. Acta 202*: 553 (1970).

220. D. T. Drewry, J. A. Lomax, G. W. Gray, and S. G. Wilkinson, *Biochem. J.* *133*:563 (1973).

221. Y. Kamio, K. C. Kim, and H. Takahashi, *J. Biochem. 70*:187 (1971).

222. D. Shaw, O. Luderitz, and E.Th. Rietschel (in preparation).

223. D. J. M. Wright and M. P. I. Weller, *J. R. Soc. Med. 73*:431 (1980).

224. E.Th. Rietschel, W. J. Palin, and D. W. Watson, *Eur. J. Biochem. 37*:116 (1973).

225. W. Erler, H. Feist, and K. D. Flossmann, *Arch. Exp. Vet. Med. (Leipzig) 31*:203 (1977).

226. O. Luderitz, Ch. Galanos, V. Lehmann, H. Mayer, E.Th. Rietschel, and J. Weckesser, *Naturwissensch. 65*:578 (1978).

227. B. Jann, K. Reske and K. Jann, *Eur. J. Biochem. 60*:239 (1975).

228. D. L. Kreutzer, C. S. Buller and D. C. Robertson, *Inf. Immun. 23*:811 (1979).

229. K. H. Schleifer and H. P. Seidl, in *Microbiology—1977* (D. Schlessinger, ed.), Am. Soc. Microbiol., Washington, D.C., 1977, pp. 339–343.

230. D. Malchow, O. Luderitz, B. Kickhofen, O. Westphal, and G. Gerisch, *Eur. J. Biochem. 7*:239 (1969).

231. St. Melberg, Thesis, Technical University of Denmark, Copenhagen, 1979.

232. S. Kanegasaki, K. Tanamoto, S. Kobayashi, Y. Kojima, J. Y. Homma, and E.Th. Rietschel, *J. Bacteriol.* (to be submitted).

233. H. Formanek, *Hoppe-Seylers Z. Phys. Chem. 359*:1083 (1978).

234. S. Schramek, J. Kazar, and E. Sadecky, *Acta Virol. 24*:223 (1980).

235. J. L. Hartley, G. A. Adams, and T. G. Tornabene, *J. Bacteriol. 118*:848 (1974).

236. J. L. Ryan, A. J. Brude, and M. Turck, *Inf. Immun. 7*:476 (1973).

237. E.Th. Rietschel, in *Methods of Carbohydrate Chemistry*, vol. 9 (J. N. DeMiller, ed.), (in press).

238. J. P. Voets, E. J. Vandamme, and E. Maerteleire, *Experientia 29*:730 (1973).

239. B. G. Schuster, M. Neidig, B. M. Alving, and C. R. Alving, *J. Immunol. 122*:900 (1979).

240. J. Mattsby-Baltzer and B. Kaijser, *Inf. Immun. 23*:758 (1979).

241. L. S. Young, in *Principles and Practice of Infectious Diseases*, vol. 1 (G. L. Mandell, R. G. Douglas, Jr., and J. E. Bennet, eds.), John Wiley, New York, 1979, pp. 571-608.

242. D. Rowley, *J. Infect. Dis. 123*:317 (1971).

243. L. van Alphen, A. Verkleij, E. Burnell, and B. Lugtenberg, *Biochim. Biophys. Acta 597*:502 (1980).

244. M. Vaara, T. Vaara, and M. Sarvas, *J. Bacteriol. 139*:664 (1979).

245. P. D. Rick, L. W.-M. Fung, C. Ho, and M. J. Osborn, *J. Biol. Chem. 252*:4904 (1977).

246. M. J. Osborn, in *Bacterial Outer Membrane* (M. Inouye, ed.), Wiley-Interscience Publication, New York, 1979, pp. 15-34.

247. G. Simon, S. Reindke, and W. Marget, *Infection 2*:178 (1979).

248. D. Blake, A. Hamlyn, S. Procto, and E. N. Wardle, *Experientia 36*:254 (1980).

249. M. Kiso, H. Nishiguchi, S. Murase, and A. Hasegawa, *Carb. Res. 88*:C5-C9 (1981).

250. M. Inage, H. Chaki, S. Kusumoto, and T. Shiba, *Tetrahedr. Lett.*, p. 3889, (1980).

251. D. Blache, M. Bruneteau, and G. Michel, *Biochimie 62*:191 (1980).

252. M. Vaara, T. Vaara, M. Jensen, J. Helander, M. Nurminen, E.Th. Rietschel, and P. H. Makela, *FEBS Lett. 129*:145 (1981).

253. H. Nakayama, T. Mitsui, M. Nishihara, and M. Kito, *Biochim. Biophys. Acta 601*:1 (1980).

254. R. Girard, R. Chaby, and G. Bordenare, *Infect. Immun. 31*:122 (1981).

255. A. Nowotny, A. Nowotny, and U. Behling, in *Bacterial Endotoxins and Host Response* (M. K. Agarwal, ed.), Elsevier, Amsterdam, 1980, pp. 3-9.

256. S. Ulitzur, B. Kagen, and S. Rottem, *Appl. Envir. Microbiol. 37*:782 (1980).

257. K. Bock and C. Petersen, *Acta Chem. Scand. Ser. B 29*:258 (1975).

258. M. A. Nashed and L. Anderson, *Carb. Res. 92*:C5-C9 (1981).

259. M. Kiso, H. Nishiguchi, A. Hasegawa, H. Okumura, and J. Azuma, *Agric. Biol. Chem. 45*:1523-1526 (1981).

10

Lipopolysaccharide and the Immune Response

DIANE M. JACOBS   Schools of Medicine and Dentistry, State
University of New York at Buffalo, Buffalo, New York

The interaction of lipopolysaccharide (LPS), a major component of the
outer membrane of gram-negative bacteria, with the immune system is
reflected in a number of characteristic effects which have been most
intensively studied in parallel with recent advances in our knowledge
of the cellular basis of the immune response. The extent to which LPS
has been used as a probe in such studies has been well documented
by Morrison and Ryan (1). What follows is an exploration and discussion of some studies carried out in my laboratory with various colleagues since the mid 1970s which serve as an example of, and introduction to, the wide spectrum of activities resulting from the interaction of LPS with the immune system.

I. Response of the B Cell System

A. *Immunogenicity of TNP-LPS*

Our initial interest in LPS resulted from a practical need for a T-
independent antigen which is easily prepared, effective in vitro, and
stimulates a response of limited specificity which is easily measured.
LPS had been shown to be a potent immunogen and a T-independent
(TI) antigen; it is also a polyclonal activator of B cells, stimulating
DNA synthesis and Ig synthesis and secretion. It was thus thought
likely that chemical coupling of the trinitrophenyl (TNP) group to LPS
would result in production of a molecule which would stimulate a T-
independent anti-TNP response; this was confirmed in early experiments. The response was specifically stimulated by low doses of antigen and was clearly more effective when TNP was coupled to LPS;
simultaneous addition to cultures of TNP-sheep red blood cells (SRBC)

TABLE 1 Specificity and T Independence of TNP-PFC
Response to TNP-LPS

Additions to culture	TNP-PFC per culture, day 4	
	Normal cells	ATxBM cells
0.1 µg TNP-LPS	480	600
2×10^6 TNP-SRBC	5	7
0.1 µg LPS	20	50
0.1 µg LPS + 2×10^6 TNP-SRBC	20	15
None	15	20

Note: There were 2×10^6 BDF$_1$ spleen cells cultured in 1 ml medium,
harvested, and assayed.

Source: Data from Ref. 2.

and LPS did not stimulate an anti-TNP response, and LPS at these
doses did not stimulate appreciable polyclonal responses (Table 1) (2).
TNP-LPS was an effective immunogen both in vitro and in vivo, stimulating a response in cultures of spleen cells from ATxBM mice (Fig.
1), nude mice, or anti-thymocyte-treated normal spleen cells, and in
their in vivo counterparts (Table 2) (2,3). Because TNP-LPS is an
active immunogen in CBA/N mice which possess an X-linked genetic
deficiency in B cell maturation, this antigen has been characterized as
a TI-1 antigen, in contrast to many polysaccharide antigens which
are TI-2 (4).

TNP is covalently attached to the LPS, most probably to the amino
groups of the phosphorylethanolamine of LPS; protein contaminants do
not have to be present in the LPS preparation for conjugation. Our
initial procedure (2) used a cacodylate buffer adjusted to pH 11.5, but
0.1% potassium carbonate or 0.1 M sodium borate, pH 10.5 (5), are now
routinely used. The alkaline pH is necessary, probably more for its
ability to make more amino groups accessible to the reactive hapten
than for its effect on the chemical reaction itself which can occur at
neutral pH. LPS has also been conjugated with fluorescein isothiocya-
nate (FITC) (6) and 4-hydroxy-3, 5-dinitrophenylacetic acid (NNP)
(7) and used to generate TI antihapten responses.

B. *Structural Requirements*

As an immunogen, TNP-LPS prepared from commercially available or
purified LPS possessed some of the same requirements for activity as

LPS alone. The structure of LPS and the evidence for the importance of the lipid A moiety in the biological activity of the macromolecule have been presented in detail in the preceding chapter. LPS from *Salmonella minnesota* Re595, containing only lipid A and KDO, is also active as a B cell mitogen and inducer of Ig secretion (8). When conjugated with TNP, it induces an anti-TNP-plaque-forming cell (PFC) response (Table 3). Alkali treatment of LPS, which removed the ester-linked fatty acids of lipid A, results in a product with reduced toxicity (9) and a loss of the ability to stimulate mitogenesis and polyclonal Ig secretion (8). Such material can be conjugated with TNP in the same manner as native LPS but can no longer induce an anti-TNP response (Table 3) (3). Thus the immunogenicity of TNP-LPS requires that the carrier portion have an intact, biologically active lipid A.

While the immunogenicity of TNP-LPS as reflected in the antihapten response appears to reflect the generalization that lipid A is the biologically relevant portion of LPS, it is not a direct reflection of the response to the LPS itself. The antibody response to the O antigens of LPS can be induced by the polysaccharide portion of LPS alone. VonEschen and Rudbach induced a primary antibody response to the O antigen using both native protoplasmic polysaccharide (NPP), the polysaccharide portion of LPS made in excess by some strains of *Escherichia coli*, and alkali-treated LPS in which the lipid A has been rendered biologically inactive (10,11). Thus the immunogenicity of LPS

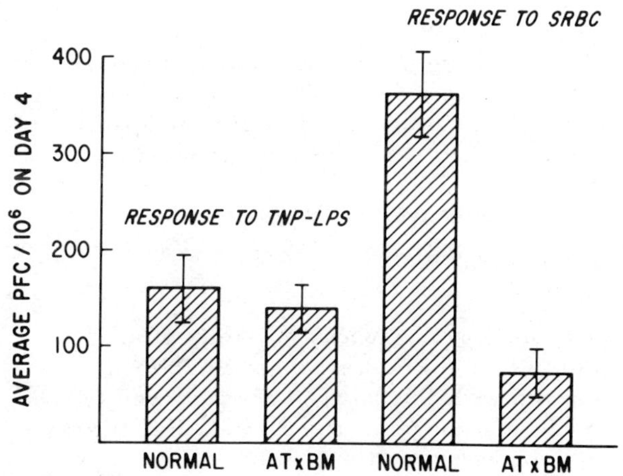

FIG. 1 Responses of normal and ATxBM (adult thymectomized irradiated, bone-marrow reconstituted) spleen cells to TNP-LPS and SRBC. Cultures contained 10^7 cells/ml and either 0.1 μg TNP-LPS or 6×10^6 SRBC. The data are a composite of 9 separate experiments. The error bars indicate standard errors of the mean. (From Ref. 2.)

TABLE 2 Responses to TNP-LPS in T Cell-depleted Mice

| | | | | PFC/10^6, Day 4 | |
Exp.	Strain	Treat-ment	Antigen	TNP-PFC	SRBC-PFC
1	CBA/H	NNTx	0.01 µg TNP-LPS	53 ± 15	
			0.1 µg TNP-LPS	363[a]	
			1.0 µg TNP-LPS	1163 ± 270	
		Normal	0.01 µg TNP-LPS	72 ± 23	
			0.1 µg TNP-LPS	388 ± 89	
			1.0 µg TNP-LPS	339 ± 54	
		NNTx	0.2 ml 1% SRBC		40 ± 13
			0.2 ml 10% SRBC		80 ± 45
		Normal	0.2 ml 1% SRBC		238 ± 106
			0.2 ml 10% SRBC		547 ± 63
2	Nu/Nu		10 µg TNP-LPS	504 ± 105	
	BALB/C		10 µg TNP-LPS	394 ± 31	

[a]One mouse in this group.

Note: CBA/H mice of both sexes were used 7 weeks after neonatal thymectomy (NNTx). Nu/Nu mice were 6-8-week-old males and BALB/C mice were 10-week-old females. All immunizations were intraperitoneal and plaque-forming cell (PFC) assays were carried out on spleens 4 days later. PFC are means ±SEM. TNP = trinitrophenyl; SRBC = sheep erythrocytes; TNP-LPS = trinitrophenylated lipopolysaccharide.

Source: Ref. 3.

is not completely dependent on lipid A. Recently, Skelly et al. (5) measured the anti-TNP and anti-LPS PFC responses to TNP-LPS. Some strains of mice immunized with this antigen respond well to the TNP moiety but poorly to the O antigens of the carrier, but the same mice respond normally when LPS alone is the immunogen.

C. Genetic Requirements

TNP-LPS has also been used to explore the genetic requirements for LPS immunological activity. In 1968, Sultzer (12) observed that the inflammatory response induced by LPS in C3H/HeJ mice was different

TABLE 3 In Vivo Responses to Various Preparations of TNP-LPS in BDF$_1$ Mice

Antigen	Dose (µg)	No. of mice	TNP-PFC/10^6, Day 4
TNP-LPS	0.1	8	424 ± 54
(commercial)	1.0	4	685 ± 102
	10.0	2	336 ± 71
TNP-LPS	0.1	15	151 ± 27
(purified)	10.0	4	933 ± 68
TNP-LPS	0.1	4	72 ± 34
(R595)	10.0	4	467 ± 29
TNP-LPS	0.1	11	1.5 ± 0.3
(base-hydrolyzed)	10.0	14	2.0 ± 0.3
LPS	10	4	24 ± 4

Note: The source of the LPS carrier is indicated in parentheses under each preparation—see text for details.

Source: Ref. 3.

from that induced in other strains, and this strain was resistant to LPS-induced toxicity. Further examination indicated that LPS did not induce mitogenicity in spleen cells from this strain, although other conventional B and T cell mitogens were effective (13). The immune response to TNP-LPS is markedly reduced in this strain, although other substrains of C3H as well as other strains with a variety of H2 haplotypes gave good responses (Table 4). Hybrid offspring of the nonresponder C3H/HeJ and other responder strains also responded to TNP-LPS, but the level of the response appeared to be lower than that of the responder parent (3). These results suggested that LPS responsiveness was controlled by an autosomal codominant gene (5). Extensive studies by Watson et al. (14,15) demonstrated that the response to LPS is controlled by a single autosomal gene (LPS) which maps to chromosome four of the mouse. Thus far, all the various types of LPS biological activities examined have been found to be under the same genetic control. Detailed studies carried out by McGhee et al. (16) have confirmed our early impression that the expression of the gene is codominant.

TABLE 4 Correlation Between Toxicity of LPS and PFC Response to TNP-LPS in Responder and Nonresponder Strains and Hybrids

Exp.	Strain	Toxicity test (survivors at 3 days)		Response to TNP-LPS ($TNP\text{-}PFC/10^6$, day 4)	
1	C3H/HeJ		4/4		12 ± 1
	C3HeB/FeJ		1/4		444 ± 19
	C3H/St		0/4		558 ± 53
	BDF_1		1/4		336 ± 71
	$C3D_2F_1/J$		0/4		560 ± 19
2	C3H/HeJ × C3H/St		ND	(♂)	113 ± 11
	BDF_1		ND	(♂)	154 ± 15
3	C3H/HeJ × C3H/St	(♂)	0/5	(♀)	263 ± 21
	C3H/St	(♀)	0/4	(♀)	343 ± 80
4	C3H/HeJ		8/8		2 ± 1
	DBA		0/8		606 ± 105
	$C3D_2F_1$		1/8		285 ± 19

Note: Toxicity studies were carried out by administration of 1 μg LPS and 12.5 μg actinomycin D i.p. Mice were immunized with 10 μg TNP-LPS, i.p. (Exps. 1 and 2) and 1 μg TNP-LPS (Exps. 3 and 4), and TNP-PFC was measured 4 days later. Average $TNP\text{-}PFC/10^6 \pm$ SEM are given. All mice in experiments 1 and 4 were females.

Source: Ref. 3.

D. *Polymyxin B*

The use of alkali-treated LPS as a technique for evaluating the requirements for lipid A in LPS responses has practical limitations. The conditions of treatment are critical and not always reproducible in different laboratories. Often, the mitogenic response appears to increase rather than decrease (17,18), and responses tested in vitro may be affected by the presence or absence of serum (17). Furthermore, it is wise to confirm that ester-linked fatty acids have been removed as predicted, and this is not always convenient for individual investigators. Finally, the molecular size of treated LPS is often changed, and this change alone may be responsible for observed differences in LPS activity. We therefore explored other methods to modify LPS activity. The cyclic peptide antibiotic polymyxin B (PB) shown by Neter et al. (19) to prevent LPS attachment to erythrocytes, also inhibited a number of LPS-induced toxic responses (20,21). We found that polymyxin B has profound effects on a number of LPS-induced effects on the immune system.

Addition of low doses of PB to cultures of spleen cells stimulated by a variety of mitogens resulted in selective inhibition of LPS-induced responses (Fig. 2). Inhibition was not due to PB toxicity, because the same result was obtained when LPS-PB complexes were prepared by mixing the two materials and removing the free PB by dialysis (22). This complex has a much reduced mitogenicity and prevents the induction of mitogenensis by free LPS. Similarly, the LPS-induced polyclonal response is reduced in the presence of PB (Table 5).

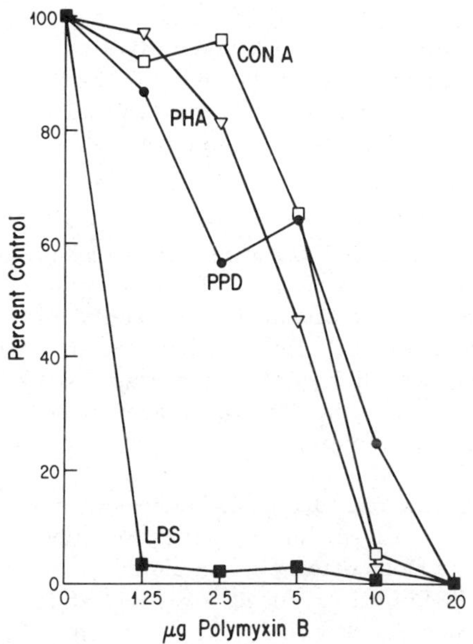

FIG. 2   Effect of polymyxin B on mitogenic response of mouse spleen cells. The indicated amount of polymyxin B was added to cultures containing 0.5 μg ConA, 0.25 μg PHA, 20 μg PPD, and 1 μg LPS. Cultures to which no polymyxin B had been added (100% response) responded as follows: ConA, 39,287 ± 1172 cpm; PHA, 33,930 ± 1362 cpm; PPD, 3,965 ± 906 cpm; LPS, 8,994 ± 508 cpm. Cultures were pulsed with ^{125}IUdR for 18 hr beginning 48 hr after initiation of culture. (From Ref. 22.)

TABLE 5   Suppression of Polyclonal Response by Polymyxin B

	Cells cultured (TNP-PFC/culture)	
Additions to culture	nu/nu	CBA/Wehi
1 µg LPS	38	240
1 µg LPS + 1 µg PB	4	68
5 µg LPS	47	262
5 µg LPS + 5 µg PB	3	82
None	1	26
1 µg PB	2	18

Note: Spleen cells were cultured in 0.2 ml RPMI-1640 containing 5% fetal calf serum in flat-bottomed microtest plates at a concentration of 10^7 cells/ml. The indicated additions were made at Day 0, and the cultures harvested and assayed 3 days later on heavily haptenated TNP-HRBC. The data are averages of results from 3 experiments.

In contrast, the immune response to TNP-LPS in our hands appeared initially to be enhanced. We interpreted these results to mean that, contrary to our earlier findings, mitogenicity of LPS was not a requirement for immunogenicity of its haptenated derivative (23). Similar experiments carried out by Smith et al. (24) were at variance with ours, finding instead that PB simply shifted the dose response of derivatized LPS and suggesting that mitogenicity was indeed necessary. This point was relevant to the one nonspecific signal model of B cell triggering proposed by Möller (25) and Coutinho (26) and has been somewhat clarified recently. We have now found that enhancement can be obtained when some batches of fetal calf serum are used and cultures carried for 4 days before assay. Most often the result is suppression when standard amounts of TNP-LPS are used for stimulation and cells are assayed after $2\frac{1}{2}$ days of culture (Table 6). When the entire range of antigen doses are examined, the response to low doses of antigen is suppressed by PB; but the usual low responses achieved in the presence of high antigen doses is reversed and enhancement of the response occurs (Fig. 3). These results are consistent with our recently developed allosteric model of B cell triggering which integrated one-signal and two-signal models with the matrix model. The mathematical basis of this general model and the experimental verification are discussed at length elsewhere (27).

To confirm that the effect of PB on LPS-induced responses was due to PB interaction with LPS, we examined the changes in the physical properties resulting from this interaction. We observed that there was an increase in the apparent molecular size and a decrease in the isopycnic density of the PB-LPS complex by comparison to the native material (28). PB interacted with LPS Re595 as well as with LPS conventionally prepared from the wild-type smooth organisms, indicating that PB was most likely bound to lipid A. By direct measurement of the bound material we determined that the interaction was stoichiometric, with one molecule of PB bound per monomer subunit of LPS (28). This amount was estimated to inhibit mitogenesis by addition to cultures directly stimulated by LPS—a good correlation considering the widely different methods used for measurement (22,28).

We then went on to examine the effect of PB on responses induced by LPS prepared by butanol extraction (Bu-LPS) for comparison to results obtained using phenol-extracted LPS (P-LPS). Bu-LPS had

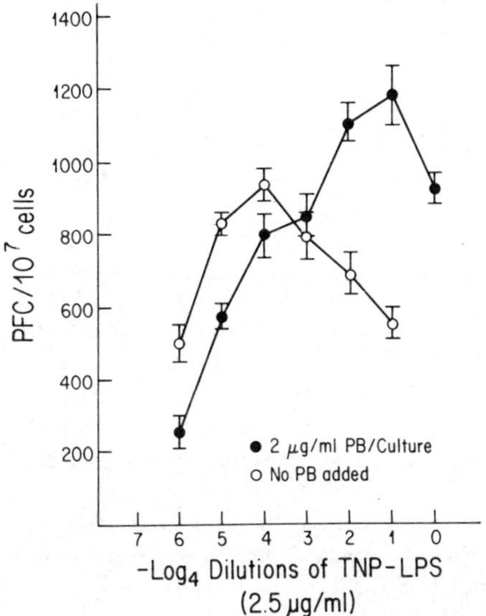

FIG. 3   The effect of polymyxin B on the PFC response to TNP-LPS. Each point represents the averaged response from three identical experiments in each of which 8 replicate cultures were set up containing 2×10^6 CBA/J spleen cells in 0.2 ml medium, and assays were carried out after $2\frac{1}{2}$ days of cultures. Adjusted PFC/10^7 added cells are given. (From Ref. 27.)

TABLE 6   Effect of Polymyxin B on Anti-TNP Response to TNP-LPS

Additions to culture		TNP-PFC/culture ± SD	
Serum	TNP-LPS (μg/ml × 10^{-3})	−PB	+PB (10 μg/ml)
None	0.63	51.5 ± 12.7	15.6 ± 8.0
	2.5	47.9 ± 6.0	36.0 ± 5.4
#759	0.63	63.1 ± 16.0	21.4 ± 11.0
	2.5	87.1 ± 9.6	72.3 ± 5.8
#420	0.63	67.4 ± 14.2	92.5 ± 14.5
	2.5	64.4 ± 12.9	69.0 ± 6.2
#997	0.63	53.0 ± 2.5	71.7 ± 20.5
	2.5	63.0 ± 4.9	61.7 ± 8.0
#024	0.63	72.3 ± 17.9	117.0 ± 7.2
	2.5	73.4 ± 6.8	85.0 ± 5.6

Note: Each number represents the average of 8 microcultures, each
of which contained 2 × 10^6 CBA/J spleen cells in a total volume of
0.2 ml medium. Assays were carried out after 4 days of culture.

been shown to be an effective mitogen in the C3H/HeJ nonresponders
(29) and we hoped to learn something about the structure of this LPS
which would account for this property. To our surprise PB had no
effect on the mitogenicity of this material, regardless of the strain of
mice used for the assay. Furthermore, neither the molecular weight
nor the density were in any way altered in the presence of excess PB
(30).

One of the possible explanations for these results was that Bu-LPS
contained a contaminant tightly bound to lipid A which prevented PB
binding to the same site. If such a contaminant were mitogenic it
would explain the activity of Bu-LPS in LPS nonresponders. Such material could in fact be recovered from a phenol extract of Bu-LPS which
is mitogenic for both responder and nonresponder strains of mice
(Table 7). Since the PB data implies association with lipid A, we have
called this material lipid A-associated protein (LAP) (30). A similar
material has been identified in LPS prepared by extraction with tri-
chloroacetic acid (TCA) (Boivin LPS) and has been termed endotoxin
protein (EP) by Sultzer and Goodman (31). The presence of LAP, EP,
and other contaminants in most commercial preparations of LPS, as

TABLE 7 Mitogenic Responses of Splenic Lymphocytes to Phenol-soluble Extract of Butanol-extracted LPS

Additions (µg)	C3H/St	C3H/HeJ
	cpm	
Control	4,100	1,100
Phenol-extracted LPS		
20 µg	16,100	1,500
0.2 µg	8,800	1,300
Butanol-extracted LPS		
20 µg	43,900	22,100
0.2 µg	12,700	3,000
Phenol-soluble extract		
20 µg	38,500	23,600
0.2 µg	11,000	3,600

Note: 5×10^5 spleen cells were cultured in microtest wells in 0.2 ml RPMI-1640 containing 5% fetal bovine serum for 24 hr in the presence of the indicated amount of mitogen. They were then pulsed with 0.5 µCi ^{3}[H]thymidine for an additional 24 hr and harvested.

Source: Ref. 30.

well as in other preparations which have not been carefully purified, pose problems for investigators whose primary interest is in the mechanism of LPS activation of cells. Acceptance of the C3H/HeJ as a true LPS nonresponder was slow, due in part to the use of LPS prepared by the Boivin method in attempts to confirm the initial observation. Whether or not such materials are important in the activity of LPS released naturally from gram-negative organisms resident in the host remains to be determined.

II. Immunomodulatory Effects of LPS

A property of LPS which has been of interest to immunologists for many years is its ability to act as an adjuvant in enhancing the antibody response when administered at the same time as, or shortly after, antigen (32). By comparison, LPS administered before antigenic challenge profoundly suppressed the induction of an antibody response (33). Our studies on both aspects of immunomodulation have indicated that LPS has multifocal effects on cells participating in antibody formation.

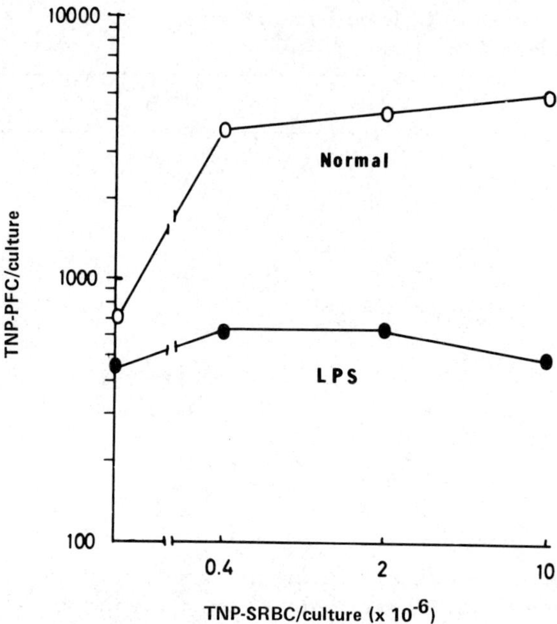

FIG. 4   Spleen cells from normal mice or mice treated with LPS 3 days previously were cultured at a concentration of 2×10^7/ml with the addition of increasing numbers of TNP-SRBC. Cultures were assayed for TNP-PFC 4 days later. (From Ref. 34.)

A. Suppression by LPS

Animals treated with LPS before antigenic stimulation give poor primary immune responses. Similarly, spleen cells removed from LPS-treated mice give poor primary immune responses in vitro (34). Thus suppression in vivo cannot be attributed solely to some physical factor preventing antigen interaction with the immune system. Unresponsiveness of splenic cell populations is dependent on the dose of LPS administered, occurring at doses of LPS between 2 and 50 μg per mouse. Recovery begins 5 days after administration and cannot be hastened by increasing the dose of antigen to which the cells are exposed (Fig. 4). Unresponsiveness resides in splenic nonadherent cells and can be attributable in part to the presence of an irradiation-sensitive suppressor cell component which inhibits the activity of normal cells (34).

Treatment of LPS spleen cells with antithymocyte serum and complement and restoration with normal T cells allows a partial recovery of the response, suggesting that suppression is due to a T cell. In

addition, however, B cells from LPS-treated mice cooperated poorly
with normal T cells, and nylon wool-enriched T cells from the same
source cooperate poorly with normal B cells. In contrast to the report
of Persson (35), we found no evidence that LPS induced suppressor B
cells. Recently, work from McGhee and his colleagues support the notion of LPS-induced suppressor T cells. They found that the immune
response to TNP-LPS in vitro, as well as the mitogenic response to
LPS, was higher in spleen cells from germ-free mice than from conventionally reared mice. These higher responses could be reduced by
addition of T cells prepared from spleens or Peyer's patches of conventionally reared mice (36). The suggested explanation of this

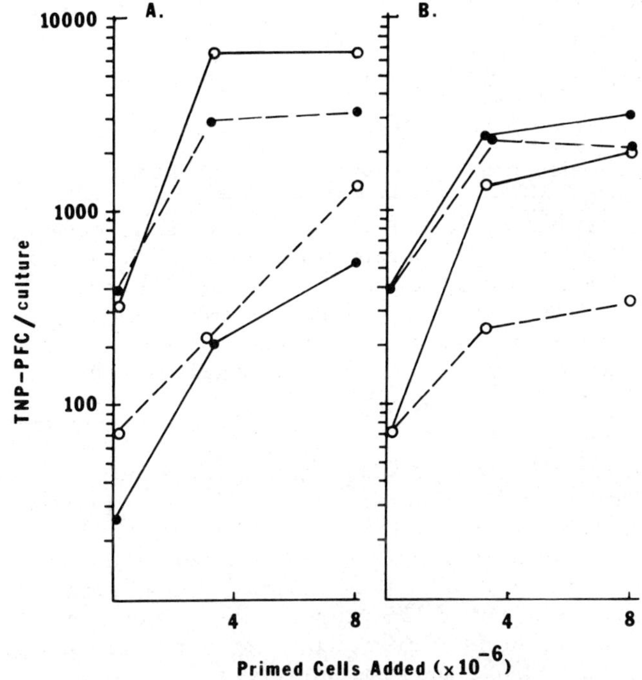

FIG. 5   SRBC-primed spleen cells (A), or nylon-wool enriched primed
T cells (B) with (----) or without (——) irradiation were added to
8×10^6 normal spleen cells. Total cell number in each culture was adjusted to 1.6×10^7 by adding normal spleen cells (when unirradiated
SRBC-primed spleen cells were added) or irradiated normal spleen
cells (in all other cases). Cell mixtures were stimulated with 3×10^6
of TNP-SRBC in the presence (●) or absence (○) of 20 µg LPS. Anti-
TNP antibody responses were assessed on day 3 of the culture. (From
Ref. 39.)

TABLE 8   Strain Dependence of LPS-induced Suppression of
Primary Antibody Response In Vitro

| Strain | Additions | | TNP-PFC/ |
	Cells	LPS	culture
C57BL/6	Primed	None	2500
	Primed	4 μg	380
	Irradiated primed	None	1800
	Irradiated primed	4 μg	2450
C57BL/10ScCR	Primed	None	3100
	Primed	4 μg	4600
	Irradiated primed	None	6000
	Irradiated primed	4 μg	5300

Note: The LPS was purified by phenol-water extraction and column
chromatography (41) and did not stimulate mitogenesis in spleen cells
from LPS nonresponders. Cultures of 1 ml contained 5×10^6 normal
cells from the indicated strain and the same number from primed syngeneic mice. TNP-SRBC were added to all cultures and LPS as indicated. PFC assays were carried out 4 days later. Irradiated cells were
exposed to 2000 rads.

phenomenon was that normal gram-negative intestinal flora induced a
population of suppressor T cells. Additional evidence that suppressor
cell activity could be due to LPS from these organisms was found in
studies using LPS nonresponder strains. Tolerance could be induced
by oral antigen administration to LPS responder mice, but immunity
resulted from the same treatment of LPS nonresponders. Backcross
analysis of F_1 and the F_2 generation from matings of responders and
nonresponders revealed that tolerance was linked to the LPS gene
(37). That is, there was a correlation between the presence of tolerance and lack of LPS responsiveness. Furthermore, tolerance was
dependent on the presence of a suppressor T cell which was induced
only in LPS responders (38). Since these experiments were carried
out without administration of LPS and there are no other apparent de-
fects relating to the immune response in this strain which are linked
to the LPS locus, the results are consistent with the possibility that
natural exposure of LPS in the mouse induces suppressor T cells.
     Addition of LPS to cultures of normal lymphoid cells also results
in suppression of an in vitro induced response (39,40). We evaluated

TABLE 9   Antigen Dependence of Synergy between LPS and TRF

| | SRBC-PFC/culture | | | |
| | Exp. 1 | | Exp. 2 | |
Additions	-SRBC	+SRBC	-SRBC	+SRBC
None	0	8 ± 3	0	0
1:2 TRF	7 ± 1	28 ± 3	0	2
10 µg LPS	23 ± 3	26 ± 4	10	40
1:2 TRF + 10 µg LPS	13 ± 1	104 ± 18	12	143

Note: There were 1×10^6 unfractionated C57B1/6 spleen cells (Exp. 1) or 5×10^5 nu/nu spleen cells (Exp. 2) cultured in the presence and absence of SRBC, LPS, and T cell-replacing factor (TRF). Values given are the mean PFC for 6 cultures (±SEM for Exp. 1). TRF used was the supernatate of 5×10^6/ml each of C57B1/6 and DBA/2 spleen cells cultured together in 10 ml volumes for 24 hr.

Source: Ref. 9.

the effect of LPS added to cultures of spleen cells or splenic B cells which had been supplemented with carrier-primed spleen cells and stimulated with hapten-conjugated erythrocytes. The antihapten response achieved in the presence of LPS was appreciably lower than in its absence. However, when the primed cells had been irradiated, the anti-TNP response was stimulated by the addition of LPS (Fig. 5). Suppressive and stimulatory effects were removed by treatment of the cells with ATS and complement; suppression was therefore due to neither a B cell nor a macrophage. Suppressive activity was also removed by passage of cells through nylon wool (Fig. 5). Thus, helper cell activity could be increased by LPS, but this was only detectable after inactivation or removal of suppressor activity, which was dependent on an irradiation-sensitive nylon-wool-adherent suppressor T cell. Suppression of the PFC response occurs in C57BL/6 cells cultured with primed syngeneic cells and purified LPS but not in similar cultures of the LPS nonresponder C57BL/10ScCR (Table 8). LPS-induced suppression is thus dependent on the genetic capacity of the host to respond to LPS.

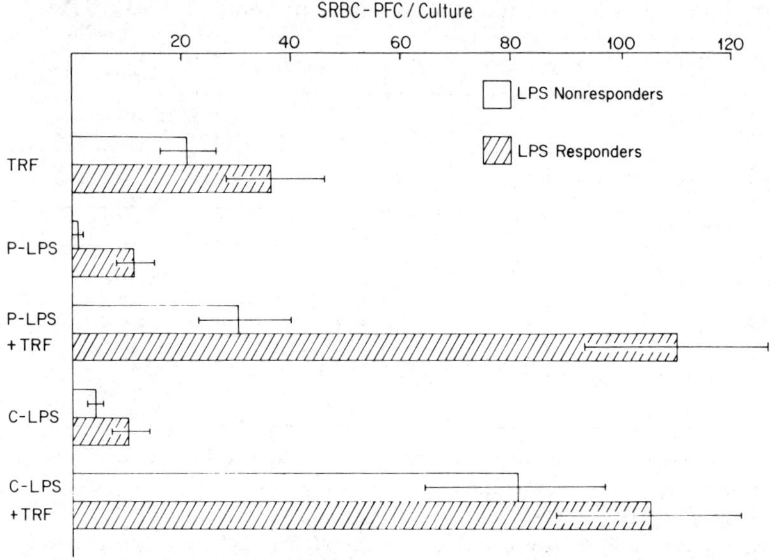

FIG. 6 Synergy of LPS and TRF in LPS responder and nonresponder strains. P-LPS—purified LPS from Dr. D. Morrison, C-LPS—Commercial LPS,TRF—allogeneic supernate (BL/6 or BL/10ScCR versus DBA/2) or ConA supernate. LPS nonresponders—C57BL/10 ScCR. LPS responders—C57BL/6 or C57BL/10Sn. 5×10^5 ATS-treated spleen cells or G-10 passed, ATS-treated spleen cells were cultured in microtest wells in the presence of 5×10^5 SRBC and 10 μg LPS or the optimal dilution of supernate, or both. In each experiment, 6 wells of each line were tested. The data shown are the geometric means ± SEM of PFC responses obtained in 14 experiments.

B. Stimulation by LPS

The involvement of helper T cells in LPS-stimulated antibody responses in vitro is consistent with observations that LPS-induced adjuvanticity in vivo may require T cells. LPS does not promote the antibody response to T-dependent antigens in nude mice (42). Adjuvanticity in ATxBM mice in vivo and similar effectiveness in vitro in the apparent absence of T cells prompted Parks et al. (42) to suggest that the nude mouse has a defective B cell; the apparent inconsistency could as well be due to residual T cells in ATxBM mice and T cell-replacing factors in the serum used for cell culture. We have argued that LPS-induced adjuvanticity and the suppressive effects observed in vitro could result if the interaction of LPS with B cells rendered these cells more sensitive to regulatory T cells, and that

TABLE 10   Increased Frequency of B Cells
Responding to SRBC in Presence of TRF and LPS

Additions	Frequency $\times 10^{-6}$
TRF	4.8–22.3
LPS	0.8–7.3
TRF + LPS (observed)	16.0–76.7
TRF + LPS (expected)	5.6–25.8

Note: Limiting dilution analyses were carried out
using techniques described in Ref. 45. ATS-
treated spleen cells were cultured in flat-bottomed
microtest plates in the presence of SRBC and the
indicated additions, and SRBC-PFC assays carried
out 4 days later. The range indicates the frequencies obtained in 7 experiments. For each experiment, the expected frequency was the sum of the
frequencies obtained for each separate addition.
When the expected and observed frequencies were
compared for these experiments by the Mann-
Whitney test, they were found to be significantly
different with P = .006.

the eventual outcome of such an interaction would depend on the activity and proportion of helper and suppressor cells present in the
system studied (39). Although there is some evidence that there is
an LPS-T cell interaction mediating adjuvanticity (43), it need not be
necessary.

One approach to examining this question is to determine whether
LPS-induced adjuvanticity can be demonstrated when a soluble T cell-
replacing factor is substituted for potential T cell targets. We examined the PFC response to SRBC of T-depleted cultures to which
had been added LPS and/or T cell-replacing factor (TRF). The PFC
response obtained in the presence of both LPS and TRF was higher
than that obtained with the addition of either TRF or LPS alone. The
synergistic response is antigen dependent and does not depend on
the presence of T cells (Table 9). Furthermore, such results are seen
with either commercial LPS or purified LPS (44). We examined the
PFC responses obtained with TRF and these types of LPS in both LPS
responder and nonresponder strains. Both LPS preparations induced
synergy in LPS responders, but purified LPS was ineffective in LPS
nonresponders (Fig. 6). Thus the effect we observed would appear
to be under the same genetic control as other LPS biological effects.

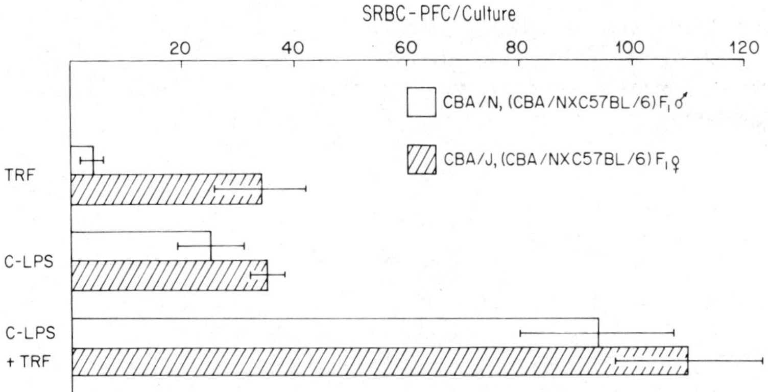

FIG. 7 Synergy of LPS and TRF in cells from CBA/N or (CBA/N ×
C57BL/6) F_1♂ mice. Controls are CBA/J or CBA/N × C57BL/6) F_1♀.
TRF--CBA/J-DBA/2 allogeneic supernatant (used on CBA/J and CBA/N
cells) or C57BL/6 ConA supernatant (used on F_1 cells). C-LPS—10 μg
commercial LPS. 5×10^5 ATS-treated spleen cells were cultures with
the indicated additions. TRF was used at the optimal concentration.
Data given are the arithmetic means ± SD of PFC responses obtained
in 6 experiments. Synergy was also obtained with purified LPS.

We concluded from the above experiments that LPS adjuvanticity
towards a T-dependent antigen was T dependent only in that it reflected the requirements of the B cells responding to a T-dependent
antigen, and this requirement could be obviated with TRF. Using a
limiting dilution analysis, we were able to demonstrate that a higher
number of PFC precursors were triggered in the presence of LPS and
TRF than would be expected from the simple additive effects of clones
stimulated by antigen and LPS or antigen and TRF alone (Table 10).
Thus adjuvanticity may be a reflection of triggering PFC precursors
which do not respond to either signal alone. Further evidence that
LPS induces functional differentiation of B cells to a state in which
they are susceptible to T cell help comes from studies on CBA/N
mice. This strain possesses an X-linked recessive defect in B cell
maturation which is reflected in a characteristic spectrum of cell surface marker distributions, including the absence of Lyb5+ cells (46).
It has been demonstrated that Lyb5+ cells are necessary for the
antigen-directed response to TRF and appear to be the cells responding to antigen presentation by accessory cells (47). It is thus of
some interest that synergy can be obtained in cells of this strain with
LPS and TRF, although they do not respond to TRF alone (Fig. 7),
suggesting the interesting possibility that LPS can induce the maturation of B cells to Lyb5+ cells in this strain.

We have not been able to demonstrate a role for macrophages in LPS-mediated adjuvanticity in vitro (44). Results from other laboratories do, however, implicate these cells in such LPS-induced responses (43). Macrophages from LPS responder strains, or a factor produced by LPS responder macrophages stimulated with LPS, rendered nonresponder B cells responsive to antigen (48). This factor appears to be interleukin 1 (IL-1), which induces functional differentiation of B cells, inducing them to mature to a state in which they are sensitive to soluble T helper factors (IL-2) (49). The possibility has not been excluded that two mechanisms are at work, based in one case on direct interaction of LPS with B cells and in the second upon LPS interaction with macrophages, which induces a factor interacting with B cells.

The most easily discernible and characteristic results of interaction of LPS with the immune system is the activation of B cells to DNA synthesis and Ig secretion. LPS as an antigen or carrier for chemically defined haptens induces a T-independent antibody response. Antibody responses to unrelated T-dependent antigens are also modulated by LPS. Such regulation can be explained by increased susceptibility of B cells to regulation after interaction with LPS, as well as by increased activity of regulatory cells resulting from their interaction with LPS. Study of these mechanisms has exploited the availability of several strains of mice which do not respond to LPS and have helped to define the genetic basis of LPS responses. In addition, they have demonstrated the existence of other bacterial cell wall components which have some of the properties of LPS but are not under the same genetic control. Future studies on the molecular nature of the interaction of LPS with target cells and the biochemical basis of cell triggering should yield information on the cell biology of cell activation.

Acknowledgments

This work was supported in part by Cancer Research funds from the University of California and United States Public Health Service Grants CA-17025, CA-20078, and AI16915.

1.   D. C. Morrison and J. L. Ryan, *Adv. Immunol.* 28:293 (1979).
2.   D. M. Jacobs and D. C. Morrison, *J. Immunol.* 114:360 (1975).
3.   D. M. Jacobs, *J. Immunol.* 115:988 (1975).
4.   D. E. Mosier, J. J. Mond, and E. A. Golding, *J. Immunol.* 119: 1874 (1977).
5.   R. R. Skelly, P. Munkenbeck, and D. C. Morrison, *Inf. Immun.* 23:287 (1979).

6. D. W. Scott, M. Venkataraman, and J. J. Jandinski, *Immunol. Rev.* **43**:241 (1979).

7. A. Coutinho, E. Gronowicz, W. W. Bullock, and G. Möller, *J. Exp. Med.* **139**:74 (1974).

8. J. Andersson, F. Melchers, G. Galanos, and O. Lüderitz, *J. Exp. Med.* **137**:943 (1973).

9. E. Neter, O. Westphal, O. Lüderitz, E. A. Gorzynski, and E. Eichenberger, *J. Immunol.* **76**:377 (1956).

10. K. B. Von Eschen and J. A. Rudbach, *J. Exp. Med.* **140**:1604 (1974).

11. K. B. Von Eschen and J. A. Rudbach, *J. Immunol.* **116**:8 (1976).

12. B. M. Sultzer, *Nature (Lond.)* **219**:1253 (1968).

13. B. M. Sultzer and B. S. Nilsson, *Nature (New Biol.)* **240**:198 (1972).

14. J. Watson, R. Riblet, and B. A. Taylor, *J. Immunol.* **118**:2088 (1977).

15. J. Watson, K. Kelley, M. Largen, and B. A. Taylor, *J. Immunol.* **120**:422 (1978).

16. J. R. McGhee, S. M. Michalek, R. N. Moore, S. E. Mergenhagen, and D. L. Rosenstreich, *J. Immunol.* **122**:2052 (1979).

17. G. W. Goodman and B. M. Sultzer, *Inf. Immun.* **17**:205 (1977).

18. S. J. Betz and D. C. Morrison, *J. Immunol.* **119**:1475 (1977).

19. E. Neter, E. A. Gorzynski, O. Westphal, and O. Lüderitz,. *J. Immunol.* **80**:66 (1958).

20. D. Rifkind, *J. Bacteriol.* **93**:1463 (1967).

21. D. Rifkind and J. D. Palmer, *J. Bacteriol.* **92**:815 (1966).

22. D. M. Jacobs and D. C. Morrison, *J. Immunol.* **118**:21 (1977).

23. D. M. Jacobs and D. C. Morrison, *J. Exp. Med.* **141**:1453 (1975).

24. E. Smith and L. Hammarström, *Pathol. Microbiol. Scand. Sect. C,* **84**:495 (1976).

25. G. Möller, *Transplant. Rev.* **23**:126 (1975).

26. A. Coutinho, *Transplant Rev.* **23**:49 (1975).

27. A. J. Rosenspire and D. M. Jacobs, *Cell. Biophys.* **3**:89 (1981).

28. D. C. Morrison and D. M. Jacobs, *Immunochemistry* **13**:813 (1976).

29. B. J. Skidmore, J. M. Chiller, D. C. Morrison, and W. O. Weigle, *J. Immunol.* **114**:770 (1975).

30. D. C. Morrison, S. J. Betz, and D. M. Jacobs, *J. Exp. Med.* **144**:840 (1976).

31. B. M. Sultzer and G. W. Goodman, *J. Exp. Med.* **144**:821 (1976).

32. A. G. Johnson, S. Gaines, and M. Landy, *J. Exp. Med.* **103**:225 (1956).

33. R. E. Franzl and P. D. McMaster, *J. Exp. Med.* **127**:1087 (1968).

34. T. Uchiyama and D. M. Jacobs, *J. Immunol.* **121**:2340 (1978).

35. U. Persson, *J. Immunol.* **118**:789 (1977).

36. J. R. McGhee, H. Kiyono, S. M. Michalek, J. L. Babb, D. L. Rosenstreich, and S. E. Mergenhagen, *J. Immunol. 124*:1603 (1980).

37. S. M. Michalek, H. Kiyono, J. L. Babb, and J. R. McGhee, *J. Immunol. 125*:2220 (1980).

38. J. R. McGhee, S. M. Michalek, H. Kiyono, J. L. Babb, M. P. Clark, and L. M. Mosteller, in *Recent Advances in Mucosal Immunity*, (W. Strober, L. Hanson, and K. Sell, eds.), Raven Press, New York, in press.

39. T. Uchiyama and D. M. Jacobs, *J. Immunol. 121*:2347 (1978).

40. M. K. Hoffman, O. Weiss, S. Koenig, J. A. Hirst, and H. F. Oettgen, *J. Immunol. 114*:738 (1975).

41. D. C. Morrison and L. Leive, *J. Biol. Chem. 250*:2911 (1975).

42. D. E. Parks, M. V. Doyle, and W. O. Weigle, *J. Immunol. 119*:1923 (1977).

43. J. R. McGhee, J. J. Farrar, S. M. Michalek, S. E. Mergenhagen, and D. L. Rosenstreich, *J. Exp. Med. 149*:793 (1979).

44. D. M. Jacobs, *J. Immunol. 122*:1421 (1979).

45. I. Lefkowits and H. Waldman, *Limiting Dilution Analysis of Cells in the Immune System*, Cambridge University Press, 1979.

46. A. Ahmed and I. Scher, in *B Lymphocytes in the Immune Response*, (M. Cooper, D. E. Mosier, I. Scher, and E. Vitetta, eds.), Elsevier North-Holland, New York, 1979, p. 117.

47. H. S. Boswell, A. Ahmed, I. Scher, and A. Singer, *J. Immunol. 125*:1340 (1980).

48. M. K. Hoffman, C. Galanos, S. Koenig, and H. F. Oettgen, *J. Exp. Med. 146*:1640 (1977).

49. M. K. Hoffman, *J. Immunol. 125*:2076 (1980).

11

Endogenous and Exogenous Modulation
of Complement Activity

ALAN M. REYNARD   School of Medicine, State University of New York
at Buffalo, Buffalo, New York

I. Introduction

Our ability to modulate the activities of the immune system as a whole
has increased greatly in recent years as a result of an increased
understanding of the mechanisms involved in immune activity. This is
also true of one part of the immune system, complement, for which
the past decade has yielded a large body of information.

There are two general categories of modulation of physiologic
systems, endogenous and exogenous. The complement system is modulated endogenously at several stages of its activity. Examples of these
are the inhibition of C1 activity by C1-INH and the inhibition of C3
activity by β1H and C3b-INA. There are also endogenous activators of
complement. Exogenous modulation can be subdivided into two broad
categories: pharmacologic and nonpharmacologic. Some modulators are
too toxic for human use. Exogenous modulators useful in humans are
very few in number, although a variety of agents have effects on
complement which are incidental to their use in medicine. A pharmacologic agent with usefulness in modulating complement is danazol, a
steroid that inhibits action of C1-INH, itself an endogenous inhibitor.
A number of agents inadvertently modulate the complement system as
a side-effect to their actions. These include gold sodium thiomalate,
penicillamine, heparin, and some radiocontrast media. Agents with
actions on the complement system, but too toxic for human use, include NH_3, KSCN, and other metabolic inhibitors.

These categories of agents will be discussed with a minimum of
description of the complement system itself, because complement has
been described in a number of reviews (1,2,3,11) and books (4,5).
Other recent reviews have stressed specific aspects of complementology,
including synthesis of complement components (6) and complement

253

deficiencies (7, 8). Pharmacologic modulation of complement has been covered in two reviews (9, 10).

References given in this chapter will be largely to more recent work. This means that a number of citations of original findings must be omitted for which apologies are extended to the authors.

II. Endogenous Regulation

A. *C1-Inhibitor (C1-INH)*

The activity of the first component of complement, C1, is regulated in vivo by a natural inhibitor, C1-INH (sometimes referred to as C1-INA or C1-In). C1 is composed of three subunits, C1q, C1r, and C1s, in the ratio of 1:2:4. The complex is held together by Ca^{2+} and is therefore sensitive to chelators of divalent cations. The binding of the C1q component to an antigen-antibody complex causes a conformation change in C1q, leading to a subsequent conformation change in C1r. C1q has no proteolytic activity, but C1r becomes activated to C1r, a serine protease, accompanied by the autocatalytic splitting of a peptide bond in C1r. The natural substrate of C1r is C1s, which is converted from proenzyme to enzyme form by proteolytic cleavage. These are the initial steps in setting off the classic pathway of complement.

C1q is of lesser interest because it is not an enzyme, and its function will be more difficult to regulate than the other members of the C1 complex. C1r and C1s, however, are of great interest because (1) they are involved in both normal and pathologic complement activity and (2) their activities can be regulated.

Although C1r has been shown to activate C1s to C1s̄ (12), it has been more convenient to assay C1r activity with synthetic substrates such as N-carbobenzyloxy-L-tyrosine-*p*-nitrophenyl ester (N-Z-L-tyr-ONp). Andrews and Baillie (13) used this ester substrate to show that C1r could be inhibited by diisopropylfluorophosphate (DFP), phenylmethanesulfonylfluoride, or *p*-tosyl-L-lysine-chloromethyl ketone, but not by other esterase inhibitors such as Trasylol, hirudin, leupeptin, or C1-INH. This result suggests that the binding of C1-INH to C1r must not be at the esterolytic site. Arlaud et al. (14) demonstrated that C1-INH inhibits the activation of C1s by C1r̄, in contrast to the above results with small synthetic substrates. Furthermore, Arlaud et al. (15) demonstrated that when C1 was bound to insoluble immune aggregates, C1-INH could bind to both C1r and C1s and that DFP could inhibit the binding of C1-INH. It was proposed that C1-INH may modulate the activation of C1s by C1r as well as modulate activation of C4 and C2 by C1s̄.

C1s̄ functions to hydrolyze C4 and C2 with the eventual formation of C4bC2a change and like other serine proteases, C1s̄ can be inhibited by N-α-blocked tyrosines and bensamidines (18) and DFP (16, 17).

C1-INH, a protein of 106,000 mol wt, promotes the dissociation of
C1 by binding to both subunits C1r and C1s (19). C1-INH deficiency
in humans leads to recurrent episodes of edema localized to the skin
and the mucous membranes of the GI tract, a condition known as
hereditary angioneurotic edema (HANE). Decreased C1-INH activity
can be caused by synthesis of nonfunctional C1-INH protein, but
more commonly is due to decreased synthesis of the C1-INH protein
itself. The normal individual with adequate C1-INH activity does not
have detectable C1 activity in the serum despite continuing conversion of C1 to C$\overline{1}$. In attacks of HANE there is extensive conversion of
C1 to C$\overline{1}$, enhanced by various factors largely unknown but including
trauma and nervous stress, leading to splitting of C4 and C2. The
split products of C4 and C2, along with plasmin, have been implicated in the production of a kinin-like polypeptide with the ability to
produce vasopermeability (20). Epsilon-aminocaproic acid (EACA) inhibits the conversion of C1 to C$\overline{1}$ (21) and plasminogen to plasmin (22).
EACA was the first compound used in the treatment of HANE, but it
has serious adverse effects which limit its usefulness (23). The occurrence of adverse effects with EACA as well as with other agents to be
mentioned later are especially important because of the long-term nature of treatment of HANE. In fact, treatment of HANE is virtually
synonymous with prophylaxis. Tranexamic acid (trans-4-aminoethyl-
cyclohexane-1-carboxylic acid), an analogue of EACA with decreased
adverse effects, has also been used in therapy of HANE (24,25).

Androgens increase serum levels of C1-INH and have been used
in treatment of HANE. Use of methyltestosterone, the first androgen
to be employed in treatment of HANE (26), was restricted by adverse
effects, especially masculinization. Oxymetholone and fluoxymesterone,
synthetic androgens, have been used with less production of masculinization (27). Danazol (Danocrine), a derivative of ethinyltestoster-
one with 1/100 the virilization activity of methyltestosterone, has more
recently been used for treatment of HANE (28,29).

B. C3b-INA, C4b-Binding Proteins, and β1H

C4 contributes to the complement cascade after it is split into two
fragments, of which C4b is part of C4bC2a, the enzyme that splits
C3 into C3b and C3a. It is also part of C4bC2aC3b, the enzyme that
splits C5. The activity of these enzymes is regulated, in part, by the
natural rate of dissociation of C2a from the complex. In addition,
there are proteins in serum which contribute to the regulation of the
two enzymes. C3b-INA (C3b inactivator) is an enzyme that catalyzes
proteolysis of both C4b and C3b. In the case of C4b, an additional
protein, C4-binding protein (C4-bp), first described in mouse serum,
has been isolated and characterized (30,31). In the case of C3b,
C4-bp serves as a cofactor for C3b-INA in the proteolysis of fluid-
phase but not cell-bound molecules, and even in the fluid-phase,

C4-bp has 20-fold less activity on a weight basis than does β1H (32).
In the mouse, C4-bp levels in serum have been shown to be under
testosterone control (33). Other mouse complement components have
been shown to be regulated by sex hormones (34,35); and steroid
control of C1-INH levels in serum of humans has been mentioned
above.

In summary, degradation of C4b appears to be controlled by
C3b-INA and C4-bp, whereas degradation of C3b is controlled by
C3b-INA and β1H.

Regulation of the activity of C3 is pivotal to development of complement activity through the classic and alternate pathways. The
fluid-phase splitting of C3 permits deposition of C3b on cell surfaces
where formation of C4bC2aC3b, the classic C5 convertase, takes
place. Cell-bound C3b additionally functions as an opsonin. C3b also
combines with Bb to form C3bBb, the amplification convertase of the
alternative pathway, an enzyme that splits C3 into C3a and C3b. As
more C3b is produced by action of C3Bb more C3Bb is formed, hence
the name "amplification convertase."

In the normal course of events, C3bBb is formed at a relatively
slow rate but is partially stabilized by properdin (P). The amount of
C3bBb present at any time is regulated by (1) a natural dissociation
of Bb from the complex and subsequent conversion of the dissociated
Bb to an inactive form (36,37), (2) a displacement of Bb from the
complex by β1H (38-40), and (3) proteolysis of C3b by C3b-INA subsequent to removal of the Bb (C3b in the C3bBb complex is protected
from C3b-INA) (41-44).

In membranoproliferative glomerulonephritis there is an increased
consumption of C3 by the alternate pathway. This occurs because of
production of C3 nephritic factor (C3NeF). C3NeF protects C3Bb
from dissociation by β1H thereby causing a pathologic increase in alternate pathway activity (45-47). Although there has been considerable controversy it now seems clear that C3NeF is an immunoglobulin,
probably an IgG, and possibly an autoantibody directed against
C3bBb (48-50).

An inhibitor of immune hemolysis that operates at the level of C3
has been found in the sera of patients with acute lymphoblastic leukemia (51) and in patients undergoing transplant rejection (52). The
inhibitor is effective in reduction of complement-mediated killing of
normal human peripheral lymphocytes (53). It appears to act by binding to cell-bound C3b, rather than to the cell surface, and by stabilizing the C3b to the proteolytic attack of C3b-INA and β1H. It has
recently been found (54) that the inhibitor is present in normal human serum and, thus, may represent one more natural control
mechanism.

C. Cell Surfaces

In addition to control of complement activity by single molecules, there is control of complement by cell surfaces. It has been found that certain particles, such as zymosan, and certain cell surfaces, such as rabbit erythrocytes, are able to activate the alternate pathway. These surfaces lack or have greatly reduced quantities of sialic acid. In contrast, sheep erythrocytes, which are relatively rich in surface sialic acid, are poor activators of the alternate pathway but can be made better activators by removal of sialic acid with neuraminidase. Furthermore, activation of the alternative pathway by erythrocytes from various inbred strains of mouse has been shown to be inversely proportional to their sialic acid content. It now appears that sialic acid provides a microenvironment for C3bBb on the cell surface that protects it from β1H (55-58).

Complement-mediated killing of gram-negative bacteria is also regulated by the cell surface. Some strains are resistant to complement because of the presence of a capsule surrounding their surfaces, probably a mechanical effect. That is, the complement components are simply prevented from reaching the outer membrane of the cells. Many strains do not have capsules and their susceptibility to complement varies according to the lipopolysaccharide (LPS) contained in their outer membrane. Strains that have LPS molecules with a complete polysaccharide side chain (the O-specific side chain) are quite resistant to complement, whereas strains that have LPS molecules without an O side chain are relatively sensitive. Specific antibody to the O side chain can initiate the classic pathway activity responsible for the bactericidal activity. Since O-specific side chains are 20-30 monosaccharides in length, it is possible that complement activity is initiated too far from the surface of the cell to be effective. It has been shown that killing of bacterial cells, constructed with the target antigen separated from the cell surface by various spacer molecules, decreased as the distance of the antigen from the cell increased (59). It is also possible that the LPS protects cells by hindering access of the complement components to the cell surface.

D. Bacterial Plasmids

Bacterial plasmids specify the production of a variety of proteins that have a role in bacterial physiology. Their most well-known role is to provide their host cells with resistance to antibiotics. A number of effects of bacterial plasmids are manifested at the cell surface. It has been shown that some bacterial plasmids provide their host cells with resistance to both rabbit (60,61) and human (62,63) sera. More recently, plasmid-mediated resistance to complement has been shown to be due to a major outer membrane protein (64), a finding that is consonant with the widely held view that the initial point of attack of

complement on gram-negative organisms is at the outer membrane.
Plasmid-mediated resistance to serum has, furthermore, been shown
to affect both the classic and alternate pathways and appears to affect the complement sequence in the region past C3, i.e., in the
attack phase (62).

E. The Attack Phase

The attack phase of the complement sequence involves preparation,
on a cell surface, of a macromolecular complex containing C5b, C6,
C7, C8, and C9. C5b is the product of the final enzymatic step in the
complement sequence; none of the above components have enzymatic
activity. Accordingly, there is less opportunity for external control
of either the formation or the activity of this part of the sequence.
Nevertheless there are some controls intrinsic to its formation and
interaction with membranes. C5b, inherently labile, decays quickly
in the fluid phase. The presence of C6 stabilizes C5b, and the C5bC6
complex represents the first stage in the formation of the attack phase
complex. At present there are no ways to modulate the C5b-C6 interaction. Surface (cell, particle, artificial membrane, and vesicle) properties influence the effectiveness of the attack phase. The attack
phase complex forms a membrane channel, originally described as the
doughnut hypothesis (65), with hydrophobic areas of the C5b-C9
proteins facing outward to interact with membrane lipids and hydrophilic areas of the proteins facing inward to form the channel that
allows passage of small hydrophilic molecules across the membrane
(2,66). That the attack phase complex interacts with membrane lipids
has been shown in a number of ways, including alteration of membrane
fluidity and organization following complement attack (67-73). There
have also been demonstrations that the lipid composition of membranes
controls the effectiveness of the attack phase unit (74,75).

   Reactive lysis involves the formation of C567 complexes which are
subsequently transferred to the target cell (76,77). The cell may
then be lysed upon addition of C8 and C9. This has proven to be a
convenient way to study the attack phase without participation of the
early complement components. It has recently been shown, using
reactive lysis, that C8, in addition to participating in the attack phase
complex, serves to regulate the attack phase by inhibiting attachment
of C567 to the cell surface (78). It had previously been demonstrated
that serum contains several other proteins that function as inhibitors
of C567 (79,80). The significance of the dual role of C8 remains to be
clarified.

III. Exogenous Regulation

A number of chemicals have been found to influence the activity of the
complement system in some fashion, but very few are in use in human

medicine. Mentioned above were EACA and several steroids used in the treatment of HANE. There is a somewhat greater number of chemicals used in human medicine which have effects on complement incidental to their use. These include some radiocontrast media, gold sodium thiomalate, and penicillamine.

A. Radiocontrast Media

Radiocontrast media (RCM) (derivatives of tri-iodobenzoic acid) are used extensively in diagnostic medicine and cause a variety of adverse reactions ranging from mild shock (3-8% of patients) to hypotensive shock (1 in 2000-14,000) and death (1 in 10,000-40,000) (81). A similarity has been noted between the complement profiles in HANE and in RCM reactions (82). However, changes in levels of C3, C4, and C5 (83), C3, C4, C5, and C6 (81), and C3 and factor B, and no change in C1-INH (84), have been noted.

B. Gold Sodium Thiomalate and Penicillamine

Gold salts, used in treatment of rheumatoid arthritis, affect a variety of processes that contribute to inflammation, including complement. The initial observation was that gold sodium thiomalate (AuTM) inactivates C1 and purified C1s, and that the inactivation cannot be reversed by dialysis (85). More recently it has been demonstrated that AuTM inhibits formation of the amplification convertase, C3bBb, without inhibiting its activity once formed nor accelerating its dissociation (86). Kinetic studies suggested that the action of AuTM is directed toward the binding site for B on C3b. Penicillamine, another agent used in treatment of rheumatoid arthritis, has been reported to inhibit hemolytic complement, but only at high concentration (87). It does not reduce CH50 in human serum at therapeutic doses. However, reduction of C3 deposits on synovial membranes have been observed after penicillamine treatment, and it may be that penicillamine concentrations in synovial fluid are higher than in serum.

C. Cyclic AMP

Cyclic AMP (cAMP) appears to play a role in complement-mediated cell damage as it does in many other cellular processes. When the cAMP content of rat mast cells was elevated by incubation of the cells with prostaglandin E, an activator of adenylate cyclase, or with aminophylline, an inhibitor of cyclic nucleotide phosphodiesterase, or with dibutyryl cAMP, there was a decrease in complement-mediated histamine release (88). It has also been observed that incubation of line-1 guinea pig hepatoma cells with cAMP resulted in decreased cytotoxicity (89). In the same experiments cAMP had no effect on hemolysis, suggesting that the effect of cAMP was not directly on the cell membrane. There is a question of the accessibility of the interior of the cell to the cAMP. It has been shown that complement attack on mouse

mastocytoma cells proceeds with an initial release of small molecules
from the cells prior to osmotic lysis (90). It is thus possible that an
initial attack by complement made the hepatoma cells more permeable
to cAMP. In an additional study it was shown that a number of inhibitors of macromolecular synthesis, adriamycin, puromycin, mitomycin
C, and actinomycin D, all of which decreased cellular concentration
of cAMP, increased the susceptibility of line-10 hepatoma cells to complement (91). Two inhibitors that did not alter intracellular concentration of cAMP also did not sensitize line-10 cells to complement. Decreased complement-mediated killing has also been observed when
mouse lymphocytes were incubated with cAMP (92).

A number of agents have been found to affect complement and are
used as tools in complementology. These include both natural products
and synthetic chemicals.

D. *Cobra Venom Factor*

Cobra venom has been known for years to be anticomplementary, and
was one of the principle tools used in unraveling the mechanism of the
alternative pathway. It is now used for decomplementing serum and for
preparing serum that is relatively rich in C1, C4, and C2 but deficient in C3 and C5. A high molecular weight protein in cobra venom
inhibits the early acting components of the classic pathway. More
commonly employed is a low molecular weight protein (144,000 mol wt)
referred to as cobra venom factor (CVF). CVF is now known to be
cobra C3b and as such can substitute for human C3b in the human
amplification convertase (93,94). CVF functions as added C3b to ac-
celerate the formation of C3bBb and has the added property of being
relatively resistant to C3b-INA. Examples of the use of CVF to de-
complement animals include studies of the role of complement in virus
infection (95,96), allograft rejection (97), and renal disease (98).
The use of CVF in whole animals may be limited by the appearance of
antibodies to it (96,99).

E. *Chelating Agents*

Metal chelating agents are important in complement research because
of the requirements for Ca^{2+} and Mg^{2+} at several stages of the complement sequence. Ca^{2+} is required for maintenance of an intact C1
complex. Mg^{2+} is required for the attachment of C2 to the EAC14b
complex and also for the function of the amplification convertase of
the alternative pathway. Treatment of serum with 10 mM EDTA eliminates all complement activity by blocking both pathways. In contrast to EDTA, which has an equal affinity for Ca^{2+} and Mg^{2+}, EGTA
(ethyleneglycol-tetraacetate) has a strong affinity for Ca^{2+}, but a
much weaker affinity for Mg^{2+}. Thus, treatment of serum with 10 mM
EGTA blocked classic pathway activity while permitting the alternative

pathway to function (100). EGTA, however, has too great an affinity for Mg^{2+}, albeit less than for Ca^{2+}, to be used by itself for optimal results. It has been demonstrated that 10 mM EGTA in solution with 10 mM Mg^{2+}, usually referred to as 10 mM MgEGTA, yields better alternative pathway activity while still blocking classic pathway activity (101-104). It has been recommended that a better reagent is 5mM Mg^{2+} combined with 10 mM EGTA (105).

References

1. M. M. Mayer, *Sci. Am.* **229**:54 (1973).
2. H. J. Muller-Eberhard, *Ann. Rev. Biochem.* **44**:697 (1975).
3. R. R. Porter and K. B. M. Reid, *Nature (Lond.)* **275**:699 (1978).
4. H. J. Rapp and T. Borsos, *Molecular Basis of Complement Action*, Appleton-Century-Crofts, New York, 1970.
5. A. G. Osler, *Complement: Mechanisms and Functions*, Prentice-Hall, Englewood Cliffs, 1976.
6. M. Adinolfi, *Am. J. Dis. Child.* **131**:1015 (1977).
7. V. Agnello, *Medicine* **57**:1 (1978).
8. C. A. Alper and F. S. Rosen, in *Mechanisms of Immunopathology* (S. Cohen, P. A. Ward, and R. M. McKluskey, eds.), John Wiley, New York, 1979.
9. B. J. Johnson, *J. Pharmaceut. Sci.* **66**:1367 (1977).
10. A. M. Reynard, *J. Immunopharmacol.* **2**:1 (1980).
11. K. F. Austen et al., *Bull. W.H.O.* **39**:935 (1968).
12. K. Sakai and R. Stroud, *Immunochemistry* **11**:191 (1974).
13. J. M. Andrews and R. D. Baillie, *J. Immunol.* **123**:1403 (1979).
14. R. J. Arlaud, A. Reboul, R. B. Sim, and M. G. Colomb, *Biochim. Biophys. Acta* **576**:151 (1979).
15. R. J. Arlaud, A. Reboul, and M. G. Colomb, *Biochim. Biophys. Acta* **485**:227 (1977).
16. I. Gigli and K. F. Austen, *J. Exp. Med.* **130**:833 (1969).
17. I. Gigli, R. R. Porter, and R. B. Sim, *Biochem. J.* **157**:541 (1976).
18. J. M. Andrews, D. P. Roman, Jr., and D. H. Bing, *J. Med. Chem.* **21**:1202 (1978).
19. R. J. Ziccardi and N. R. Cooper, *J. Immunol.* **123**:788 (1979).
20. K. Willms, F. S. Rosen, and V. H. Donaldson, *Immunol. Immunopathol.* **4**:174 (1975).
21. N. A. Soter, K. F. Austen, and I. Gigli, *J. Immunol.* **114**:928 (1975).
22. A. P. Kaplan and K. F. Austen, *J. Exp. Med.* **136**:1378 (1972).
23. I. M. Nilsson, L. Anderson, and S. E. Bjorkman, *Acta Med. Scand.* **448**:(Suppl.) 21 (1966).

24. B. Lundh, A.-B. Laurell, H. Wetterqvist, T. White, and G.
     Granerus, *Clin. Exp. Immunol. 3*:733 (1968).
25. A. L. Sheffer, K. F. Austen, and F. S. Rosen, *N. Engl. J.
     Med. 287*:452 (1972).
26. W. B. Spaulding, *Ann. Int. Med. 53*:739 (1960).
27. P. J. Davis, F. B. Davis, and P. Charache, *Johns Hopkins
     Med. J. 135*:391 (1974).
28. J. A. Gelfand, R. J. Sherins, D. W. Alling, and M. M. Frank,
     N. Engl. J. Med. 295:1444 (1976).
29. S. W. Hosea and M. M. Frank, *Drugs 19*:370 (1980).
30. J. Scharfstein, A. Ferreira, I. Gigli, and V. Nussenzweig,
     J. Exp. Med. 148:207 (1978).
31. T. Fujita, I. Gigli, and V. Nussenzweig, *J. Exp. Med. 148*:
     1044 (1978).
32. T. Fujita and V. Nussenzweig, *J. Exp. Med. 150*:267 (1979).
33. A. Ferreira, P. Weiz-Carrington, and V. Nussenzweig, *J.
     Immunol. 121*:1213 (1978).
34. R. M. Weintraub, W. H. Churchill, C. Crisler, H. J. Rapp,
     and T. Borsos, *Science 152*:783 (1966).
35. W. H. Churchill, R. M. Weintraub, T. Borsos, and H. J.
     Rapp, *J. Exp. Med. 125*:657 (1967).
36. D. T. Fearon, K. F. Austen, and S. Ruddy, *J. Exp. Med.
     138*:1305 (1973).
37. D. T. Fearon and K. F. Austen, *J. Exp. Med. 142*:856 (1975).
38. J. M. Weiler, M. R. Daha, K. F. Austen, and D. T. Fearon,
     Proc. Natl. Acad. Sci. U.S.A. 73:3268 (1976).
39. K. Whaley and S. Ruddy, *J. Exp. Med. 144*:1147 (1976).
40. S. K. Law, D. T. Fearon, and R. P. Levine, *J. Immunol.
     122*:759 (1979).
41. N. Tamara and R. A. Nelson, *J. Immunol. 99*:582 (1967).
42. P. J. Lachmann and H. J. Muller-Eberhard, *J. Immunol. 100*:
     691 (1968).
43. S. Ruddy and K. F. Austen, *J. Immunol. 107*:742 (1971).
44. C. A. Alper, F. S. Rosen, and P. J. Lachmann, *Proc. Natl.
     Acad. Sci. U.S.A. 69*:2910 (1972).
45. M. R. Daha, D. T. Fearon, and K. F. Austen, *Immunology 31*:
     789 (1976).
46. M. R. Daha, D. T. Fearon, and K. F. Austen, *J. Immunol.
     116*:1 (1976).
47. M. R. Daha, K. F. Austen, and D. T. Fearon, *J. Immunol.
     119*:812 (1977).
48. M. R. Daha, K. F. Austen, and D. T. Fearon, *J. Immunol.
     120*:1389 (1978).
49. D. M. Scott, N. Amos, J. G. P. Sissons, P. J. Lachmann,
     and D. K. Peters, *Clin. Exp. Immunol. 32*:12 (1978).
50. M. R. Daha and L. A. van Es, *J. Immunol. 123*:755 (1979).

51. D. K. Kalwinsky, J. R. Urmson, A. E. Stitzel, and R. E. Spitzer, *J. Lab. Clin. Med. 88*:745 (1976).

52. R. Spitzer, A. Stitzel, L. Florio, and J. Urmson, *Immunochemistry 13*:395 (1976).

53. G. H. Bock, A. E. Stitzel, K. W. Rittenhouse, and R. E. Spitzer, *Transplantation 26*:415 (1978).

54. R. E. Spitzer, A. E. Stitzel, and G. L. Hoffman, *J. Ped. 96*:564 (1980).

55. D. T. Fearon and K. F. Austen, *J. Exp. Med. 146*:22 (1977).

56. D. T. Fearon and K. F. Austen, *Proc. Natl. Acad. Sci. U.S.A. 74*:1683 (1977).

57. M. K. Pangburn and H. J. Muller-Eberhard, *Proc. Natl. Acad. Sci. U.S.A. 75*:2416 (1978).

58. U. E. Nydegger, D. T. Fearon, and K. F. Austen, *Proc. Natl. Acad. Sci. U.S.A. 75*:6078 (1978).

59. D. Rowley and K. J. Turner, *Nature (Lond.) 217*:657 (1968).

60. A. M. Reynard and M. E. Beck, *Inf. Immun. 14*:848 (1976).

61. A. M. Reynard, M. E. Beck, and R. J. Cunningham, *Inf. Immun. 19*:861 (1978).

62. A. Fietta, E. Romero, and A. G. Siccardi, *Inf. Immun. 18*:278 (1977).

63. R. T. Ogata and R. P. Levine, *J. Immunol. 125*:1494 (1980).

64. A. P. Moll, A. Manning, and K. N. Timmis, *Inf. Immun. 28*:359 (1980).

65. M. M. Mayer, *Proc. Natl. Acad. Sci. U.S.A. 69*:2954 (1972).

66. S. Bhakdi and J. Tranum-Jensen, *Proc. Natl. Acad. Sci. U.S.A. 75*:5655 (1978).

67. R. P. Mason, E. B. Giavedoni, and A. P. Dalmasso, *Biochemistry 16*:1196 (1977).

68. E. B. Giavedoni, R. P. Mason, and A. P. Dalmasso, *J. Immunol. 120*:2003 (1978).

69. A. E. Esser, R. M. Bartholomew, J. W. Parce, and H. M. McConnell, *J. Biol. Chem. 254*:1768 (1979).

70. A. E. Esser, W. P. Kolb, E. R. Podack, and H. J. Muller-Eberhard, *Proc. Natl. Acad. Sci. U.S.A. 76*:1410 (1979).

71. E. R. Podack, G. Biesecker, and H. J. Muller-Eberhard, *Proc. Natl. Acad. Sci. U.S.A. 76*:897 (1979).

72. S. J. Shattil, D. B. Cines, and A. D. Schreiber, *J. Clin. Invest. 61*:582 (1978).

73. M. Nakamura, S. Ohnishi, H. Kitamura, and S. Inai, *Biochemistry 15*:4838 (1976).

74. M. M. Mayer, C. H. Hammer, D. W. Michaels, and M. L. Shin, *Immunochemistry 15*:813 (1979).

75. M. L. Shin, W. A. Paznekas, and M. M. Mayer, *J. Immunol. 120*:1996 (1978).

76. R. A. Thompson and D. S. Rowe, *Immunology 14*:745 (1968).

77. R. A. Thompson and P. J. Lachmann, *J. Exp. Med.* *131*:629 (1970).

78. G. R. Nemerow, K.-I. Yamamoto, and T. F. Lint, *J. Immunol.* *123*:1245 (1979).

79. B. C. McLeod, P. Baker, and H. Gewurz, *Int. Arch. Allergy Appl. Immunol.* *47*:643 (1974).

80. B. C. McLeod, P. Baker, and H. Gewurz, *Immunology* *28*:133 (1975).

81. G. Till, U. Rother, and D. Gemsa, *Int. Arch. Allergy Appl. Immunol.* *56*:543 (1978).

82. E. C. Lasser, J. H. Lang, S. G. Lyon, and A. E. Hamblin, *J. Allergy Clin. Immunol.* *64*:105 (1979).

83. P. Lieberman and R. L. Siegle, *J. Allergy Appl. Immunol.* *64*:13 (1979).

84. C. M. Arroyave, M. Schatz, and R. A. Simon, *J. Allergy Clin. Immunol.* *63*:276 (1979).

85. D. R. Schultz, J. E. Volanakis, P. I. Arnold, N. L. Gottlieb, K. Sakai, and R. M. Stroud, *Clin. Exp. Immunol.* *17*:395 (1974).

86. J. J. Burge, D. T. Fearon, and K. F. Austen, *J. Immunol.* *120*:1625 (1978).

87. O. J. Mellbye and E. Munthe, *Ann. Rheum. Dis.* *36*:453 (1977).

88. M. Kaliner and K. F. Austen, *Science* *183*:659 (1974).

89. M. D. P. Boyle, S. H. Ohanian, and T. Borsos, *J. Immunol.* *116*:1276 (1976).

90. E. Martz, S. J. Burakoff, and B. Benacerraf, *Proc. Natl. Acad. Sci. U.S.A.* *71*:177 (1974).

91. T. N. Lo and M. P. D. Boyle, *Cancer Res.* *39*:3156 (1979).

92. P. Ebbesen and K. M. Arnung, *Transplantation* *16*:476 (1973).

93. P. J. Lachmann and P. Nichol, *Lancet* *1*:465 (1973).

94. C. A. Alper and D. Balavitch, *Science* *191*:1275 (1976).

95. R. L. Hirsch, D. E. Griffin, and J. Winkelstein, *J. Immunol.* *121*:1276 (1978).

96. J. T. Hicks, F. A. Ennis, E. Kim, and M. Verbonitz, *J. Immunol.* *121*:1437 (1978).

97. R. D. C. Forbes, M. Pinto-Blonde, and R. D. Guttman, *Laboratory Inv.* *39*:463 (1978).

98. U. H. Rudofsky, R. W. Sterblay, and B. Pollara, *Clin. Immunol. Immunopath.* *3*:396 (1975).

99. C. G. Cochrane, H. J. Muller-Eberhard, and B. S. Aikin, *J. Immunol.* *105*:55 (1970).

100. D. P. Fine, S. R. Marney, D. G. Colley, J. S. Sergent, and R. M. Des Prez, *J. Immunol.* *109*:807 (1972).

101. T. A. E. Platts-Mills and K. Ishizaka, *J. Immunol.* *113*:348 (1974).

102. C. S. Bryan, *Proc. Soc. Exp. Biol. Med.* *145*:1431 (1974).
103. A. Forsgren and P. G. Quie, *J. Immunol.* *26*:1251 (1974).
104. R. M. Des Prez, C. S. Bryan, J. Hawiger, and D. G. Colley, *Inf. Immun.* *11*:1235 (1975).
105. J. E. May and M. M. Frank, *J. Immunol* *111*:1668 (1973).

Author Index

Numbers in parentheses are reference numbers and indicate that an author's work is referred to although the name is not cited in text. Italic numbers give page on which the complete reference is listed.

Subject Index